CURRENT CLINICAL PATHOLOGY

AF167326

ANTONIO GIORDANO, MD, PhD
Philadelphia, PA, USA

SERIES EDITOR

More information about this series at http://www.springer.com/series/7632

Antonio Russo • Antonio Giordano
Christian Rolfo
Editors

Liquid Biopsy in Cancer Patients

The Hand Lens for Tumor Evolution

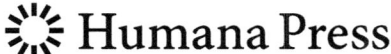 Humana Press

Editors
Antonio Russo
Surgical and Oncological Sciences
University of Palermo School
   of Medicine
Palermo, Italy

Antonio Giordano
College of Science and Technology
Temple University Sbarro Institute
   for Cancer Research
Philadelphia, Pennsylvania, USA

Christian Rolfo
Oncology
University Hospital Antwerp
Edegem, Antwerpen, Belgium

ISSN 2197-781X   ISSN 2197-7828   (electronic)
Current Clinical Pathology
ISBN 978-3-319-85719-0   ISBN 978-3-319-55661-1   (eBook)
DOI 10.1007/978-3-319-55661-1

Printed on acid-free paper

This Humana Press imprint is published by Springer Nature
The registered company is Springer International Publishing AG
The registered company address is: Gewerbestrasse 11, 6330 Cham, Switzerland

Contents

The original version of this book was revised. An erratum to this book can be found at
DOI 10.1007/ 978-3-319-55661-1_20

Contributors

Estíbaliz Alegre Department of Biochemistry, Clínica Universidad de Navarra, IDISNA, Pamplona, Spain

Riccardo Alessandro Department of Biopathology and Medical Biotecnologies, University of Palermo, Palermo, Italy

Sevilay Altintas Multidisciplinary Oncologic Centre Antwerp (MOCA), Edegem, Belgium

Walter Arancio Tumor Immunology Unit, Human Pathology Section, Department ProSaMI (Dipartimento per la Promozione della Salute e Materno Infantile "G. D'Alessandro"), Palermo University School of Medicine, Palermo, Italy

Mariamena Arbitrio ISN-CNR, Roccelletta di Borgia, Catanzaro, Italy

Giuseppe Badalamenti Department of Surgical, Oncological and Oral Sciences, Section of Medical Oncology, University of Palermo, Palermo, Italy

Nadia Barraco Department of Surgical, Oncological and Oral Sciences, Section of Medical Oncology, University of Palermo, Palermo, Italy

Viviana Bazan Department of Experimental Biomedicine and Clinical Neurosciences, University of Palermo, Palermo, Italy

Institute for Cancer Research and Molecular Medicineand Center of Biotechnology, College of Science and Biotechnology, Philadelphia, PA, USA

Beatrice Belmonte Tumor Immunology Unit, Human Pathology Section, Department ProSaMI (Dipartimento per la Promozione della Salute e Materno Infantile "G. D'Alessandro"), Palermo University School of Medicine, Palermo, Italy

Valentina Calò Department of Surgical, Oncological and Oral Sciences, Section of Medical Oncology, University of Palermo, Palermo, Italy

Stefano Caruso Génomique Fonctionnelle des Tumeurs Solides, INSERM, Paris, France

Marta Castiglia Department of Surgical, Oncological and Oral Sciences, Section of Medical Oncology, University of Palermo, Palermo, Italy

Alex Le Cesne Department of Cancer Medicine, Gustave Roussy Cancer Campus, Villejuif, France

V. Chiantera Department of Gynaecology, Charité University, Hindenburgdamm, Berlin, Germany

Department of Gynecology Oncology, University Hospital "Paolo Giaccone", Palermo, Italy

M. Ciaccio Section of Clinical Biochemistry and Clinical Molecular Medicine, Department of Biopathology and Medical Biotechnology, University of Palermo – U.O.C. Laboratory Medicine – CoreLab, Policlinico University Hospital, Palermo, Italy

Domenico Ciliberto Department of Experimental and Clinical Medicine, Magna Graecia University, Catanzaro, Italy

Amanda J. Craig Division of Liver Diseases, Liver Cancer Program, Department of Medicine, Tisch Cancer Institute, Icahn School of Medicine at Mount Sinai, New York, NY, USA

Daniele Fanale Department of Surgical, Oncological and Oral Sciences, Section of Medical Oncology, University of Palermo, Palermo, Italy

Simona Fontana Department of Biopathology and Medical Biotecnologies, University of Palermo, Palermo, Italy

Juan Pablo Fusco Department of Oncology, Clínica Universidad de Navarra, IDISNA, Pamplona, Spain

A. Galvano Department of Surgical, Oncological and Oral Sciences, Section of Medical Oncology, University of Palermo, Palermo, Italy

Marco Giallombardo Department of Biopathology and Medical Biotecnologies, University of Palermo, Palermo, Italy

Ignacio Gil-Bazo Department of Oncology, Clínica Universidad de Navarra, IDISNA, Pamplona, Spain

Program of Solid Tumors and Biomarkers, Center for Applied Medical Research, IDISNA, Pamplona, Spain

Antonio Giordano Sbarro Institute for Cancer Research and Molecular Medicine, Center for Biotechnology, College of Science and Technology, Temple University, Philadelphia, PA, USA

E. Giovannetti Department of Medical Oncology, VU University Medical Center, Cancer Center Amsterdam, HV, Amsterdam, The Netherlands

AIRC Start Up Unit, University of Pisa, Pisa, Italy

Álvaro González Department of Biochemistry, Clínica Universidad de Navarra, IDISNA, Pamplona, Spain

Antonella Ierardi Department of Experimental and Clinical Medicine, Magna Graecia University, Catanzaro, Italy

Lorena Incorvaia Department of Surgical, Oncological and Oral Sciences, Section of Medical Oncology, University of Palermo, Palermo, Italy

Juan Lucio Iovanna Centre de Recherche en Cancérologie de Marseille (CRCM), INSERM U1068, CNRS UMR 7258, Aix-Marseille Université et Institut Paoli-Calmettes, Parc Scientifique et Technologique de Luminy, Marseille, France

Anthony H. Kong Institute of Head and Neck Studies (InHANSE), Institute of Cancer and Genomic Sciences, University of Birmingham, Birmingham, UK

Ismail Labgaa Division of Liver Diseases, Liver Cancer Program, Department of Medicine, Tisch Cancer Institute, Icahn School of Medicine at Mount Sinai, New York, NY, USA

Division of Visceral Surgery, University Hospital of Lausanne (CHUV), Lausanne, Switzerland

A. Listì Department of Surgical, Oncological and Oral Sciences, Section of Medical Oncology, University of Palermo, Palermo, Italy

Umberto Malapelle Department of Public Health, University of Naples Federico II, Naples, Italy

Maria Teresa Di Martino Department of Experimental and Clinical Medicine, Magna Graecia University, Catanzaro, Italy

Daniela Massihnia Department of Surgical, Oncological and Oral Sciences, Section of Medical Oncology, University of Palermo, Palermo, Italy

Arianna Di Napoli Department of Clinical and Molecular Medicine, Sant'Andrea Hospital, Sapienza University, Rome, Italy

K. Papadimitriou Department of Oncology, Antwerp University Hospital, Edegem, Belgium

Francesco Passiglia Department of Surgical, Oncological and Oral Sciences, Section of Medical Oncology, University of Palermo, Palermo, Italy

Patrick Pauwels Center for Oncological Research, Faculty of Medicine and Health Sciences, University of Antwerp, Wilrijk, Belgium

Department of Pathology, Antwerp University Hospital, Edegem, Belgium

M. Peeters Department of Oncology, Antwerp University Hospital, Edegem, Belgium

Alessandro Perez Department of Surgical, Oncological and Oral Sciences, Section of Medical Oncology, University of Palermo, Palermo, Italy

Pasquale Pisapia Department of Public Health, University of Naples Federico II, Naples, Italy

Natalia Ramírez Oncohematology Research Group, Navarrabiomed, Miguel Servet Foundation, IDISNA (Navarra's Health Research Institute), Pamplona, Spain

Pablo Reclusa Phase I-Early Clinical Trials Unit, Oncology Department, Antwerp University Hospital, Edegem, Belgium

Center for Oncological Research (CORE), Antwerp University, Antwerp, Belgium

Center for Oncological Research, Faculty of Medicine and Health Sciences, University of Antwerp, Wilrijk, Belgium

Department of Pathology, Antwerp University Hospital, Edegem, Belgium

Christian Rolfo, MD, PhD Department of Oncology, Antwerp University Hospital, Edegem, Belgium

Phase I-Early Clinical Trials Unit, Oncology Department, Antwerp University Hospital, Edegem, Belgium

Center for Oncological Research (CORE), Antwerp University, Antwerp, Belgium

Antonio Russo, MD, PhD Department of Surgical, Oncogical and Oral Sciences, Section of Medical Oncology, University of Palermo, Palermo, Italy

Sbarro Institute for Cancer Research and Molecular Medicine and Center of Biotechnology, College of Science and Biotechnology, Philadelphia, PA, USA

Pierluigi Scalia, MD, PhD Sbarro Institute for Cancer Research & Molecular Medicine, Philadelphia, PA, USA

Caltanissetta, ISOPROG, Caltanissetta, Italy

M.J. Serrano GENYO, Centre for Genomics and Oncological Research (Pfizer/University of Granada/Andalusian Regional Government), PTS Granada Av. de la Ilustración, Granada, Spain

Laure Sober Center for Oncological Research, Faculty of Medicine and Health Sciences, University of Antwerp, Wilrijk, Belgium

Department of Pathology, Antwerp University Hospital, Edegem, Belgium

A.B. Di Stefano Department of Surgical, Oncogical and Oral Sciences, Section of Medical Oncology, University of Palermo, Palermo, Italy

Pierosandro Tagliaferri Department of Experimental and Clinical Medicine, Magna Graecia University, Catanzaro, Italy

Pierfrancesco Tassone Department of Experimental and Clinical Medicine, Magna Graecia University, Catanzaro, Italy

Claudio Tripodo Tumor Immunology Unit, Human Pathology Section, Department ProSaMI (Dipartimento per la Promozione della Salute e Materno Infantile "G. D'Alessandro"), Palermo University School of Medicine, Palermo, Italy

Giancarlo Troncone Department of Public Health, University of Naples Federico II, Naples, Italy

Augusto Villanueva, MD, PhD Division of Liver Diseases, Liver Cancer Program, Department of Medicine, Tisch Cancer Institute, Icahn School of Medicine at Mount Sinai, New York, NY, USA

Division of Hematology/Medical Oncology, Department of Medicine, Icahn School of Medicine at Mount Sinai, New York, NY, USA

Stephen J. Williams Sbarro Institute for Cancer Research & Molecular Medicine, Philadelphia, PA, USA

Caltanissetta, ISOPROG, Caltanissetta, Italy

Leyre Zubiri Department of Oncology, Clínica Universidad de Navarra, IDISNA, Pamplona, Spain

Liquid Biopsy in Cancer Patients: The Hand Lens to Investigate Tumor Evolution

A. Russo, A. Giordano, and C. Rolfo

Introduction

In recent years the treatment of cancer patients has profoundly changed, thanks to the study and the comprehension of the biological processes underlying tumor development and progression. Almost 20 year ago was first used the term "oncogene addiction" to describe the phenomenon where the activation of a specific oncogene is required for cancer cell survival and proliferation [1]. It was then supposed that a pharmacological agent, able to specifically target the hyperactivated oncogene, was efficient to selectively kill cancer cells sparing normal cells from toxicity. This is no longer a dream, but it has become part of clinical real life for oncologists and their patients. Since then clinicians have changed the way to treat and select patients for a specific treatment, moving from one-size-fits-all strategy to the so-called precision medicine that is based on a correct patient's selection. Patient's selection is based on a series of molecular biology procedures able to define a specific molecular profile for the tumors [2]. Therefore, until now, the path of cancer patients' survival is tissue dependent (Fig. 1.1). The identification of a specific gene status in a precise tumor type (e.g., *c-KIT* for gastrointestinal stromal tumors or *EGFR* in non-small cell lung cancer) enables the selection of the patient for a targeted therapy [3–5]. If considered the above-mentioned examples, for those patients in which the molecular analysis does not provide any information (wild-type patients), the strategy is the standard treatment indicated for their disease. Moreover, we are now witnessing another revolution brought from immunotherapy, but that's another story beyond the scope of this volume [6].

As previously mentioned the path of patients' survival is tissue dependent, but this may have several limitations (Fig. 1.2). Indeed a single tissue biopsy represents only a snapshot limited in time and space, but we are learning that tumor evolves and thus the initial molecular portrait may dramatically change over time. This means that metastatic lesion or even the primary tumor itself may be considered as a completely new "molecular disease," for which it might be needed a different therapeutic approach. Last but not the

A. Russo (✉)
Department of Surgical, Oncological and Oral Sciences, Section of Medical Oncology, University of Palermo, Via del Vespro 129, 90127 Palermo, Italy
e-mail: antonio.russo@usa.net

A. Giordano
Sbarro Institute for Cancer Research and Molecular Medicine, Center for Biotechnology, College of Science and Technology, Temple University, Philadelphia, PA 19122, USA

C. Rolfo
Phase I-Early Clinical Trials Unit, Oncology Department, Antwerp University Hospital, Wilrijkstraat 10, 2650 Edegem, Belgium

Center for Oncological Research (CORE), Antwerp University, Antwerp, Belgium
e-mail: christian.rolfo@uza.be

© Springer International Publishing AG 2017
A. Giordano et al. (eds.), *Liquid Biopsy in Cancer Patients*, Current Clinical Pathology,
DOI 10.1007/978-3-319-55661-1_1

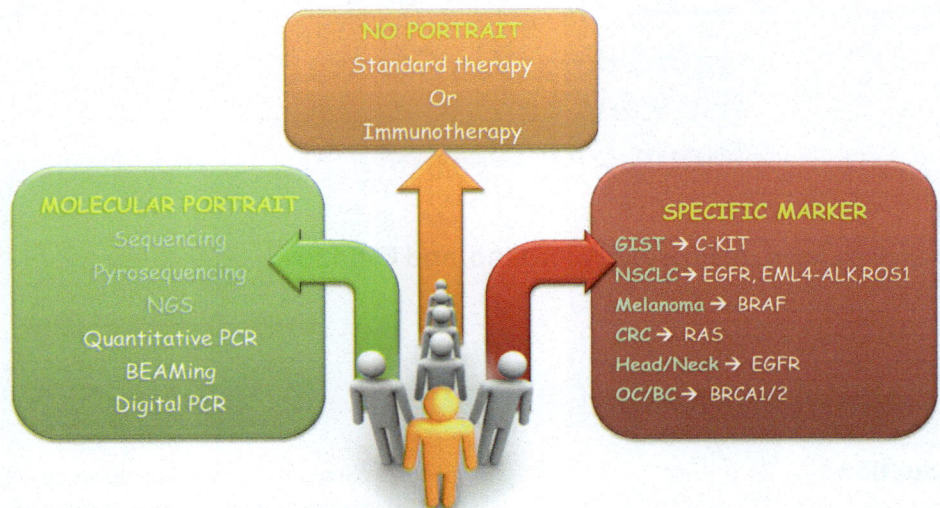

Fig. 1.1 The molecular portrait of tumors can be obtained through different molecular biology techniques such as sequencing approaches (sanger sequencing, pyrosequencing, next-generation sequencing, and its various applications) and real-time PCR-based approaches (quantitative PCR, beaming, and digital PCR). Using these techniques it is possible to identify specific markers in different tumor types and to select patients for a targeted treatment. When a tumor is defined as wild type, the treatment is based on standard chemotherapy. Therefore, the path of survival in cancer patients is tissue dependent

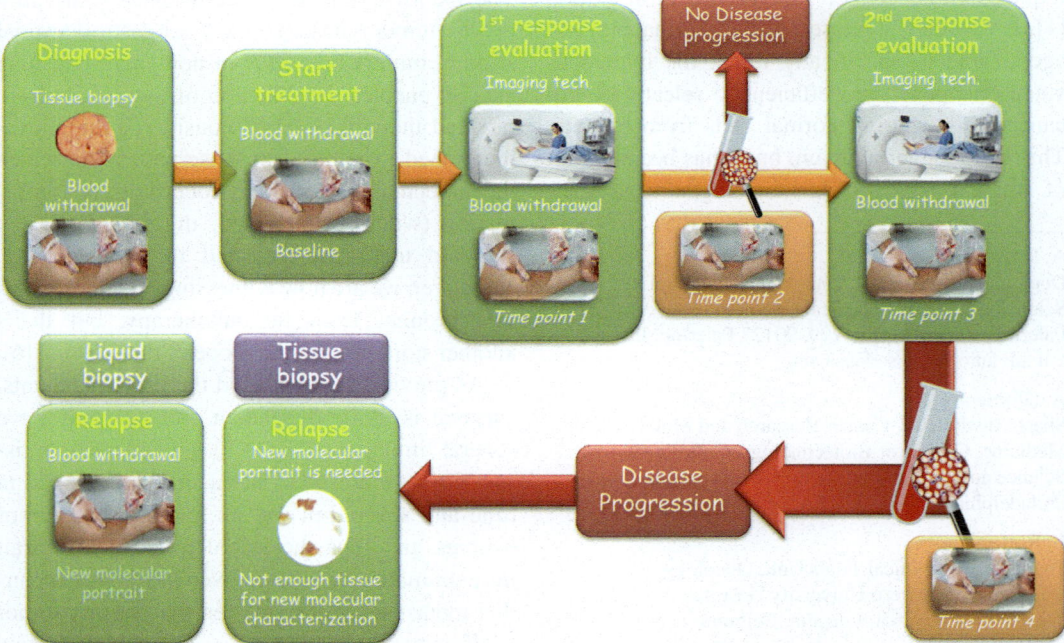

Fig. 1.2 The neoplastic tissue path from diagnosis to relapse. At diagnosis tissue biopsy is fundamental for a proper histological characterization. From this moment the same tissue will be used for several molecular tests, e.g., for NSCLC. At relapse it might be needed a new molecular portrait, but the initial tissue is not enough for a new molecular characterization. Liquid biopsy can be repeated at different time points, and therefore it can complement both tissue biopsy and imaging techniques, during the disease course. Moreover, liquid biopsy could anticipate disease progression even months before radiological progression

least, there is the problem of tumor heterogeneity that may be very difficult to overcome especially when the lesion is not easily accessible and thus multiple tissue biopsies are not feasible [7].

For all these reasons, it became necessary to search for new noninvasive or minimally invasive markers that can allow a strict patients' follow-up at different time points. Here comes the concept of *liquid biopsy*, i.e., a liquid biomarker that can be easily isolated from many body fluids (blood, saliva, urine, ascites, pleural effusion, etc.) and, as well as a tissue biopsy, is representative of the tissue from which it is spread [8]. The term liquid biopsy encompasses several components: circulating tumor cells (CTCs), cell-free DNA (cfDNA) and circulating tumor DNA (ctDNA), exosomes, and circulating cell-free nucleic acids (cfNAs, such as microRNA, mRNA, and long noncoding RNAs). We are just at the beginning

and we still have to investigate and understand the different components of liquid biopsy. Despite the promising expectations, not everything that glitters is gold, and for some components, such as exosomes, we are still far away from clinical applications [9, 10]. Moreover also for CTCs and ctDNA, we can list a series of pros and cons that are reported in Fig. 1.3. Notwithstanding, in some cases liquid biopsy is already a valid tool that can be used in clinical practice. This is the case of ctDNA testing in non-small cell lung cancer and CTCs enumeration in breast, prostate, and colon cancer [11–16], as it will be explained in the following chapters.

There are several possible clinical applications for liquid biopsies (Fig. 1.4): early diagnosis, prognostic information, surrogate endpoint biomarker and real-time monitoring of the disease (Fig. 1.5), identification of therapeutic

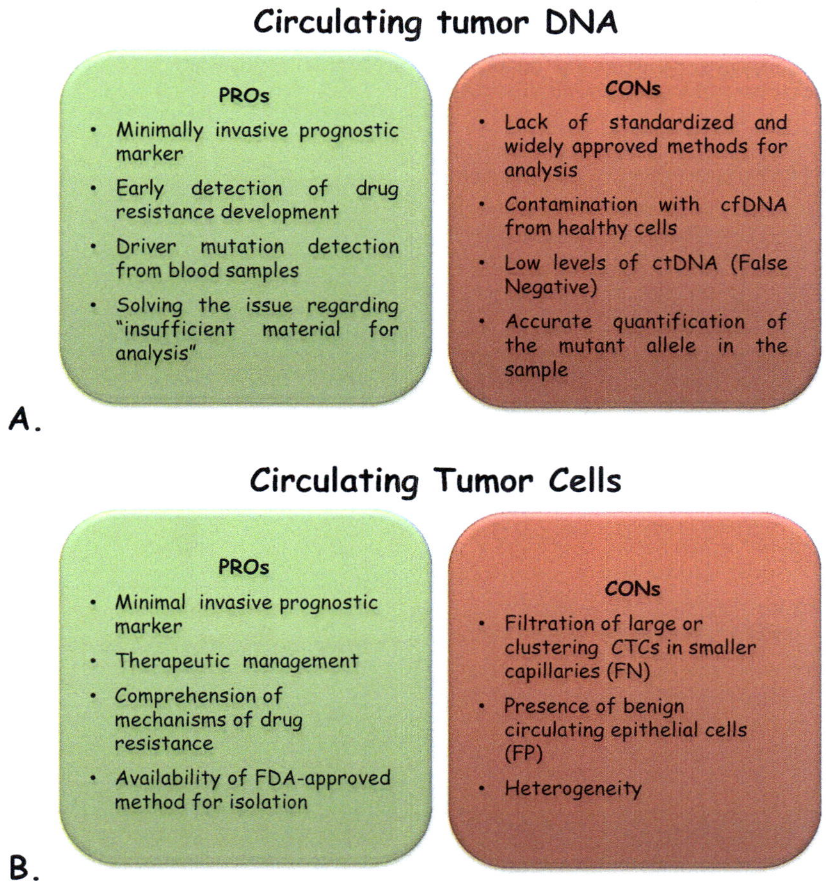

Circulating tumor DNA

PROs
- Minimally invasive prognostic marker
- Early detection of drug resistance development
- Driver mutation detection from blood samples
- Solving the issue regarding "insufficient material for analysis"

CONs
- Lack of standardized and widely approved methods for analysis
- Contamination with cfDNA from healthy cells
- Low levels of ctDNA (False Negative)
- Accurate quantification of the mutant allele in the sample

A.

Circulating Tumor Cells

PROs
- Minimal invasive prognostic marker
- Therapeutic management
- Comprehension of mechanisms of drug resistance
- Availability of FDA-approved method for isolation

CONs
- Filtration of large or clustering CTCs in smaller capillaries (FN)
- Presence of benign circulating epithelial cells (FP)
- Heterogeneity

B.

Fig. 1.3 Overview of the main pros and cons of both ctDNA (**a**) and CTCs (**b**)

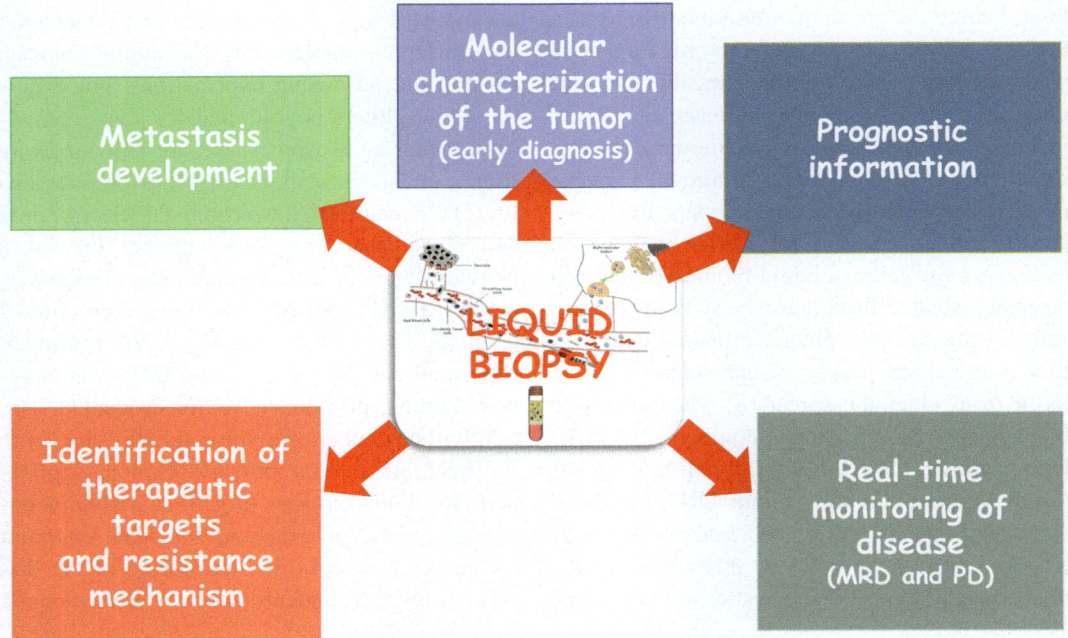

Fig. 1.4 The possible clinical applications of liquid biopsy: (i) early diagnosis, (ii) prognostic information, (iii) real-time monitoring of disease, (iv) identification of therapeutic targets and resistance mechanism, and (v) metastasis development

Fig. 1.5 Liquid biopsy as surrogate endpoint biomarker. This term refers to a single or combination of factors related to the patients or the tumors, whose changes during the treatment reflect the antitumor activity. For example, the progressive reduction of surrogate biomarker during targeted therapies can be associated with treatment response. Accordingly, an increased level of the same biomarker could imply the onset of resistance

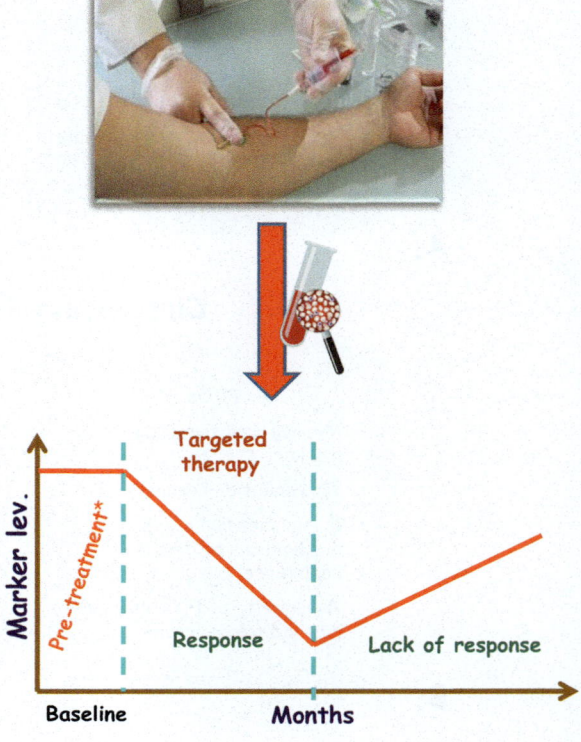

targets and resistance mechanisms, and metastasis development.

Therefore, both biologists and medical doctors (oncologists and pathologists) must work together, for a better comprehension on how patients can benefit the most from liquid biopsy application in clinical practice.

The aim of this volume is to shed light on the role of liquid biopsy in the clinical management of different tumor types. Along the volume, the readers will find the most updated results of CTC, ctDNA, and exosome investigation in the main solid tumors, trying to point out their relevance as diagnostic, prognostic, and predictive tools. The liquid biopsy revolution has started, and with this volume we want to contribute to understand its clinical relevance but also its weakness.

References

1. Weinstein IB. Cancer. Addiction to oncogenes – the Achilles heal of cancer. Science. 2002;297:63–4.
2. Batth IS, Mitra A, Manier S, Ghobrial IM, Menter D, Kopetz S, Li S. Circulating tumor markers: harmonizing the yin and yang of CTCs and ctDNA for precision medicine. Ann Oncol. 2016. pii: mdw619. doi:10.1093/annonc/mdw619.
3. Bronte G, Franchina T, Alù M, et al. The comparison of outcomes from tyrosine kinase inhibitor monotherapy in second- or third-line for advanced non-small-cell lung cancer patients with wild-type or unknown EGFR status. Oncotarget. 2016;7:35803–12.
4. Russo A, Rizzo S. Biomarkers and efficacy: are we nearly there yet? Ann Oncol. 2011;22(7):1469–70.
5. Corsini LR, Bronte G, Terrasi M, et al. The role of microRNAs in cancer: diagnostic and prognostic biomarkers and targets of therapies. Expert Opin Ther Targets. 2012;16:103–9.
6. Rolfo C, Sortino G, Smits E, et al. Immunotherapy: is a minor god yet in the pantheon of treatments for lung cancer? Expert Rev Anticancer Ther. 2014;14: 1173–87.
7. Santini D, Loupakis F, Vincenzi B, et al. High concordance of KRAS status between primary colorectal tumors and related metastatic sites: Implications for clinical practice. Oncologist. 2008;13(12): 1270–5.
8. Rolfo C, Castiglia M, Hong D, et al. Liquid biopsies in lung cancer: the new ambrosia of researchers. Biochim Biophys Acta. 1846;2014:539–46.
9. Giallombardo M, Chacartegui Borras J, Castiglia M, et al. Exosomal miRNA analysis in non-small cell lung cancer (NSCLC) patients' plasma through qPCR: a feasible liquid biopsy tool. J Vis Exp. 2016;(111). doi:10.3791/53900
10. Reclusa P, Giallombardo M, Castiglia M, et al. P2.06: exosomal miRNA analysis in non-small cell lung cancer: new liquid biomarker?: track: biology and pathogenesis. J Thorac Oncol. 2016;11:S219–20.
11. Hayes DF, Cristofanilli M, Budd GT, et al. Circulating tumor cells at each follow-up time point during therapy of metastatic breast cancer patients predict progression-free and overall survival. Clin Cancer Res. 2006;12:4218–24.
12. Danila DC, Heller G, Gignac GA, et al. Circulating tumor cell number and prognosis in progressive castration-resistant prostate cancer. Clin Cancer Res. 2007;13:7053–8.
13. Cohen SJ, Punt CJ, Iannotti N, et al. Relationship of circulating tumor cells to tumor response, progression-free survival, and overall survival in patients with metastatic colorectal cancer. J Clin Oncol. 2008;26: 3213–21.
14. Andreyev HJ, Benamouzig R, Beranek M, et al. Mutant K-ras2 in serum. Gut. 2003;52(6):915–6.
15. Bazan V, Bruno L, Augello C, et al. Molecular detection of TP53, ki-ras and p16 INK4A promoter methylation in plasma of patients with colorectal cancer and its association with prognosis, results of a 3-year GOIM prospective study. Ann Oncol. 2006;17: 84–90.
16. Russo A, Rizzo S, Bronte G, Silvestris N, Colucci G, Gebbia N, Bazan V, Fulfaro F. The long and winding road to useful predictive factors for anti-egfr therapy in metastatic colorectal carcinoma: the KRAS/BRAF pathway. Oncology. 2010;77:57–68.

Precision Oncology: Present Status and Perspectives

2

Pierosandro Tagliaferri, Mariamena Arbitrio,
Antonella Ierardi, Domenico Ciliberto,
Maria Teresa Di Martino,
and Pierfrancesco Tassone

Introduction

Recent advancements in medical research brought to a better understanding of the molecular bases of diseases and the interindividual variability in drug response, opening a new era in the management of patient care, known as the *precision medicine*. In this view, new approaches to patient diagnosis, monitoring or treatment can benefit from the integration of information deriving from different technologic approaches such as high-throughput *omics* (next-generation sequencing, metabolomics, proteomics, epigenomics, bioinformatics, system biology, and medicine biobanks) in order to allow the implementation of a truly tailored therapy [1]. In fact, for a specific disease, a multidisciplinary approach will allow a more accurate prediction of treatment and strategy, differently from the traditional "one-size-fits-all" approaches [2]. Systems pharmacology and pharmacogenomics (PGx) helped the understanding of the clinical impact of genetic-determined interindividual differences in pharmacokinetics (PK) of many drugs especially

for antineoplastic agents, in which the patient risk is due to the narrow therapeutic index. On the other hand, in the era of precision medicine, the understanding of the tumor molecular profile has the potential to drive clinical decisions for tailored treatment options with improved efficacy. Consequently, the interindividual variability in drug response, in terms of efficacy and toxicity, due to the interaction of genetic, pathophysiological and environmental factors, has a relevant effect on cancer treatment. Cancer is not a single disease but is a series of genome-based diseases and its treatment activity is conditioned by disease diffusion and individual patient-related factors. In fact, genomic deregulation at different levels is involved in tumorigenesis and includes different events such as gene inactivation (promoter silencing, deletion, mutations), alterations in gene expression (copy number variation, methylation), and mutations or rearrangements responsible of protein activation [3]. The transition from conventional cytotoxic drugs to molecular biomarkers-driven decision for the selection of cancer therapeutic options improved the management of many advanced-stage tumors. In fact, the identification of somatic and germline genetic biomarkers provides information about the likelihood of response to treatment and offers therefore predictive and prognostic information for the selection of patients. The frequent exposure to endogenous and exogenous reactive chemicals can alter the DNA sequence as well as

P. Tagliaferri (✉) • A. Ierardi • D. Ciliberto
M.T. Di Martino • P. Tassone
Department of Experimental and Clinical Medicine,
Magna Graecia University, Catanzaro, Italy
e-mail: tagliaferri@unicz.it

M. Arbitrio
ISN-CNR, Roccelletta di Borgia, Catanzaro, Italy

© Springer International Publishing AG 2017
A. Giordano et al. (eds.), *Liquid Biopsy in Cancer Patients*, Current Clinical Pathology,
DOI 10.1007/978-3-319-55661-1_2

chromatin structure and bring to somatic genomic and epigenomic abnormalities. In most cases, no cellular abnormalities occurs, while in some cases in a prone tissue, the clonal transformation of a cell takes place and consequently begins the development process, which will finally drive to a malignant lesion. In many cancers, including chronic myeloid leukemia, colon, breast, lung and melanoma, predictive biomarkers are currently in use to select patients, which might benefit of targeted therapy and avoid toxic side effects of chemotherapy. Biomarkers, providing information on cancer molecular signatures, may allow treatment tailoring and are distinguished into: diagnostic, prognostic, treatment and prevention subgroups. Key mutations and molecular pathways involved in tumor development and proliferation can be identified by predictive biomarkers, which are measurable and linked to relevant clinical outcomes. They have undergone a validation process for use as predictive tool within clinical trials. Instead, prognostic biomarkers identify somatic and germline mutations, alterations in DNA methylation, microRNA (miRNA) and circulating tumor cells (CTC) in blood and provide information on tumor outcome independent from treatment. Today, diagnostic companion assays undergo validation for biomarker value for treatment decision-making. High-throughput technologies provided the opportunity to identify genomic changes conditioning development and progression of a tumor ("driver" lesions) with a selective growth advantage and *addiction* of the cancer cell to a particular molecular pathway, despite other quantitatively preponderant and concomitant armless *passenger* alterations [4]. Consequently, genes identified to have a driver role in at least one cancer type are considered oncogenes [5]. A subset of the driver aberrations could have significantly diagnostic, prognostic or therapeutic potential and are often indicated as *actionable*; a subset of mutations may also be *druggable* as target for drug development [6]. Today, tumors molecular characterization and predictive/prognostic biomarker discoveries have allowed better understanding of the complex mechanisms of carcinogenesis and have fueled the development

of novel drug targets and new treatment strategies to enhance patient care. The hallmarks of precision medicine rely on genomics and clinical data integration based on cancer molecular characteristics in order to personalize oncology and to design new clinical trials. In order to study targeted therapies in different tumor types expressing low-frequency mutations (<5%) it is possible to design *basket trials* where are enrolled a small number of patients with different kind of cancer expressing the same genetic alteration, while in an alternative approach, *umbrella trials* recruit patients with a single cancer type but different actionable mutations. Drug structure analysis allows the design of new studies to test new drugs and biomarkers. In *basket trials*, a hypothesis-driven strategy is implemented and can be the proof-of-principle validation of a putative target and offer the opportunity to integrate a classical clinical trial design with the knowledge of molecular expression at tumor level. The limit of this trial design is that a mutation can act differently as driver druggable target in a given tumor, while it can be a passenger lesion in other tumor contexts. Another aspect emerging and in contrast with the performance of basket and umbrella trials is the role of tumor stroma in conditioning therapeutic choices and future drug development [7, 8].

In our chapter, as a prototypical condition, we will discuss the current scenario of personalized treatment of colon–rectal cancer, including molecular cancer-related and patient-related biomarkers, the emerging molecular landscapes and finally we will discuss the new approach of integrative genomics, as emerging vision based on large biological annotated datasets and bioinformatics tools.

Current Status: The Case of Colorectal Cancer (CRC)

Metastatic colorectal cancer (mCRC) is characterized by several molecular lesions involving activation or loss-of-function mutations, which occur in receptor tyrosine kinases (RTKs) and more frequently in downstream components of

RTK-activated intracellular pathways. Therefore, treatment effects of the target therapy can be considered as strictly related to specific molecular alterations.

The epidermal growth factor receptor (EGFR), expressed on the cell surface, belongs to the ERbB-family, a subfamily of RTKs. The anti-EGFR cetuximab and panitumumab mAbs prevent activation of EGFR [9, 10]. They block ligand-stimulated EGFR signaling and they probably stop activation of phosphatidylinositol 3-kinase (PI3K)/AKT and RAS/MAP2K (also called MEK)/MAPK1/3 (also called ERK2/1) signaling pathways, leading to inhibition of cellular proliferation and induction of apoptosis [11].

One of the most important molecular mechanisms of primary resistance to EGFR mAbs (cetuximab and panitumumab) is KRAS mutation. In fact, the mutation in KRAS appears to hold a negative predictive value for the response of anti-EGFR therapy [12, 13]. At the beginning, only the mutation in exon 2 of KRAS was considered [14, 15] and then the research for mutations was expanded to the exons 3, 4 of KRAS and 2,3,4 of NRAS, also involved in the resistance to anti-EGFR drugs [16].

In patients with mCRC the efficacy of chemotherapy can be, in fact, implemented by biological drugs based on the molecular status of RAS, in particular cetuximab and panitumumab for wild-type RAS status and bevacizumab for both RAS wild type and mutated [17–22].

The correlation between the molecular status of KRAS and the survival endpoints in first-line mCRC treated with cetuximab and standard chemotherapy regimens was initially demonstrated by a retrospective analysis of the Crystal study [23].

In patients with PAN–RAS mutations the best standard first-line treatment is represented by the association of chemotherapy with bevacizumab [17–20], whereas in mutated patients has not been established the best sequence for the use of anti-EGFR drugs in first line rather than in the second one [24–26].

During the carcinogenesis trajectory, genetic aberrations accumulate and this process leads to the so-called genetic heterogeneity resulting in the selection of clones with different functions including the ability to respond to a specific treatment and to generate metastases [27]. For this reason, patients with RAS wild-type mCRC could present mutated subclones that induce resistance to treatment with anti-EGFR under the selective therapy pressure [28, 29].

It is known that in patients RAS wild-type molecular alterations of BRAF [30, 31] and PIK3CA [32, 33] genes might be present, which may cause primary resistance to anti-EGFR.

BRAF is a human gene that encodes a protein called BRAF and it is a member of the RAF gene family. BRAF protein is a serine–threonine protein kinase involved in RAS-activated pathway. BRAF mutation is found in 15% of colorectal cancers, and it is known that this alteration is linked to a poor prognosis [31, 34].

The most frequent BRAF mutation is V600E, located in the kinase activation domain and it leads to an increased activity of MAPK1/3 pathway. BRAF-mutant tumors have dissimilar clinical and histological characteristics from RAS-mutant tumors [35]. It was found that the CpG island methylator phenotype (CIMP) and microsatellite instability are observed in BRAF-mutated tumors [31, 35].

In a retrospective consortium analysis it was revealed that only two patients out of a total of 24 patients with BRAF-mutated cancer responded to the treatment with cetuximab [32].

Only a small sample of patients with BRAF-mutated cancer benefit from treatment with panitumumab or cetuximab [35].

PIK3CA is part of lipid kinase family involved in various cellular processes regarding growth, proliferation, differentiation, motility, survival and intracellular trafficking [36].

PIK3CA mutations can occur more frequently (80%) in exon 9 (60–65%) and 20 (20–25%) [32]. In a study it was shown that only mutation in exon 20 of PIK3CA is associated to a resistance to cetuximab activity in population KRAS wild-type [32]. Moreover, PIK3CA has a negative prognostic value because it is associated with a shorter survival in tumors RAS wild-type stage I–III [37].

Another important molecular lesion involves PTEN gene that encodes the phosphatase and tensin homolog protein. PTEN mutations are present in nearly 5% with high microsatellite instability. PTEN role in colorectal cancer is not clear, but it was shown that PTEN loss is associated with a reduced response to cetuximab [30, 38–40].

Other important factors are prognostic for survival in colorectal cancer in addition to defined molecular defects [41, 42].

The importance of the clinical and biological difference between proximal and distal cancer is becoming now clear. Right- and left-sided CRCs are characterized by different carcinogenesis trajectories, mucosal immunologic microenvironment and gut microbiota [43]. Right-sided cancer is most frequently diploid and has a mucinous histology, high microsatellite instability, CpG island methylation and BRAF mutations [44, 45], while the left-sided one is characterized by chromosomal instability. These peculiarities reflect a different embryonic origin [46, 47].

The analysis of the correlation among tumor sidedness and survival after chemotherapy+/− bevacizumab was performed in three independent cohorts in a study. According to this, patients with right colon cancer have a lower recurrence, but they show a more aggressive behavior in relapsed disease [48]. In this group of patients, the role of BRAF is clear as a negative prognostic factor [49] in a more advanced phase of the carcinogenesis process and, with other factors, might play a role in chemoresistance, while the left colon cancers have an increased benefit from treatment on activity and efficacy endpoints [48].

About the benefit of the biological treatment according to the tumor site, it was found an increased activity of anti-EGFR drugs in the left-sided primary tumor location, demonstrated in terms of PFS [50].

It is important to consider that the tumor microenvironment is different between the left and right colon. Indeed the right colon cancers have a higher share of eosinophils and intraepithelial T cells [51, 52].

It has been speculated that this could be the result of a homeostatic balance in T cells between tolerance for the commensal microbiota and the immune response against pathogens [53].

Currently major attention is focused on the mismatch repair (MMR) gene deficiency, which can be sporadic or occurs within the Lynch syndrome. It is found in 1 out of 35 patients with colon–rectal cancer [54] and it leads to microsatellite instability (MSI) represented by alterations in the length of tandem nucleotide repeats [55, 56].

MSI overall predicts for a better prognosis. The correlation between the microenvironment rich in lymphocyte cells, the immune-score and the favorable outcome in tumors with MSI needs additional investigation [57].

The immune-score is characterized by the determination of the number of cytotoxic and memory T cells represented in intra-tumor and peri-tumor infiltration and it is considered a biomarker with prognostic relevance [58, 59].

The presence of high levels of CD8 + lymphocytes in the microenvironment that express the chemokine-receptor-7 (CCR7) is found to influence the prognosis increasing the overall survival and progression-free survival after a first-line chemotherapy [60].

Moreover, high levels of FOXP3+ T lymphocyte correlate with the outcome of patients who undergo chemotherapy or chemo-immunotherapy [61].

All together, these findings open a new biological scenario where the immune system plays a substantial role. In fact, there is now a renewed interest for the immunotherapy which has opened the way for immune checkpoint inhibitors development that modulate immune response against tumor cells. While in some tumors, such as malignant melanoma, immunotherapy has produced highly successful results, in others unfortunately did not reach the same activity, such as in mCRC. In fact, only a small subgroup of mCRC patients with deficiency of the MMR mechanism benefit from treatment with programmed death-1 (PD-1) checkpoint inhibitors (5–10% of all mCRC patients) [62].

A phase 2 trial showed the efficacy of treatment with pembrolizumab in tumors with MMR deficiency [63]. Tumors with defective MMR are more responsive to the PD1 block confirming the successful advantage of high density of immune system cells in the microenvironment and the mismatch repair deficiency [64–66].

Another potential predictive biomarker is represented by mutation in exonuclease domain of DNA polymerase epsilon (Pol-ε). This mutation correlates with a higher immune infiltrate (like MMR deficiency) and a better disease-free survival in MSI-proficient tumors. Both MMR deficiency and Pol-ε mutation lead to increased tumor mutation burden and to the onset of tumor specific neo-antigens, which could activate the immune system in a tumor specific response [67].

Recently, it has been focused on HER2 gene alterations (HER2 over-expression or amplification) that make the cancer sensitive to a specific combination of direct molecular targeted drugs against this target [68].

To conclude, the selection of the most appropriate treatment should be based on the patient, on the biological characteristics of the tumor, on the objectives to be achieved, on the toxicity of the treatment, and finally on the continuum of care, which indeed needs to be also considered.

At present only negative predictors of response to various treatments are available and validated for the clinical scenario. The biomarker that has demonstrated a deep impact in the history of colorectal cancer is the RAS mutational status, which is indeed a negative predictor.

To guide the oncologist in the decision-making process of treatment of colorectal cancer, positive predictive biomarkers are eagerly awaited for treatment individualization and need validation in prospective trials (Fig. 2.1).

Future Perspective: Molecular Landscape of Colorectal Cancer

Genomic Classificationof Colorectal Cancer

Surgery is the mainstay treatment for CRC patients although, at the time of diagnosis, CRC is often a systemic disease and therefore adjuvant chemotherapy is the best choice for preventing disease relapse. The standard classification of CRC considers pathological staging a clinical prognostic factors to select patients for adjuvant chemotherapy.

For this lethal disease, with an estimated heritability of approximately 5%, exists a classification based on molecular profiling and linkage studies. In fact, germline mutations on APC gene and DNA MMR genes characterized the hereditary colorectal cancer syndromes, while other low penetrance genetic variants have been correlated to approximately 20% of the familial association in CRC [69]. Inherited CRC syndromes are classified based on the presence of large numbers of adenomatous polyps like familial adenomatous polyposis (FAP), attenuated FAP and MUT-Y-homolog-associated polyposis (MAP) and the presence of hamartoma polyps like primary lesions in Peutz–Jeghers syndrome (PJS) and juvenile polyposis syndrome (JPS) as well as non-adenoma syndromes Lynch 1 and 2. Hyperplastic polyposis (HPP) is a condition that produces substantially increased cancer risk. Somatic mutations and polymorphic features in TP53 gene impact susceptibility to sporadic CRC, prognosis and response to therapy [70].

According to gene expression profile, supervised approaches contributed to identify signatures related to relevant outcomes such as recurrence, metastasis and overall survival, while semi-supervised approaches refined outcome prediction according to patients selection based on stage disease [71, 72].

Recently, an unsupervised analysis considers inherent molecular subtypes for CRC classification and correlates them to prognosis [73, 74], while recent studies proposed a consensus classification system identifying three groups: the Goblet/Inflammatory group, the TA/Enterocyte group, and the stem/serrated/mesenchymal (SSM) group [75, 76]. However, it has been proposed also a sub-classification of CRC that distinguishes those with MSI (which arises on a hereditary and sporadic basis, located primarily in the right colon and associated with the CpG island methylator phenotype (CIMP) and hypermutation) and those that are microsatellite stable (MSS) but chromosomally unstable (CIN) [77]. Barat et al. utilized microarray-based gene expression and methylation dataset to identify

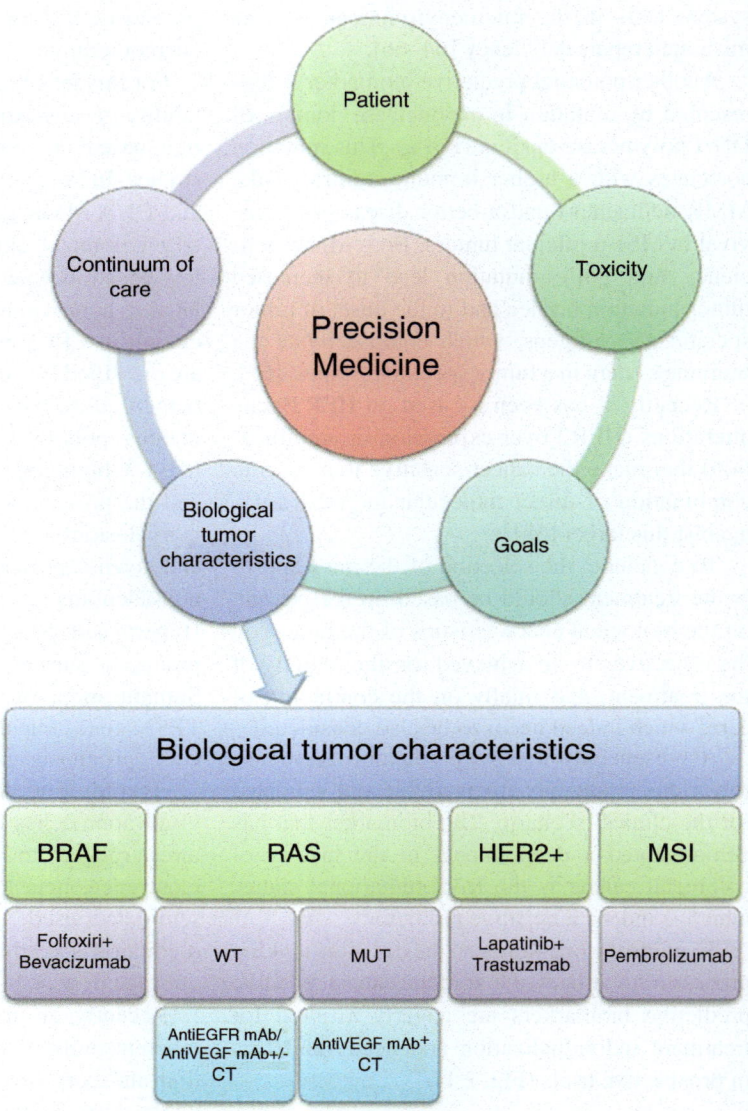

Fig. 2.1 This chart describes the possible molecular alterations that lead to the therapy's customization based on the molecular profile of each patient. The center of our attention is precision medicine that has to guide the oncologist's decision in order to provide the best choice based on the characteristics of patient, tumor, and treatment

methylation-based subgroups and distinguished three main clusters: highly methylated (HM), intermediately methylated (IM) and large clusters with both lower and rarer locus-specific methylation (LM) [78]. The study provides evidence that integration and combination of gene expression and methylation datasets analyses could better described the CRC subtypes. Gene expression profiles and genomic characterization influence CRC outcome (Fig. 2.2).

Critical genes and pathways, including the WNT, RAS–MAPK, PI3K, TGF-b, P53 and DNA MMR pathways, are involved in the initiation and progression of CRC [77, 79]. They are associated with different mutation frequencies of the main oncogenes RAS, BRAF, APC and other genetic events, whose expression redefines treatment selection. With the exception of hypermutated cancers, CRC have similar patterns of genomic alteration, and there is evidence of sig-

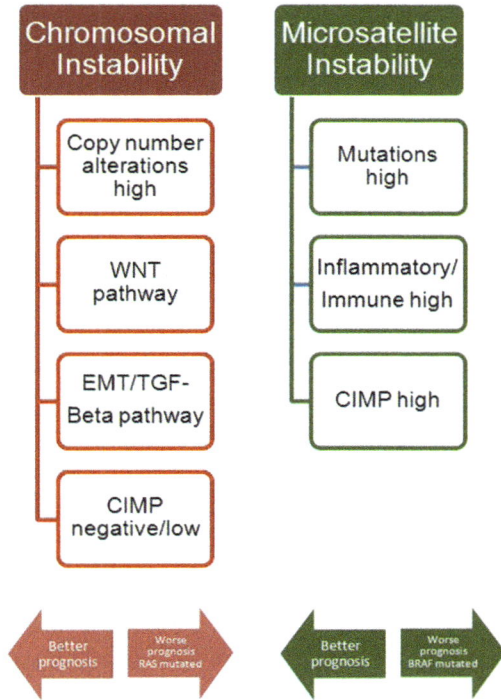

Fig. 2.2 Diagram of gene alteration pathways based on genomic characterization: the related outcome according to CRC subtypes

nificant intra-tumor genetic heterogeneity due to variations in localized somatic mutations and copy number abnormalities [80].

Through bioinformatics tools in 750 patients with stage I to IV CRC, undergone to surgical treatment, it has been possible to stratify CRC by transcriptomic-based classification on the bases of clinical-pathological features and common DNA markers [76]. In fact, six prognostic molecular subgroups of CRC sample have been identified and validated on the bases of gene expression data, associated with clinical and pathological characteristics, molecular alterations, specific gene expression signatures and deregulated signaling pathways. Today, although official guidelines indicate a risk stratification, no clear recommendations for adjuvant chemotherapy in stage II disease are available, and molecular technologies are strictly required to improve the selection of individualized therapeutics [81]. Promise derives now from validation clinical trials evaluat-

ing two prognostic tests, based on the expression of different gene panels like ColoPrint (Agendia, Amsterdam, the Netherlands), which are based on 18 genes, and Oncotype DX (Genomic Health, Redwood City, CA) which includes 12 genes (seven recurrence risk genes and five reference genes) and represents the individual prognostic score most widely retrospectively evaluated with a little overlapping [82, 83]. Until now ColoPrint and Oncotype DX were available to improve risk prediction in early-stage CRC [83, 84] and have been investigated in three independent datasets of stage II–IIIA CC and as a prognostic score in the QUASAR and CALGB9581 trials, respectively [76]. Presently current pathological staging is not able to predict recurrence in a phase of curable disease, so it is necessary to take benefit from additional tools. Nomograms such as "Adjuvant Online" or Memorial Sloan Kettering Cancer Center (MSKCC) and Bayesian Belief Network (BBN) can be used in clinical practice to show outcome of patients in the same disease condition and predict the probability of CRC patient's to 5 years OS after surgical removal of all cancerous tissue [85]. Another prognostic nomograms was developed by Peng et al. for predicting outcome in patients with locally advanced rectal cancers without preoperative treatment, while no nomogram can predict long-term outcome after CRC surgery for all disease stages [86, 87].

It is clear that all the above-described tools represent sound decision supporting instruments but cannot be defined bona fide precision medicine approaches, taking into account the intrinsic heuristic nature. Despite this complex scenario, presently there isn't an integrated view of the CRC genetic and genomic changes in initiation and subsequent different stages of disease progression. Further insight may help the understanding of CRC pathophysiology and the identification of potential therapeutic targets.

Recently, Dalerba et al. identified a subgroup of stage II CRC patients who might benefit from adjuvant chemotherapy for the lack of caudal-type homeobox transcription factor 2 (CDX2) expression in their cancer stem cells [88]. By a bioinformatics approach, the authors, in order to identify a single prognostic biomarkers for stratification of

CRC undifferentiated tumors, have analyzed a large database of gene expression arrays obtained from populations of stem and progenitor cells and searched for genes associated with differentiation processes. Among the 16 selected candidate genes for identification of predictive biomarkers, negatively linked to the activated leukocyte–cell adhesion molecule (ALCAM/CD166) in CRC patients with stage II or stage III, they selected the homeobox transcription factor CDX2 strictly correlated to ALCAM expression and tested for the association with disease-free survival and a benefit from adjuvant chemotherapy. In particular, it was identified that subgroup of high-risk stage II CRC patients benefit from adjuvant chemotherapy and was characterized by lack of CDX2 expression and high levels of ALCAM.

The translation of this knowledge in CRC has had an important impact into drug development and biomarker discovery for the different subtypes and examples of molecular targeted therapies are tyrosine kinase inhibitors, regorafenib and bevacizumab.

Pharmacogenomicsand Irinogenomics

In CRC, despite the standard chemotherapy and novel targeted drugs provided an improvement in terms of response rate and patient's survival, toxicity remains an unsolved problem and PGx has helped the routinely administration of drugs in CRC patients [89]. In CRC as well as in other cancers, the treatment paradigm is to give the dose which achieves the best drug exposure and effectiveness, with an acceptable risk of toxicity [90]. Unluckily, the inter-patient PK variability is a limiting factor due not only to differences in body size but also to variability in absorption, metabolism, distribution and/or excretion (ADME) of the drug and metabolites. In fact, several enzymes and transporters that are part of the ADME processes can condition drug efficacy and toxicity because their expression and activity are highly variable between patients, partially due to germline genetic variability. Germline variants in the coding region can change protein

activity, while variations outside of the coding region could influence protein expression [91]. Another important aspect to consider is patient's germline variation underlying sensitizing condition that mimics the toxicity and can be worsened by the drug. Thus, a patient who carries a sensitizing germline variant would not be able to tolerate the dose required for treatment efficacy and might require to receive a dose adjustment or the selection of an alternative treatment agent. The most frequent type of genetic variants among people (10 million in the human genome) associated with the interindividual variability in drug response are the single nucleotide polymorphisms (SNPs) which represent a difference in a single nucleotide in certain stretch of DNA sequence between two genes. Frequently they are devoid of a functional role but, if a SNP occurs within a gene or in a regulatory region near a gene, they could play a more direct role in disease or in drug metabolism by affecting gene's function. Most of identified SNPs are in linkage disequilibrium with gene variants with higher or lower activity and serve therefore as markers predictive of activity or toxicity due to different enzyme function. SNPs linked to genes coding for enzymes involved in drug metabolism and transport affect therefore the body response and PK profile influencing the efficacy and toxicity of treatment. The possibility to identify SNPs as predictive biomarkers of response to antineoplastic agents by classical approaches like candidate-gene-based research and the genome-wide association study (GWAS) or by technologic advances like the Affymetrix (Santa Clara, California, USA) Drug Metabolizing Enzymes and Transporters (DMET™) microarray platform will allow an improvement of patient care in the optic of personalized therapy. In particular by DMET™ platform is possible to investigate 1931 SNPs and five copy number variations (CNV) in 231 genes related to drugs metabolism contributing to discover polymorphic variants associated to the individual risk of adverse drug reactions (ADRs) and to drug efficacy. By this technology, in case-control studies we identified several polymorphic variants associated with toxicity in different diseases and added novel information on irinogenomics (see below) [92–97]. DMET™ platform offers wide opportunity to identify and validate biomarkers of drug sensitivity for tailored treatment of CRC patients.

Pharmacological treatment of CRC is based on cytotoxic agents like fluoropyrimidines (FdUMP (fluorodeoxyuridine monophosphate, fluorouracil (5-FU), and its oral precursor, capecitabine), irinotecan (IRI, CPT-11), and oxaliplatin (OX), used either alone or in combinations in FOLFIRI (folinic acid, fluorouracil (5-FU), and irinotecan) and FOLFOX (folinic Acid, 5-FU, and oxaliplatin) regimens, and novel targeted agents. Recently, CRC treatment has benefited of novel biological agents as monoclonal antibodies (mAbs) targeting VEGF (i.e. bevacizumab, aflibercept) and EGFR (i.e. cetuximab, panitumumab) pathways or agents leading to a multiple-kinase inhibition (regorafenib) [98]. Cytotoxic drugs have a narrow therapeutic index and strictly dose-related effect also conditioned by interindividual variability in their metabolism. Therefore PGx knowledges, validated biomarkers, integrative genomic approaches and the availability of genetic testing could allowed the identification of subgroups of CRC patients with benefits in terms of prognosis and drug efficacy in the aim of precision medicine. In cytotoxic CRC therapy, important PGx studies have been done on highly polymorphic specific targets, whose genetic or molecular deregulation might correlate to treatment efficacy. Unfortunately, the translation of PGx researches into clinical practice is presently limited with small exceptions regarding the metabolism of 5-FU/capecitabine and irinotecan. For 5-FU SNPs in two important metabolic enzymes have a relevance in clinical practice: the thymidylate synthase (TYMS) and dihydropyrimidine dehydrogenase (DPD), while for irinotecan polymorphic variants in uridine diphosphate glucuronosyltransferases (UGTs) influence variability in biliary excretion and the degradation of irinotecan is conditioned by inherited variations in metabolic pathway. 5-Fluorouracil (5-FU) or its prodrug capecitabine is a cytotoxic drug, classified as "antimetabolite," and represents the main chemotherapeutic regimen adopted in CRC treatment, having an improving impact on survival and other solid cancer [99].

The activity of this pyrimidine analog is due to the incorporation of fluoronucleotides into RNA and DNA and to the irreversible inhibition of its target enzyme the thymidylate synthase (TS). Three major active metabolites derive from 5-FU intracellular metabolism: fluorodeoxyuridine monophosphate (FdUMP), fluorodeoxyuridine triphosphate (FdUTP), and fluorouridine triphosphate (FUTP). Genetic variants in the three drug-metabolizing enzymes thymidine phosphorylate (TP), TYMS and DPD are responsible for variability in response, toxicity and overall survival (OS) in 5-FU-based treatment schedules [100].

5-FU cytotoxic activity is mediated by its methylation to dUMP with 5,10-methylenetetrahydrofolate (CH2THF) as cofactor, which forms in the cell a stable ternary complex with TYMS enzyme and supplies the only de novo source of thymidylate. Consequently, its cytotoxicity is due to the blocking access of dUMP to the nucleotide-binding site and to the inhibition and depletion of deoxythymidine monophosphate (dTMP) production, important for DNA replication and repair [101, 102]. In 5-FU metabolism in normal and cancer cells its conversion in dihydrofluorouracil (DHFU) is mediated by dihydropyrimidine dehydrogenase (DPD) and represents the rate-limiting step. DPD is abundant in the liver where is normally catabolized more than 80% of administered 5-FU [100]. The administration of the oral prodrug of 5-FU, capecitabine, has revealed a 5-FU comparable efficacy but a lower toxicity [103, 104]. In the liver, capecitabine is converted to 5'-deoxy-5-fluoruridine (DFUR) by carboxylesterase and cytidine deaminase and then converted to 5-FU by thymidine phosphorylase (TP) and/or uridine phosphorylase (UP) [105, 106]. The tumor-selective activation of capecitabine might be explained by the higher expression of both TP and UP in tumor tissue compared to normal tissue [107]. Patients with a decrease activity of catabolic enzymes in 5-FU pathway revealed an interindividual variability to cytotoxic chemotherapy with an increase in drug concentration and consequent high toxicity risk. DPD catalyzes

5-FU and eliminates >80% of administered drug. Its activity is influenced by dihydropyrimidine dehydrogenase (DPYD) gene which is variable at tumoral tissue level and can influence drug efficacy in consideration that intra-tumor drug concentration is fundamental for dug efficacy and antitumor activity. Mucositis, granulocytopenia and neuropathy are the most frequent toxic effects for which might be necessary a dose reduction [108].

In 5–10% of the general population, a partial DPD activity deficiency is demonstrated and only in 0.2% a total loss of enzyme activity [109]. However, DPD polymorphisms influenced the 23–38% of 5-FU toxicity [110]. The most common polymorphic variant recognized to be associated with partial DPD deficiency and consequent 5-FU toxicity is IVS14+1G>A mutation in intron 14 coupled with exon 14 deletion (DPYD*2A), together with the SNPs at 496A>G in exon 6, at 2846A>T in exon 22, and at T1679G (DPYD*13) in exon 13, also recognized to be associated with 5-FU toxicity [111–113].

The US Food and Drug Administration (FDA) has underlined, in the drug labels for 5-FU and capecitabine, that their use should not be allowed in carriers of high-risk alleles. The Dutch Pharmacogenetics Working Group has recommended an alternative treatment in patients homozygous for the high-risk allele and almost a dose reduction of 50% or an alternative drug in patients heterozygous for a decreased-activity allele [114, 115] (in agreement with the more recent Clinical Pharmacogenetics Implementation Consortium Guidelines for Dihydropyrimidine Dehydrogenase Genotype and Fluoropyrimidine Dosing).

Polymorphic variants in TYMS gene are responsible for an increased expression of the enzyme with a consequent high risk of 5-FU toxicity and reduced drug efficacy. TS overexpression is frequently associated with a reduced response to 5-FU treatment based both in adjuvant and in advanced CRC patients with more severe side effects [116, 117].

In CRC patients carrying low levels of TYMS gene product, a significantly higher rate of treatment response and a prolonged overall survival compared to CRC patients with higher TS expression in tumor tissue have been described [109].

Two meta-analyses supported the role of TS expression on overall response rate and overall survival [118, 119]. However, further analyses are necessary to allow a better identification of TYMS transcription regulatory mechanisms and the understanding of the role played by genetic different SNPs combinations in several metabolic enzymes and their frequency in general populations to better clarify the interindividual variability to drugs response. Until now, no recommendations are suggested according to TS phenotype in CRC patient underwent to fluoropyrimidines treatment and although an assay for DPD and TYMS polymorphisms testing is commercially available, pre-emptive testing is not recommended. No recommendations have been issued on dosing of fluoropyrimidines by TS phenotype.

Other gene polymorphisms possibly important for fluoropyrimidine efficacy and toxicity for various enzymes have currently been explored (e.g., dihydropyrimidinase, beta-ureidopropionase, methylenetetrahydrofolate reductase), but available research data are insufficient for conclusions on their potential clinical usefulness. Several other polymorphic variants in enzymes involved at different levels in 5-FU metabolic pathways probably influenced intrinsic and acquired 5-FU pharmacoresistance in CRC patients, but no translation in clinical practice is validated, until now [120].

In CRC treatment another widely used anticancer drug is irinotecan, a camptothecin analog and inactive prodrug, activated at liver level via human carboxylesterases CES1 and CES2 into the active form SN-38, subsequently inactivated through glucuronidation via members of the UDP-glucuronosyltransferase (UGT) enzyme family catalyzing also bilirubin glucuronidation. Somatic tumor-specific mutations seem to influence irinotecan toxicity and efficacy as well as interindividual variability limited its PK and PD [121–123]. Severe diarrhea and neutropenia represent dose-limiting toxicities. Despite the unequivocal confirmation of the role of somatic mutations on patient's outcome who underwent to irinotecan treatment, scientific evidences confirmed a role of polymorphic variants in UGTs family members, especially for UGT1A1 isoenzyme and other isoforms [103]. Polymorphic variants in UGT1A1 enzyme are responsible for impaired glucuronidating activity and consequent toxicity due to elevated serum levels of SN-38 and bilirubin [124, 125]. Ando et al. published the first evidence on the role of *UGT1A1*28 (UGT1A1 7/7 genotype)* in the development of irinotecan toxicity [126]. The homozygous UGT1A1*28 allele phenotype, responsible for increased risk for severe neutropenia and diarrhea, is represented in the 8–10% of the population and according to the FDA treatments in combination with other agents or as a single agent requires a reduction in the starting dose [127]. Dias et al. put in evidence an association between *UGT1A1* genotype and overall response rate in patients treated with irinotecan, but no direct evidences confirm that a dose reduction in *UGT1A1*28* homozygous phenotypes will not lead to an important reduction in overall response rate [128]. Despite FDA recommendations, in clinical practice the preemptive UGT1A1*28 allele testing is not yet applied although commercial assays for *UGT1A1* testing are available. There are other important polymorphic genes involved in irinotecan metabolic pathways under investigation for their role as putative biomarkers of hematological and gastric toxicities, but further validations are necessary for their potential clinical utility in irinogenomics [93, 129, 130].

Future Perspectives: Precision Medicine Based on Integrative Genomics

In the recent years, the development of a variety of high technology platforms has led researchers to produce large amount of data at different molecular levels and network, in different disciplines of the *omic* world. Traditionally, approaches of bioinformatics analysis were focused on the use of single classes of data (i.e. genomic data or proteomic data). The rising number of data has made clear that the integration of data at different levels could produce more relevant results. Consequently, many different approaches have pointed to such kind of integration, leading to the rise of a novel discipline, often defined as *integromics*, or integrated analysis of *omic* data, in which computer science, bioinformatics, and mathematical modeling have the main role. This discipline focuses on the elucidation of basic principles of the interplay among different biological molecules (such as proteins or genes), where the network theory plays a synergistic role [131–133]. The focus of computational integrative genomics is to identify basic principles of interplay of different molecules in order to better elucidate the molecular mechanism. This is under the assumption that the information gathered from integrated analysis is higher than in the single and separate study of any data source [131]. It usually utilized a common approach for findings that share a common flow of information. The flow starts from gathering data of different data sources. Then all data are integrated into a single network model, and the model is analyzed with different algorithms tailored to the specific application. Data sources of integrative omics mainly reside on messenger RNA (mRNA), miRNA and protein expression, DNA copy number, SNPs and may be produced in dedicated experiments or extracted from different available databases. Specifically, miRNA therapeutics is emerging as a valuable tool in translational precision oncology [134–139]. The scientific community has recently produced a large number of different databases useful for integrated analysis. In addition to academic data, pharmaceutical and biotech companies retain large amounts of "proprietary data" – inherited from their own and other sources. Most of the data is stored in older types of databases designed to manage a single type of data; therefore, the integration of these data source into a single comprehensive one is a relevant challenge [140].

From a biological point of view, it is clear that the main actors of this process are mRNAs, miR-

NAs, and transcription factors (TFs), those play an interacting role in the regulation of gene expression that results in variable levels of gene transcripts and proteins. Usually, the integration of such datasets relies on the formalism provided from graph theory. As a result, bioinformatics approaches for the integrated analysis usually build comprehensive graphs in which nodes are mRNAs, miRNAs, and TFs (or other molecules) and edges represent the interactions among them. Edges include two main categories: (i) activation edges modeling the interplay between molecules, among whose one may increase the level of another one, and (ii) inhibition edges that model the action of inhibition. The analysis of such graphs uses different algorithms tailored to the specific application. For instance, the individuation of small and connected subgraphs with three different classes of nodes is often used for the identification of loops (feedback and feed-forward) in which the regulation of the expression of a gene could be related to a synergistic action of both miRNA and TF.

All the methods of analysis available share some specific characteristics. First, the use of an internal knowledge base containing information collected from literature and from different databases. The knowledge base usually stores association among mRNAs, miRNAs, and TFs modeled as graphs. This internal knowledge base guides the analysis of experimental data. Second, the approaches enable the user to take external experimental datasets from a pool of samples extracted from patients in case-control or time-series experiments. Then, data of knowledge bases allow to build the association graph including experimental data. Finally, this association graph is mined to extract knowledge.

We here list some main approaches of integrative analysis focusing only on freely available tools.

MAGIA2 is the evolution of the precedent MAGIA web tool for the integrated analysis of both mRNA and miRNA. MAGIA receives as input, expression level data obtained by case-control or time-series experiments. In this way, it is able to integrate literature evidence, prediction algorithms, and mRNA and miRNA experimental data based on anticorrelation of miRNA-target expression, using four different relatedness measures. It is able to highlight different regulatory circuits involving either miRNA or TF as regulators: (i) a TF that regulates both a given miRNA and its target gene and (ii) a miRNA that regulates both a given TF and its regulated gene. Furthermore, this tool provides functional enrichment of the gene network using DAVID platform [141].

The *dchip GEMINI* is a freely available web server that receives as input expression levels of miRNA and mRNA obtained from time-series experiments analyzing two conditions, e.g., normal and cancer conditions. It is able to individuate Feed-Forward Loops (FFLs) consisting of TFs, miRNAs and their common target genes. The association among miRNA and their target (TF and mRNA) information is extracted from the literature and stored into the web server. TFs derived from literature used as null model to statistical ranks predicted FFLs from the experimental data [142].

mirConnX is a software tool based on a web interface to build gene regulatory networks starting from mRNA and miRNA expression data on a whole-genome scale. It based on a network built using as a priori model consisting of TF-gene associations and miRNA target predictions for human and mouse derived by computational methods and literature. Experimental data allow inference of experimental associations among TF, miRNA and genes. These associations allow to weight the predefined network and the resulting weighted network can be visualized by the user [143].

miRIN is a web application designed for the identification of the modules of protein–protein interaction networks regulated by miRNAs. The approach of analysis consists of the integration of miRNA target data from literature, protein–protein interactions between target genes from literature, as well as mRNA and miRNA expression profiles provided as data input. The output of

Table 2.1 Available software tools that integrate in a single model miRNA and mRNA data

Tool	Input	Output	Model	Website
MAGIA2	miRNA/mRNA Expression Data Time Series	Feed-forward loops (FFL) Ontological Analysis	Statistical model and literature evidence	http://gencomp.bio.unipd.it/magia2/start/
dCHIPGemini	miRNA/mRNA Expression Data Time Series	Feed-Forward Loops (FFL)	Statistical model and literature evidence	http://www.canevolve.org/dChip-GemiNi
mirConnX	miRNA, mRNA time series	Regulatory Networks	Pre-built network	http://www.benoslab.pitt.edu/mirconnx
miRIN	miRNA, mRNA	Regulatory networks of miRNA, mRNA, TFs, and proteins	Associations derived from literature	http://mirin.ym.edu.tw/

miRIN is a set of regulatory networks involving miRNAs, mRNAs, TFs, and proteins (Table 2.1).

We should note that the literature also reports an approach of integration available for Ingenuity Pathway Analysis (IPA®, Qiagen, Hilden, Germany). The IPA® platform enables the reconstruction of causal networks constructed from individual relationships providing a set of tools for inferring and scoring upstream regulators of gene expression data [144]. This approach has been presented in a previous work by Di Martino et al. and has been applied to the analysis of multiple myeloma data [145]. With respect to the prior work, the authors first applied the integrated analysis into a clinical relevant scenario by applying results to the profiling of MM patients. The workflow of analysis was based on the use of publicly available published by Wu et al. [146]. Data were, initially, preprocessed by Affymetrix proprietary software and filtered using the freely available DChip tool. Through the use of DChip, the authors identified significant differentially expressed (SDE) miRNA and mRNA in two subgroups of multiple myeloma patients: hyperdiploids (HD) MM versus non-hyperdiploids (nHD) MM. These data (SDE genes and SDE miRNAs) were integrated into a single model by using the approach of Kramer et al. implemented into the IPA® software [144]. This approach also enabled to consider the role of TFs and to extract causal relationships among them. The authors also analyzed data into a functional space looking at canonical pathways and bio-functions, carried out by SDE genes and miRNAs. The main result of this analysis was the identification of different biological events related to the two MM subtypes, while the upstream regulator analysis enabled to identify URs related to the identified transcription events, drawing a new molecular scenario of the two main disease subgroups (Fig. 2.3).

Conclusions

Precision medicine is a reality, but the shift from single gene analysis to multilayered approaches as integrative genomics is likely to produce a novel way to identify targets and individualize treatment. The growing interest for immunotherapy makes this point even more compelling taking into account that each therapeutic approach needs to be personalized based on the immunobiology of the individual patients, which will drive to another shift to tumor analysis to tumor/microenvironment axis evaluation. These perspectives need not only robust technologies but also a novel way to validate findings and novel research approaches which are mostly based on Bayesian design.

Precision medicine does not substitute for good clinics but even allow better and wiser clinics.

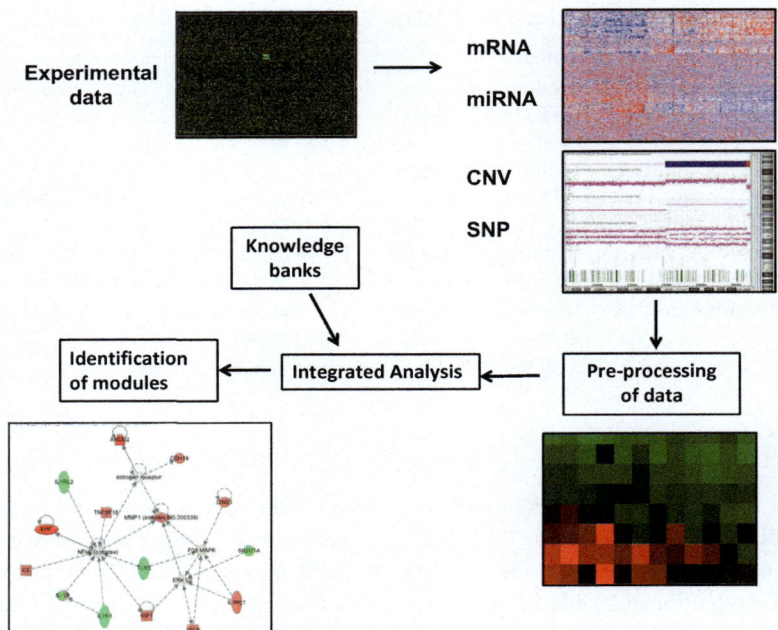

Fig. 2.3 This picture depicts the flow of data in integrative genomics. Different experimental data are collected from the investigator. The data span from classical microarray technologies (e.g. mRNA or miRNA expression) to next-generation sequencing techniques as well as genomic technologies such as CNV or SNP data. The whole set of data is then pre-processed in order to select only significant subsets of data or to evidence difference among classes. Then data are integrated into single theoretical models and analyzed with respect to data and information annotated in existing knowledge repositories. Finally, results are presented to the users by supporting models usually coming from graph theories

References

1. Personalized Medicine Coalition. Pers Med 4. 2014;66. http://www.personalizedmedicinecoalition.org/Userfiles/PMCCorporate/file/pmc_case_for_personalized_medicine.pdf. Accessed 15 Dec 2015.
2. Shah RR, Shah DR. Personalized medicine: is it a pharmacogenetic mirage? Br J Clin Pharmacol. 2012;74(4):698–721.
3. Ma QC, Ennis CA, Aparicio S. Opening Pandora's Box-the new biology of driver mutations and clonal evolution in cancer as revealed by next generation sequencing. Curr Opin Genet Dev. 2012;22:3–9.
4. Stratton MR, Campbell PJ, Futreal PA. The cancer genome. Nature. 2009;458(7239):719–24.
5. Vogelstein B, Papadopoulos N, Velculescu VE, Zhou S, Diaz Jr LA, Kinzler KW. Cancer Genome Landscapes. Science. 2013;339(6127):1546–58.
6. Dienstmann R, Rodon J, Barretina J, Tabernero J. Genomic medicine frontier in human solid tumors: prospects and challenges. J Clin Oncol. 2013;31:1874–84.
7. Biankin AV, Piantadosi S, Hollingsworth SJ. Patient-centric trials for therapeutic development in precision oncology. Nature. 2015;526(7573):361–70.
8. Peters GJ. Precision medicine in cancer: beyond wishful thinking? Expert Rev Precis Med Drug Dev. 2016;1(1):1–3.
9. Personeni N, Fieuws S, Piessevaux H, De Hertogh G, De Schutter J, Biesmans B, et al. Clinical usefulness of EGFR gene copy number as a predictive marker in colorectal cancer patients treated with cetuximab: a fluorescent in situ hybridization study. Clin Cancer Res. 2008;14:5869–76.
10. Sartore-Bianchi A, Moroni M, Veronese S, Carnaghi C, Bajetta E, Luppi G, et al. Epidermal growth factor receptor gene copy number and clinical outcome of metastatic colorectal cancer treated with panitumumab. J Clin Oncol. 2007;25(22):3238–45.
11. Ciardiello F, Tortora G, Magrassi SF, Lanzara A. EGFR antagonists in cancer treatment. N Engl J Med. 2008;358(258):1160–74.
12. Allegra CJ, Jessup JM, Somerfield MR, Hamilton SR, Hammond EH, Hayes DF, et al. American society of clinical oncology provisional clinical opinion:

testing for KRAS gene mutations in patients with metastatic colorectal carcinoma to predict response to anti-epidermal growth factor receptor monoclonal antibody therapy. J Clin Oncol. 2009;27(12):2091–6.

13. Lièvre A, Bachet JB, Le Corre D, Boige V, Landi B, Emile JF, et al. KRAS mutation status is predictive of response to cetuximab therapy in colorectal cancer. Cancer Res. 2006;66(8):3992–5.

14. Van Cutsem E, Lenz HJ, Köhne CH, Heinemann V, Tejpar S, Melezínek I, et al. Fluorouracil, leucovorin, and irinotecan plus cetuximab treatment and RAS mutations in colorectal cancer. J Clin Oncol. 2015;33(7):692–700.

15. Peeters M, Oliner KS, Price TJ, Cervantes A, Sobrero AF, Ducreux M, et al. Analysis of KRAS/NRAS mutations in a phase III study of panitumumab with FOLFIRI compared with FOLFIRI alone as second-line treatment for metastatic colorectal cancer. Clin Cancer Res. 2015;21(24):5469–79.

16. Douillard J-Y, Oliner KS, Siena S, Tabernero J, Burkes R, Barugel M, et al. Panitumumab-FOLFOX4 treatment and RAS mutations in colorectal cancer. N Engl J Med. 2013;369(11):1023–34.

17. Loupakis F, Cremolini C, Masi G, Lonardi S, Zagonel V, Salvatore L, et al. Initial therapy with FOLFOXIRI and bevacizumab for metastatic colorectal cancer. N Engl J Med. 2014;371(17):1609–18.

18. Hurwitz H, Fehrenbacher L, Novotny W, Cartwright T, Hainsworth J, Heim W, et al. Bevacizumab plus irinotecan, fluorouracil, and leucovorin for metastatic colorectal cancer. N Engl J Med. 2004;350(23):2335–42.

19. Kabbinavar FF, Schulz J, McCleod M, Patel T, Hamm JT, Hecht JR, et al. Addition of bevacizumab to bolus fluorouracil and leucovorin in first-line metastatic colorectal cancer: results of a randomized phase II trial. J Clin Oncol. 2005;23(16):3697–705.

20. Saltz LB, Clarke S, Díaz-Rubio E, Scheithauer W, Figer A, Wong R, et al. Bevacizumab in combination with oxaliplatin-based chemotherapy as first-line therapy in metastatic colorectal cancer: a randomized phase III study. J Clin Oncol. 2008;26(12):2013–9.

21. Douillard J-Y, Siena S, Cassidy J, Tabernero J, Burkes R, Barugel M, et al. Randomized, phase III trial of panitumumab with Infusional fluorouracil, leucovorin, and oxaliplatin (FOLFOX4) versus FOLFOX4 alone as first-line treatment in patients with previously untreated metastatic colorectal cancer: the PRIME study. J Clin Oncol. 2010;28(31):4697–705.

22. Van Cutsem E, Köhne C-H, Hitre E, Zaluski J, Chang Chien C-R, Makhson A, et al. Cetuximab and chemotherapy as initial treatment for metastatic colorectal cancer. N Engl J Med. 2009;360(14):1408–17.

23. Van Cutsem E, Lang I, Folprecht G, Nowacki M, Barone C, Shchepotin I, et al. Cetuximab plus FOLFIRI: Final data from the CRYSTAL study on the association of KRAS and BRAF biomarker status with treatment outcome [abstract]. J Clin Oncol. 2010;28:3570.

24. Heinemann V, Von Weikersthal LF, Decker T, Kiani A, Vehling-kaiser U, Scholz M, et al. FOLFIRI plus cetuximab versus FOLFIRI plus bevacizumab as first-line treatment for patients with metastatic colorectal cancer (FIRE-3): a randomised, open-label, phase 3 trial. Lancet Oncol. 2014;15(10):1065–75.

25. Khattak MA, Martin H, Davidson A, Phillips M. Role of first-line anti-epidermal growth factor receptor therapy compared with anti-vascular endothelial growth factor therapy in advanced colorectal cancer: a meta-analysis of randomized clinical trials. Clin Colorectal Cancer. 2015;14(2):81–90.

26. Lenz HJ, Niedzwiecki D, Innocenti F, Blanke C, Mahony MR, O'Neil BH, Shaw JE, Polite B, Hochster H, Atkins J, Goldberg R, Mayer R, Schilsky RL. CALGB/SWOG 80405: Phase III trial of FOLFIRI or mFOLFOX6 with bevacizumab or cetuximab for patients with expanded RAS analyses in untreated metastatic adenocarcinoma of the colon or rectum. Ann Oncol. 2014;25(Suppl 4).

27. De Sousa Melo FE, Vermeulen L, Fessler E, Paul MJ. Cancer heterogeneity – a multifaceted view. Nat Publ Gr. 2013;14(10):686–69592.

28. Misale S, Yaeger R, Hobor S, Scala E, Liska D, Valtorta E, et al. Emergence of KRAS mutations and acquired resistance to anti EGFR therapy in colorectal cancer. Nature. 2014;486(7404):532–6.

29. Diaz Jr LA, Williams RT, Wu J, Kinde I, Hecht JR, Berlin J, et al. The molecular evolution of acquired resistance to targeted EGFR blockade in colorectal cancers. Nature. 2012;486(7404):4–7.

30. Laurent-Puig P, Cayre A, Manceau G, Buc E, Bachet JB, Lecomte T, et al. Analysis of PTEN, BRAF, and EGFR status in determining benefit from cetuximab therapy in wild-type KRAS metastatic colon cancer. J Clin Oncol. 2009;27(35):5924–30.

31. Di Nicolantonio F, Martini M, Molinari F, Sartore-Bianchi A, Arena S, Saletti P, et al. Wild-type BRAF is required for response to panitumumab or cetuximab in metastatic colorectal cancer. J Clin Oncol. 2008;26(35):5705–12.

32. De Roock W, Claes B, Bernasconi D, De Schutter J, Biesmans B, Fountzilas G, et al. Effects of KRAS, BRAF, NRAS, and PIK3CA mutations on the efficacy of cetuximab plus chemotherapy in chemotherapy-refractory metastatic colorectal cancer: a retrospective consortium analysis. Lancet Oncol. 2010;11(8):753–62.

33. Sartore-Bianchi A, Martini M, Molinari F, Veronese S, Nichelatti M, Artale S, et al. PIK3CA mutations in colorectal cancer are associated with clinical resistance to EGFR-targeted monoclonal antibodies. Cancer Res. 2009;69(5):1851–7.

34. Samowitz WS, Sweeney C, Herrick J, Albertsen H, Levin TR, Murtaugh MA, et al. Poor survival associated with the BRAF V600E mutation in

microsatellite-stable colon cancers. Cancer Res. 2005;65(14):6063–70.

35. Roth AD, Tejpar S, Delorenzi M, Yan P, Fiocca R, Klingbiel D, et al. Prognostic role of KRAS and BRAF in stage II and III resected colon cancer: results of the translational study on the PETACC-3, EORTC 40993, SAKK 60-00 trial. J Clin Oncol. 2010;28(3):466–74.

36. Markman B, Atzori F, Pérez-García J, Tabernero J, Baselga J. Status of PI3K inhibition and biomarker development in cancer therapeutics. Ann Oncol. 2009;21:683–91.

37. Ogino S, Nosho K, Kirkner GJ, Shima K, Irahara N, Kure S, et al. PIK3CA mutation is associated with poor prognosis among patients with curatively resected colon cancer. J Clin Oncol. 2009;27(9): 1477–84.

38. Frattini M, Saletti P, Romagnani E, Martin V, Molinari F, Ghisletta M, et al. PTEN loss of expression predicts cetuximab efficacy in metastatic colorectal cancer patients. Br J Cancer. 2007;97(8): 1139–45.

39. Loupakis F, Pollina L, Stasi I, Ruzzo A, Scartozzi M, Santini D, et al. PTEN expression and KRAS mutations on primary tumors and metastases in the prediction of benefit from cetuximab plus irinotecan for patients with metastatic colorectal cancer. J Clin Oncol. 2009;27(16):2622–9.

40. Sartore-Bianchi A, Di Nicolantonio F, Nichelatti M, Molinari F, De Dosso S, Saletti P, et al. Multi-determinants analysis of molecular alterations for predicting clinical benefit to EGFR-targeted monoclonal antibodies in colorectal cancer. PLoS One. 2009;4(10):e7287.

41. Markowitz S, Bertagnolli M. Molecular basis of colorectal cancer. N Engl J Med. 2010;362(13):1246. author reply 1246-7.

42. George B, Kopetz S. Predictive and prognostic markers in colorectal cancer. Curr Oncol Rep. 2011;13(3):206–15.

43. Gill SR, Pop M, Deboy RT, Eckburg PB, Turnbaugh PJ, Samuel BS, et al. Metagenomic analysis of the human distal gut microbiome. Science. 2006; 312(5778):1355–9.

44. Tran B, Kopetz S, Tie J, Gibbs P, Jiang ZQ, Lieu CH, et al. Impact of BRAF mutation and microsatellite instability on the pattern of metastatic spread and prognosis in metastatic colorectal cancer. Cancer. 2011;117(20):4623–32.

45. Hutchins G, Southward K, Handley K, Magill L, Beaumont C, Stahlschmidt J, et al. Value of mismatch repair, KRAS, and BRAF mutations in predicting recurrence and benefits from chemotherapy in colorectal cancer. J Clin Oncol. 2011;29(10): 1261–70.

46. Glebov OK, Rodriguez LM, Nakahara K, Jenkins J, Cliatt J, Humbyrd CJ, et al. Distinguishing right from left colon by the pattern of gene expression. Cancer Epidemiol Biomark Prev. 2003;12(8):755–62.

47. Birkenkamp-Demtroder K, Olesen SH, Sørensen FB, Laurberg S, Laiho P, Aaltonen LA, et al. Differential gene expression in colon cancer of the caecum versus the sigmoid and rectosigmoid. Gut. 2005;54(3):374–84.

48. Loupakis F, Yang D, Yau L, Feng S, Cremolini C, Zhang W, et al. Primary tumor location as a prognostic factor in metastatic colorectal cancer. J Natl Cancer Inst. 2015;107(3).

49. Popovici V, Budinska E, Tejpar S, Weinrich S, Estrella H, Hodgson G, et al. Identification of a poor-prognosis BRAF-mutant-like population of patients with colon cancer. J Clin Oncol. 2012;30(12): 1288–95.

50. Brulé SY, Jonker DJ, Karapetis CS, O'Callaghan CJ, Moore MJ, Wong R, et al. Location of colon cancer (right-sided versus left-sided) as a prognostic factor and a predictor of benefit from cetuximab in NCIC CO.17. Eur J Cancer. 2015;51(11):1405–14.

51. Kirby JA, Bone M, Robertson H, Hudson M, Jones DEJ. The number of intraepithelial T cells decreases from ascending colon to rectum. J Clin Pathol. 2003;56(2):158.

52. Selby WS, Janossy G, Jewell DP. Immunohistological characterisation of intraepithelial lymphocytes of the human gastrointestinal tract. Gut. 1981;22(3): 169–76.

53. Fausto Petrelli, Gianluca Tomasello, Karen Borgonovo, Michele Ghidini, Luca Turati, Pierpaolo Dallera, Rodolfo Passalacqua, Giovanni Sgroi, Sandro Barni M. Prognostic survival associated with left-sided vs right-sided Colon cancer a systematic review and meta-analysis. JAMA Oncol 2016; 3(2):211–9.

54. Hampel H, Frankel WL, Martin E, Arnold M, Khanduja K, Kuebler P, et al. Feasibility of screening for lynch syndrome among patients with colorectal cancer. J Clin Oncol. 2008;26(35):5783–8.

55. Lynch HT, Snyder CL, Shaw TG, Heinen CD, Hitchins MP. Milestones of lynch syndrome: 1895–2015. Nat Rev Cancer. 2015;15(March):181–94.

56. Parsons R, Li GM, Longley MJ, W horng F, Papadopoulos N, Jen J, et al. Hypermutability and mismatch repair deficiency in RER+ tumor cells. Cell. 1993;75(6):1227–36.

57. Mlecnik B, Bindea G, Angell HK, Maby P, Angelova M, Tougeron D, et al. Integrative analyses of colorectal cancer show Immunoscore is a stronger predictor of patient survival than microsatellite instability. Immunity. 2016;44(3):698–711.

58. Galon J, Mlecnik B, Bindea G, Angell HK, Berger A, Lagorce C, et al. Towards the introduction of the "immunoscore" in the classification of malignant tumours. J Pathol. 2014;232:199–209.

59. Galon J, Costes A, Sanchez-Cabo F, Kirilovsky A, Mlecnik B, Lagorce-Pagès C, et al. Type, density, and location of immune cells within human colorectal tumors predict clinical outcome. Science. 2006;313(5795):1960–4.

60. Correale P, Rotundo MS, Botta C, Del Vecchio MT, Ginanneschi C, Licchetta A, et al. Tumor infiltration by T lymphocytes expressing chemokine receptor 7 (CCR7) is predictive of favorable outcome in patients with advanced colorectal carcinoma. Clin Cancer Res. 2012;18(3):850–7.

61. Correale P, Rotundo MS, Del Vecchio MT, Remondo C, Migali C, Ginanneschi C, et al. Regulatory (FoxP3+) T-cell tumor infiltration is a favorable prognostic factor in advanced colon cancer patients undergoing chemo or chemoimmunotherapy. J Immunother. 2010;33(4):435–41.

62. Correale P, Botta C, Ciliberto D, Pastina P, Ingargiola R, Zappavigna S, et al. Immunotherapy of colorectal cancer: new perspectives after a long path. Immunotherapy. 2016;8(11):1281–92.

63. Le DT, Uram JN, Wang H, Bartlett BR, Kemberling H, Eyring AD, et al. PD-1 blockade in tumors with mismatch-repair deficiency. N Engl J Med. 2015;372(26):2509–20.

64. Dolcetti R, Viel A, Doglioni C, Russo A, Guidoboni M, Capozzi E, et al. High prevalence of activated intraepithelial cytotoxic T lymphocytes and increased neoplastic cell apoptosis in colorectal carcinomas with microsatellite instability. Am J Pathol. 1999;154(6):1805–13.

65. Young J, Simms LA, Biden KG, Wynter C, Whitehall V, Karamatic R, et al. Features of colorectal cancers with high-level microsatellite instability occurring in familial and sporadic settings: parallel pathways of tumorigenesis. Am J Pathol. 2001;159(6):2107–16.

66. Kim H, Jen J, Vogelstein B, Hamilton SR. Clinical and pathological characteristics of sporadic colorectal carcinomas with DNA replication errors in microsatellite sequences. Am J Pathol. 1994;145(1): 148–56.

67. Eng C. POLE mutations in colorectal cancer: a new biomarker? Lancet Gastroenterol Hepatol. 2016; 1(3):176–7.

68. Sartore-Bianchi A, Trusolino L, Martino C, Bencardino K, Lonardi S, Bergamo F, et al. Dual-targeted therapy with trastuzumab and lapatinib in treatment-refractory, KRAS codon 12/13 wild-type, HER2-positive metastatic colorectal cancer (HERACLES): a proof-of-concept, multicentre, open-label, phase 2 trial. Lancet Oncol. 2016;17(6): 738–46.

69. Ngeow J, Eng C. New genetic and genomic approaches after the genome-wide association study era--back to the future. Gastroenterology. 2015; 149(5):1138–41.

70. Naccarati A, Polakova V, Pardini B, Vodickova L, Hemminki K, Kumar R, et al. Mutations and polymorphisms in TP53 gene – an overview on the role in colorectal cancer. Mutagenesis. 2012;27(2):211–8.

71. Sanz-Pamplona R, Berenguer A, Cordero D, Riccadonna S, Solé X, Crous-Bou M, et al. Clinical value of prognosis gene expression signatures in colorectal cancer: a systematic review. PLoS One. 2012;7(11):e48877.

72. Jorissen RN, Gibbs P, Christie M, Prakash S, Lipton L, Desai J, et al. Metastasis-associated gene expression changes predict poor outcomes in patients with Dukes stage B and C colorectal cancer. Clin Cancer Res. 2009;15(24):7642–51.

73. de Sousa E Melo F, Wang X, Jansen M, Fessler E, Trinh A, de Rooij LPMH, et al. Poor-prognosis colon cancer is defined by a molecularly distinct subtype and develops from serrated precursor lesions. Nat Med. 2013;19(5):614–8.

74. Sadanandam A, Lyssiotis CA, Homicsko K, Collisson EA, Gibb WJ, Wullschleger S, et al. A colorectal cancer classification system that associates cellular phenotype and responses to therapy. Nat Med. 2013;19(5):619–25.

75. Isella C, Terrasi A, Bellomo SE, Petti C, Galatola G, Muratore A, et al. Stromal contribution to the colorectal cancer transcriptome. Nat Genet. 2015;47(4):312–9.

76. Marisa L, de Reyniès A, Duval A, Selves J, Gaub MP, Vescovo L, et al. Gene expression classification of Colon cancer into molecular subtypes: characterization, validation, and prognostic value. PLoS Med. 2013;10(5):e1001453.

77. The Cancer Genome Network Atlas. Comprehensive molecular characterization of human colon and rectal cancer. Nature. 2012;487(7407):330–7.

78. Barat A, Ruskin H, Byrne A, Prehn J. Integrating Colon cancer microarray data: associating locus-specific methylation groups to Gene expression-based classifications. Microarrays. 2015;4(4):630–46.

79. Fearon ER. Molecular genetics of colorectal cancer. Annu Rev Pathol. 2011;6:479–507.

80. Hardiman KM, Ulintz PJ, Kuick RD, Hovelson DH, Gates CM, Bhasi A, et al. Intra-tumor genetic heterogeneity in rectal cancer. Lab Investig. 2015;96(1):4–15.

81. Maughan TS, Adams RA, Smith CG, Meade AM, Seymour MT, Wilson RH, et al. Addition of cetuximab to oxaliplatin-based first-line combination chemotherapy for treatment of advanced colorectal cancer: results of the randomised phase 3 MRC COIN trial. Lancet. 2011;377(9783):2103–14.

82. Di Narzo AF, Tejpar S, Rossi S, Yan P, Popovici V, Wirapati P, et al. Test of four colon cancer risk-scores in formalin fixed paraffin embedded microarray gene expression data. J Natl Cancer Inst. 2014;106(10).

83. Salazar R, Roepman P, Capella G, Moreno V, Simon I, Dreezen C, et al. Gene expression signature to improve prognosis prediction of stage II and III colorectal cancer. J Clin Oncol. 2011;29(1):17–24.

84. O'Connell M, Lavery I, Yothers G. Relationship between tumor gene expression and recurrence in four independent studies of patients with stage II/III colon cancer treated with surgery alone or surgery. J Clin Oncol. 2010;28(25):3937–44.

85. Walker AS, Johnson EK, Maykel JA, Stojadinovic A, Nissan A, Brucher B, et al. Future directions for

the early detection of colorectal cancer recurrence. J Cancer. 2014;5:272–80. Ivyspring International Publisher.

86. Kawai K, Sunami E, Yamaguchi H, Ishihara S, Kazama S, Nozawa H, et al. Nomograms for colorectal cancer: a systematic review. World J Gastroenterol. 2015;21(41):11877–86.

87. Peng J, Ding Y, Tu S, Shi D, Sun L, Li X, et al. Prognostic nomograms for predicting survival and distant metastases in locally advanced rectal cancers. PLoS One. 2014;9(8):e106344.

88. Dalerba P, Sahoo D, Paik S, Guo X, Yothers G, Song N, et al. CDX2 as a prognostic biomarker in stage II and stage III Colon cancer. N Engl J Med. 2016;374(3):211–22.

89. Stoehlmacher J. Prediction of efficacy and side effects of chemotherapy in colorectal cancer. Recent Results Cancer Res. 2007;176:81–8.

90. Lin JH. Pharmacokinetic and pharmacodynamic variability: a daunting challenge in drug therapy. Curr Drug Metab. 2007;8(2):109–36.

91. Hertz DL, McLeod HL. Use of pharmacogenetics for predicting cancer prognosis and treatment exposure, response and toxicity. J Hum Genet. 2013;58(6):346–52.

92. Di Martino MT, Scionti F, Sestito S, Nicoletti A, Arbitrio M, Guzzi PH, et al. Genetic variants associated with gastrointestinal symptoms in Fabry disease. Oncotarget. 2016;7(52):85895–904.

93. Arbitrio M, Di Martino MT, Scionti F, Agapito G, Guzzi PH, Cannataro M, et al. DMET TM (drug metabolism enzymes and transporters): a pharmacogenomic platform for precision medicine. Oncotarget. 2016;7(33):54028–50.

94. Arbitrio M, Di Martino MT, Barbieri V, Agapito G, Guzzi P, Botta C, et al. Identification of polymorphic variants associated with erlotinib-related skin toxicity in advanced non-small cell lung cancer patients by DMET microarray analysis. Cancer Chemother Pharmacol. 2015;77(1):205–9.

95. Guzzi P, Agapito G, Di Martino M, Arbitrio M, Tassone P, Tagliaferri P, et al. DMET-analyzer: automatic analysis of Affymetrix DMET data. BMC Bioinformatics. 2012;13(1):258.

96. Agapito G, Botta C, Guzzi P, Arbitrio M, Di Martino M, Tassone P, et al. OSAnalyzer: a bioinformatics tool for the analysis of gene polymorphisms enriched with clinical outcomes. Microarrays [Internet]. 2016;5(4):24. Available from: http://www.mdpi.com/2076-3905/5/4/24.

97. Di Martino MT, Arbitrio M, Guzzi PH, Leone E, Baudi F, Piro E, et al. A peroxisome proliferator-activated receptor gamma (PPARG) polymorphism is associated with zoledronic acid-related osteonecrosis of the jaw in multiple myeloma patients: analysis by DMET microarray profiling. Br J Haematol. 2011;154(4):529–33.

98. Schmoll H, Stein A. Towards improved drugs, combinations and patient selection. Nat Publ Gr. 2014;11(2):79–80.

99. Cassidy J, Saltz L, Twelves C, Van cutsem E, Hoff P, Kang Y, et al. Efficacy of capecitabine versus 5-fluorouracil in colorectal and gastric cancers: a meta-analysis of individual data from 6171 patients. Ann Oncol. 2011;22(12):2604–9.

100. Longley DB, Paul Harkin D, Johnston PG. 5-fluorouracil: mechanisms of action and clinical strategies. NatureCom. 2003;3(May):330–8.

101. Parker W, Cheng Y. Metabolism and mechanism of action of 5-fluorouracil. Pharmacol Ther. 1990;48(3):381–95.

102. Zhang N, Yin Y, Xu SJ, Chen WS. 5-fluorouracil: mechanisms of resistance and reversal strategies. Molecules. 2008;13:1551–69.

103. Twelves C, Wong A, Nowacki MP, Abt M, Burris H, Carrato A, et al. Capecitabine as adjuvant treatment for stage III colon cancer. N Engl J Med. 2005;352(26):2696–704.

104. Twelves C, Scheithauer W, Mckendrick J, Seitz JF, Van Hazel G, Wong A, et al. Capecitabine versus 5-fluorouracil/folinic acid as adjuvant therapy for stage III colon cancer: final results from the X-ACT trial with analysis by age and preliminary evidence of a pharmacodynamic marker of efficacy. Ann Oncol. 2012;23(5):1190–7.

105. Miwa M, Ura M, Nishida M, Sawada N, Ishikawa T, Mori K, et al. Design of a novel oral fluoropyrimidine carbamate, capecitabine, which generates 5 fluorouracil selectively in tumours by enzymes concentrated in human liver and cancer tissue. Eur J Cancer. 1998;34(8):1274–81.

106. Cao D, Russell RL, Zhang D, Leffert JJ, Pizzorno G. Uridine phosphorylase (-/-) murine embryonic stem cells clarify the key role of this enzyme in the regulation of the pyrimidine salvage pathway and in the activation of fluoropyrimidines. Cancer Res. 2002;62(8):2313–7.

107. Schüller J, Cassidy J, Dumont E, Roos B, Durston S, Banken L, et al. Preferential activation of capecitabine in tumor following oral administration to colorectal cancer patients. Cancer Chemother Pharmacol. 2000;45(4):291–7.

108. Milano G, Etienne MC, Pierrefite V, Barberi-Heyob M, Deporte-Fety R, Renée N. Dihydropyrimidine dehydrogenase deficiency and fluorouracil-related toxicity. Br J Cancer. 1999;79(3–4):627–30.

109. Turk VE. Pharmacogenetics of cytotoxic therapy in colorectal cancer. 2015;23(2):257–73.

110. Li Q, Liu Y, Zhang HM, Huang YP, Wang TY, Li DS, et al. Influence of DPYD genetic polymorphisms on 5-fluorouracil toxicities in patients with colorectal cancer: a meta-analysis. Gastroenterol Res Pract. 2014;2014.

111. Van Kuilenburg ABP, Haasjes J, Richel DJ, Zoetekouw L, Van Lenthe H, De Abreu RA, et al. Clinical implications of dihydropyrimidine dehydrogenase (DPD) deficiency in patients with severe 5-fluorouracil-associated toxicity: identification of new mutations in the DPD gene. Clin Cancer Res. 2000;6(12):4705–12.

112. Schwab M, Zanger UM, Marx C, Schaeffeler E, Klein K, Dippon J, et al. Role of genetic and nongenetic factors for fluorouracil treatment-related severe toxicity: a prospective clinical trial by the German 5-FU toxicity study group. J Clin Oncol. 2008; 26(13):2131–8.

113. Lee A, Ezzeldin H, Fourie J, Diasio R. Dihydropyrimidine dehydrogenase deficiency: impact of pharmacogenetics on 5-fluorouracil therapy. Clin Adv Hematol Oncol. 2004;2:527–32.

114. Swen JJ, Nijenhuis M, de Boer a, Grandia L, Maitland-van der Zee a H, Mulder H, et al. Pharmacogenetics: from bench to byte--an update of guidelines. Clin Pharmacol Ther. 2011;89(5): 662–73.

115. Caudle KE, Thorn CF, Klein TE, Swen JJ, McLeod HL, Diasio RB, et al. Clinical pharmacogenetics implementation consortium guidelines for dihydropyrimidine dehydrogenase genotype and fluoropyrimidine dosing. Clin Pharmacol Ther. 2013;94(6): 640–5.

116. Leichman CG, Lenz HJ, Leichman L, Danenberg K, Baranda J, Groshen S, et al. Quantitation of intratumoral thymidylate synthase expression predicts for disseminated colorectal cancer response and resistance to protracted-infusion fluorouracil and weekly leucovorin. J Clin Oncol. 1997;15(10):3223–9.

117. Paradiso A, Simone G, Petroni S, Leone B, Vallejo C, Lacava J, et al. Thymidilate synthase and p53 primary tumour expression as predictive factors for advanced colorectal cancer patients. Br J Cancer. 2000;82(3):560–7.

118. Popat S, Matakidou A, Houlston RS. Thymidylate synthase expression and prognosis in colorectal cancer: a systematic review and meta-analysis. J Clin Oncol. 2004;22(3):529–36.

119. Qiu LX, Tang QY, Bai JL, Qian XP, Li RT, Liu BR, et al. Predictive value of thymidylate synthase expression in advanced colorectal cancer patients receiving fluoropyrimidine-based chemotherapy: evidence from 24 studies. Int J Cancer. 2008;123(10): 2384–9.

120. De Mattia E, Cecchin E, Toffoli G. Pharmacogenomics of intrinsic and acquired pharmacoresistance in colorectal cancer: toward targeted personalized therapy. Drug Resist Updat. 2015;20:39–62.

121. Cortejoso L, López-Fernández LA. Pharmacogenetic markers of toxicity for chemotherapy in colorectal cancer patients. Pharmacogenomics. 2012;13(10): 1173–91.

122. Freyer G, Duret A, Milano G, Chatelut E, Rebischung C, Delord JP, et al. Pharmacogenetic tailoring of irinotecan-based first-line chemotherapy in metastatic colorectal cancer: results of a pilot study. Anticancer Res. 2011;31(1):359–66.

123. Marsh S, McLeod HL. Pharmacogenetics of irinotecan toxicity. Pharmacogenomics. 2004;5(7):835–43.

124. Mathijssen RHJ, Verweij J, De Jonge MJA, Nooter K, Stoter G, Sparreboom A. Impact of body-size measures on irinotecan clearance: alternative dosing recommendations. J Clin Oncol. 2002;20(1):81–7.

125. Innocenti F, Undevia SD, Iyer L, Chen PX, Das S, Kocherginsky M, et al. Genetic variants in the UDP-glucuronosyltransferase 1A1 gene predict the risk of severe neutropenia of irinotecan. J Clin Oncol. 2004;22(8):1382–8.

126. Ando Y, Saka H, Ando M, Sawa T, Muro K, Ueoka H, et al. Polymorphisms of UDP-glucuronosyltransferase gene and irinotecan toxicity: a pharmacogenetic analysis. Cancer Res. 2000;60(24):6921–6.

127. Marcuello E, Altés A, Menoyo A, Del Rio E, Gómez-Pardo M, Baiget M. UGT1A1 gene variations and irinotecan treatment in patients with metastatic colorectal cancer. Br J Cancer. 2004; 91(4):678–82.

128. Dias MM, McKinnon RA, Sorich MJ. Impact of the UGT1A1*28 allele on response to irinotecan: a systematic review and meta-analysis. Pharmacogenomics. 2012;13(8):889–99.

129. Marsh S, Hoskins JM. Irinotecan pharmacogenomics. Pharmacogenomics. 2010;11(7):1003–10.

130. Di Martino MT, Arbitrio M, Leone E, Guzzi PH, Rotundo MS, Ciliberto D, et al. Single nucleotide polymorphisms of ABCC5 and ABCG1 transporter genes correlate to irinotecan-associated gastrointestinal toxicity in colorectal cancer patients: a DMET microarray profiling study. Cancer Biol Ther. 2011;12(9):780–7.

131. Kristensen VN, Lingjaerde OC, Russnes HG, Vollan HK, Frigessi A, Borresen-Dale AL. Principles and methods of integrative genomic analyses in cancer. Nat Rev Cancer. 2014;14(5):299–313.

132. Guzzi PH, Agapito G, Milano M, Cannataro M. Methodologies and experimental platforms for generating and analysing microarray and mass spectrometry-based omics data to support P4 medicine. Brief Bioinform. 2016;17(4):553–61.

133. Roy S, Guzzi PH. Biological network inference from microarray data, current solutions, and assessments. Methods Mol Biol. 2016;1375:155–67.

134. Di Martino MT, Rossi M, Caracciolo D, Gullà A, Tagliaferri P, Tassone P. Mir-221/222 are promising targets for innovative anticancer therapy. Expert Opin Ther Targets [Internet] 2016;8222(March):1–10. Available from: http://www.tandfonline.com/doi/full/10.1517/14728222.2016.1164693.

135. Rossi M, Tagliaferri P, Tassone P. MicroRNAs in multiple myeloma and related bone disease. Ann Transl Med. 2015;3(21):334.

136. Rossi M, Amodio N, Martino M, Tagliaferri P, Tassone P, Cho W. MicroRNA and multiple myeloma: from laboratory findings to translational therapeutic approaches. Curr Pharm Biotechnol [Internet]. 2014 [cited 2017 Jan 30];15(5):459–67. Available from: http://www.eurekaselect.com/openurl/content.php?genre=article&issn=1389-2010&volume=15&issue=5&spage=459.

137. Rossi M, Amodio N, Martino M, Caracciolo D, Tagliaferri P, Tassone P. From target therapy to

miRNA therapeutics of human multiple myeloma: theoretical and technological issues in the evolving scenario. Curr Drug Targets [Internet]. 2013 [cited 2017 Jan 30];14(10):1144–9. Available from: http://www.eurekaselect.com/openurl/content.php?genre=article&issn=1389-4501&volume=14&issue=10&spage=1144.

138. Amodio N, Di Martino MT, Neri A, Tagliaferri P, Tassone P. Non-coding RNA: a novel opportunity for the personalized treatment of multiple myeloma. Expert Opin Biol Ther [Internet]. 2013 [cited 2017 Jan 30];13(sup1):S125–37. Available from: http://www.tandfonline.com/doi/full/10.1517/14712598.2013.796356.

139. Tagliaferri P, Rossi M, Di Martino MT, Amodio N, Leone E, Gulla A, et al. Promises and challenges of MicroRNA-based treatment of multiple myeloma. Curr Cancer Drug Targets [Internet]. 2012;12(7):838–46. Available from: http://www.ncbi.nlm.nih.gov/entrez/query.fcgi?cmd=Retrieve&db=PubMed&dopt=Citation&list_uids=22671926.

140. Venkatesh T, Harlow H. Integromics: challenges in data integration. Genome Biol. 2002;3(8):reports4027.1-reports4027.3.

141. Bisognin A, Sales G, Coppe A, Bortoluzzi S. MAGIA 2 : from miRNA and genes expression data integrative analysis to microRNA – transcription factor mixed regulatory circuits (2012 update). Nucleic Acids Res. 2012;40:W13-21 (Web Server Issue).

142. Yan Z, Shah PK, Amin SB, Samur MK, Huang N, Wang X, et al. Integrative analysis of gene and miRNA expression profiles with transcription factor-miRNA feed-forward loops identifies regulators in human cancers. Nucleic Acids Res. 2012;40(17):e135.

143. Huang GT, Athanassiou C, Benos P V. MirConnX: condition-specific mRNA-microRNA network integrator. Nucleic Acids Res. 2011;39:W416–23.

144. Kramer A, Green J, Pollard J, Tugendreich S. Causal analysis approaches in ingenuity pathway analysis. Bioinformatics. 2014;30(4):523–30.

145. Di Martino MT, Guzzi PH, Caracciolo D, Agnelli L, Neri A, Walker BA, et al. Integrated analysis of microRNAs, transcription factors and target genes expression discloses a specific molecular architecture of hyperdiploid multiple myeloma. Oncotarget. 2015;6(22):19132–47.

146. Wu P, Agnelli L, Walker BA, Todoerti K, Lionetti M, Johnson DC, et al. Improved risk stratification in myeloma using a microRNA-based classifier. Br J Haematol. 2013;162(3):348–59.

Cancer Clonal Evolution and Intra-tumor Heterogeneity

3

Daniele Fanale, Juan Lucio Iovanna,
Antonio Giordano, Christian Rolfo,
and Antonio Russo

Introduction

Despite recent advances in the understanding of cancer onset mechanisms and development of new therapeutic strategies, however, the resistance of tumor cells to different therapies represents the main obstacle to the successful treatment, resulting in poor prognosis and tumor recurrence. Since current therapies are not always able to fully eradicate the disease, understanding the causes underlying the resistance and implementing strategies to solve this issue are currently the most important objectives of the oncology research [1]. Tumors are not uniform diseases but heterogeneous entities formed by populations of cells or "cell clones," with different genetic and molecular characteristics. This variability underlies their ability to evolve and adapt to the anticancer drug therapies, by developing often resistance mechanisms [2]. Most of cancers exhibit usually a single clonal origin at the early stages of the disease, but, subsequently, in advanced stages, tumors may contain multiple cell populations with different properties, acquiring the ability to invade other tissues and develop distant metastases [3, 4]. This tumor heterogeneity causes changes in clinical patterns, by affecting the treatment effectiveness, since these tumor cell clones have acquired the ability to modulate their motility or adhesion. Also, cell clones with metastatic potential exhibit different genetic features than clones without metastatic potential [5, 6]. For this reason, in these last years, the main aim of many researchers was to identify genetic

D. Fanale
Department of Surgical, Oncological and Oral Sciences, Section of Medical Oncology, University of Palermo, Via del Vespro 129, 90127 Palermo, Italy
e-mail: fandan@libero.it

J.L. Iovanna
Centre de Recherche en Cancérologie de Marseille (CRCM), INSERM U1068, CNRS UMR 7258, Aix-Marseille Université et Institut Paoli-Calmettes, Parc Scientifique et Technologique de Luminy, Marseille, France
e-mail: juan.iovanna@inserm.fr

A. Giordano
Sbarro Institute for Cancer Research and Molecular Medicine, Center for Biotechnology, College of Science and Technology, Temple University, Philadelphia, PA 19122, USA

C. Rolfo
Phase I- Early Clinical Trials Unit, Oncology Department and Multidisciplinary Oncology Center Antwerp (MOCA), Antwerp University Hospital, Edegem, Belgium
e-mail: christian.rolfo@uza.be

A. Russo, MD, PhD (✉)
Department of Surgical, Oncological and Oral Sciences, Section of Medical Oncology, University of Palermo, Via del Vespro 129, 90127 Palermo, Italy

Sbarro Institute for Cancer Research and Molecular Medicine, Center for Biotechnology, College of Science and Technology, Temple University, Philadelphia, PA 19122, USA
e-mail: antonio.russo@usa.net

© Springer International Publishing AG 2017
A. Giordano et al. (eds.), *Liquid Biopsy in Cancer Patients*, Current Clinical Pathology,
DOI 10.1007/978-3-319-55661-1_3

markers of metastatic cell clones [7–9]. Despite little is yet known concerning this, two models have been proposed to elucidate the biological mechanisms underlying the metastases. The genetic selection model suggested that only a subset of cancer cells acquires metastatic potential and aggressive phenotype during the late stages of the multistep process of tumorigenesis, thereby hypothesizing that metastasis is an event arising from a late clonal selection process [10, 11]. Conversely, the ability by cancer cells to acquire a metastatic potential during a relatively early stage of the tumorigenesis process, depending on the genetic background, underlies another interesting model [12]. This latter hypothesis was supported by a gene expression study carried out by Ramaswamy et al. [13] on primary and metastatic tumor samples, in which a metastasis-associated molecular signature was identified.

Furthermore, a high degree of tumor heterogeneity is determined by the presence of a large number of genomic alterations found within each tumor, although most of these, such as somatic mutations or chromosomal rearrangements, seems to be not involved in tumor progression and not detected across all samples from a tumor or metastasis lesions [14]. Another determinant for the intra-tumor heterogeneity appears to be the branched evolution that occurs during tumor progression, enabling to identify phylogenetically genomic alterations that arise during tumor clonal evolution [1, 15]. Experimental evidences suggested that intra-tumor heterogeneity can vary in the space and time, determining the development of different clones that evolve independently, but not always in a divergent manner. In fact, several studies showed that different parallel mutations that accumulate in the same gene may determine a convergent clonal evolution, suggesting the significant involvement of a specific molecular pathway in the progression of a given tumor and, consequently, highlighting targets clinically useful for the development of new potential therapeutic strategies [16–19]. Since the molecular characterization of a tumor biopsy provides us only a snapshot restricted in the time and space of a given tumor, often without supplying an overview of its heterogeneity, it could be very useful to analyze the molecular alterations of a tumor over time in order to promote, accordingly, the development of personalized therapeutic approaches [20, 21].

In this chapter, we will describe the concepts of cancer clonal evolution and intra-tumor heterogeneity, discussing how these may affect the tumor recurrence, clinical outcome, therapy response, emergence of drug resistance, and biomarker validation.

Cancer Clonal Evolution

Carcinogenesis is a multistep process caused by the progressive accumulation of gene mutations and epigenetic alterations that modulate specific molecular pathways and collectively give rise to a malignant phenotype [22, 23]. The clonal evolution model involves that a spontaneous or induced genetic alteration confers a selective advantage to a cancer cell that generates a dominant subpopulation driving tumor progression. According to this model, tumor progression and diversity are driven by natural selection and genetic drift [24–26].

The initial cytogenetic studies concerning tumor clonality had led to the hypothesis that tumors have a monoclonal origin, as they originate from a single transformed somatic progenitor and all cancer cells have in common at least one primary chromosomal anomaly, subsequently followed by a clonal selection process, according to the Darwinian evolution, that develops among different cancer subclonal populations carrying secondary alterations [27]. Afterward, more detailed cytogenetic analyses and further studies performed on multiple specimens from the same patient revealed sometimes the presence of several cytogenetically independent clones, questioning the monoclonal theory and knowledge so far acquired on tumor clonality [28–33]. Several experimental evidences allowed to hypothesize four potential different mechanisms explaining the concept of cancer clonal evolution. The first model relies on the monoclonal hypothesis, suggesting that cancer cells maintain the original monoclonality during the course of the disease without acquiring further secondary alterations as those detected by karyotypic analysis. This condition is typically present in some sarcomas and leukemias, where only a single genetic aberration is observed in all cancer cells (Fig. 3.1a). The second mechanism is based on the concept of clonal divergence, confirming the monoclonality of the cancerogenesis process, but speculating a secondary clonal heterogeneity due to subsequent alterations occurring over time (Fig. 3.1b). The third hypothesis suggests the emergence of an initial polyclonality in tumor, followed by a clonal convergence process that involves a significant decrease in genomic aberrations and selection of cytogenetically independent clones during tumor growth, leading to a secondary mono- or oligoclonality (Fig. 3.1c). Lastly, the fourth model proposes a cancer polyclonal origin characterized by early clonal convergence and late clonal divergence arising from

the occurrence of further cytogenetic alterations that enabled specific clones to survive during the intermediate stages of tumorigenesis [34–36] (Fig. 3.1d). Experimental evidence showed that cancer clonal evolution is a multiple sequential event involving the coexistence and coevolution of various subclonal populations which acquire selective survival advantages during tumor progression and change spatially and temporally [37, 38]. Additionally, clonal evolution has been shown to be a highly heterogeneous process, as different evolution mechanisms may be adopted by different tumor types [39, 40]. There exist four different modalities by which tumor evolution can occur: linear evolution, clonal separation (or allopatric speciation), clonal competition (or antagonist evolution), and clonal cooperation (or symbiotic evolution). The linear evolution implicates the occurrence of sequential alterations over time and can lead to tumor heterogeneity

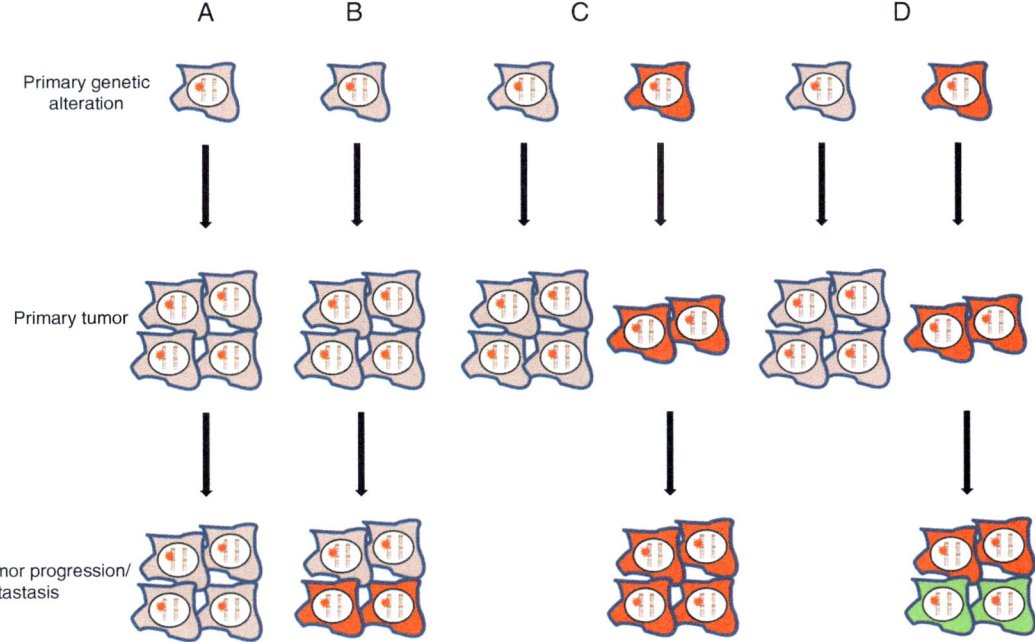

Fig. 3.1 Models of cancer clonal evolution. (**a**) The monoclonal hypothesis suggests that cancer cells maintain a monoclonal origin during the course of the disease without acquiring further secondary alterations. (**b**) The second mechanism relies on the concept of clonal divergence, confirming a monoclonal tumorigenesis process followed by a secondary clonal heterogeneity due to

subsequent alterations occurring over time. (**c**) The third model involves an initial polyclonal tumorigenesis followed by clonal convergence resulting in a secondary mono- or oligoclonality. (**d**) The last model proposes a cancer polyclonal origin characterized by early clonal convergence and late clonal divergence when a subclone is not able to overcome its predecessors. Clonal separation is an event equivalent to the allopatric speciation and involves the presence of subclonal populations geographically isolated within tumor and genetically distinct in different tumor areas [41, 42]. Recently, some studies highlighted the possibility by distinct subclones to cooperate between them during tumor evolution (clonal cooperation) [43]. This cross talk sometimes can cause tumor collapse due to clonal interference, when, for example, a subclone with higher proliferative ability and unable to survive alone overcomes an autonomous driver subclone (clonal competition). Therefore, therapeutic approaches aimed to identify and target specific subclonal populations promoting survival and growth of neighboring cells in the tumor should be developed [44].

Furthermore, evaluating the relationships between tumor clonality and phylogenetic may allow to genetically correlate a primary tumor with its metastases over time [45]. Tumor evolution may occur through two distinct pathways defined as microevolution and macroevolution. While microevolution is a gradual process, instead macroevolution involves significant, nongradual jumps along the evolutionary lines [40].

These models of cancer clonal evolution were better studied in recent years, thanks to the progresses acquired in the molecular technology field, such as the next-generation sequencing (NGS) analysis and development of more sophisticated computational methods, that allowed to obtain a high-resolution overview of the genetic alterations present in tumors, to study more deeply spatial distribution of subclones, and to better characterize tumor heterogeneity [46–52]. Furthermore, several studies showed that cancer subclonal evolution during disease progression, therapy, and acquisition of drug resistance may be predicted and tracked by analysis of circulating tumor DNA (ctDNA) [53].

Intra-tumor Heterogeneity

A crucial event in cancer clonal evolution process is the variability within individual tumors, called intra-tumor heterogeneity (ITH), which determines and drives the genetic selection mechanism of the more suitable cell clones [37, 54]. Experimental evidence clearly showed that cancer cells present in an individual tumor can exhibit genetic, morphological, and behavioral variability [55]. For the first time, in 1800s, the pathologist Rudolf Virchow and other researchers observed the cellular heterogeneity within single tumor entities by means of a compound microscope [56]. While inter-tumor heterogeneity allows to highlight the differences between tumors that hinder the eradication of the disease, instead intra-tumor heterogeneity, recently, has been shown to affect both tumor progression and therapy effectiveness [16, 57, 58]. Indeed, in 1984, Heppner suggested that patient cure and new therapeutic strategies may arise by the knowledge of factors and events that give rise to the intra-tumor heterogeneity [59]. Different genetic changes may be detected in a restricted number of biomarkers or genes from cancer specimens recruited at different stages and from diverse individuals [60]. Usually, the origin of tumor heterogeneity may be explained through two theoretical models potentially complementary between them, the clonal evolution model [61] and cancer stem cell (CSC) hypothesis [62]. These two theories, formerly considered mutually exclusive, appear to have some similarities, hypothesizing that tumors arise following the accumulation of multiple molecular alterations and acquisition of an uncontrolled proliferative capacity by individual cells and interplay with (micro)environmental factors [63]. Among the main discrepancies, we can include that concerning the tumor cell organization that is considered hierarchical in CSC model and stochastic in clonal evolution model. Furthermore, the source of heterogeneity is represented by aberrant differentiation processes and mutations in the CSC theory, instead by epigenetic and genetic changes followed by natural selection in other models [64]. Additionally, according to the CSC hypothesis, tumor progression and therapy resistance seem to be driven by a small cell subset only, whereas, in the case of the clonal evolution, they depend on the genetic instability (mutation frequency), cell population size, proliferation rate, and selective pressure determined by

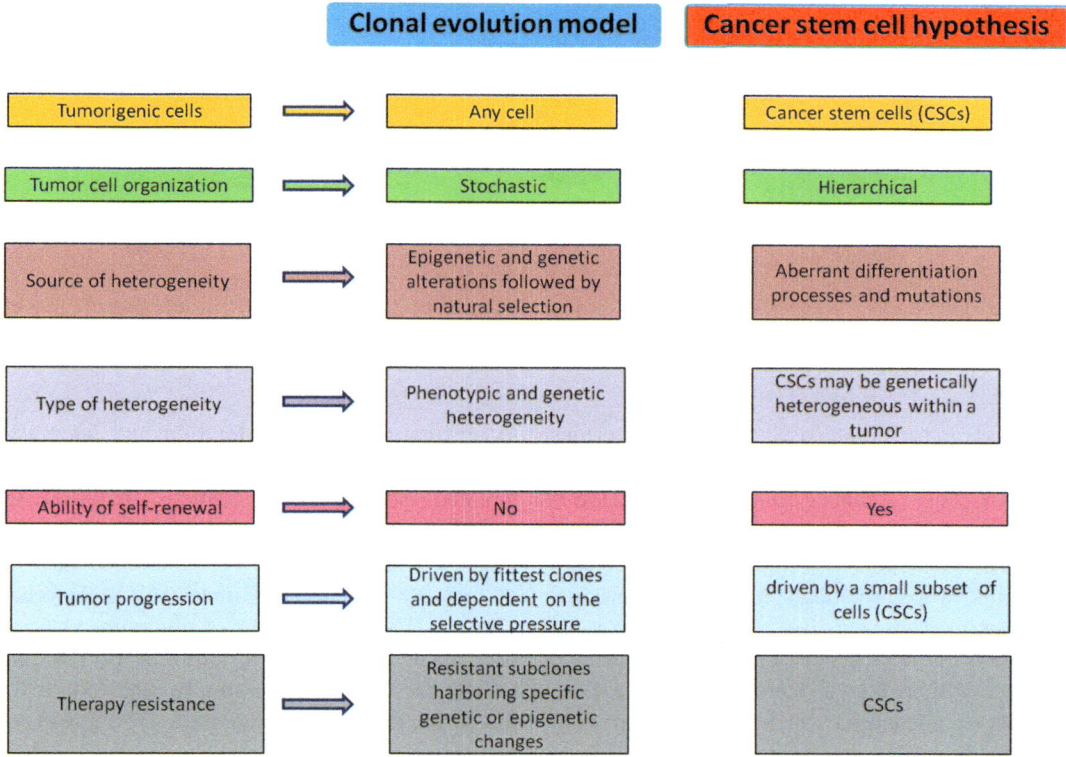

Fig. 3.2 Differences between clonal evolution model and cancer stem cell (CSC) hypothesis. The origin of tumor heterogeneity may be explained through these two theoretical models potentially complementary

external selective forces, according to the Darwinian evolutionary theory [65] (Fig. 3.2).

The intra-tumor heterogeneity detected in most of tumors has been shown to restrict therapy response and induce drug resistance in advanced disease, promoting the selection of resistant subclones, sometimes detectable prior to treatment [66] (Fig. 3.3). Therefore, the success of the anticancer therapies depends on the understanding of the contribution that tumor heterogeneity gives to therapeutic response, investigating the correlation between clonal heterogeneity and clinical significance of subclonal driver mutations [67–70]. Usually, the presence of target driver mutations detected in the primary tumor by means of histological or molecular analyses drives the clinical decision to use a specific targeted therapy. Nevertheless, intra-tumor heterogeneity and clonal evolution within each tumor represent the main hurdle to the

successful treatment, because not all cancer cells may harbor target mutation in the primary tumor or metastatic lesions [71]. In fact, the microenvironment of the metastatic site may affect the evolution of metastatic disease, causing, in some cases, the selection and enrichment of some tumor subclones and conferring a phenotypic and genomic variability between primary tumor and metastases in different tumors [17]. In other cases, instead, it was observed the maintenance of the same genetic alterations both in primary tumor and metastatic lesions [3, 6].

Models of Intra-tumor Heterogeneity: Melanoma and NSCLC

Among tumors, melanoma and non-small cell lung cancer (NSCLC) can provide an interesting example of intra-tumor heterogeneity.

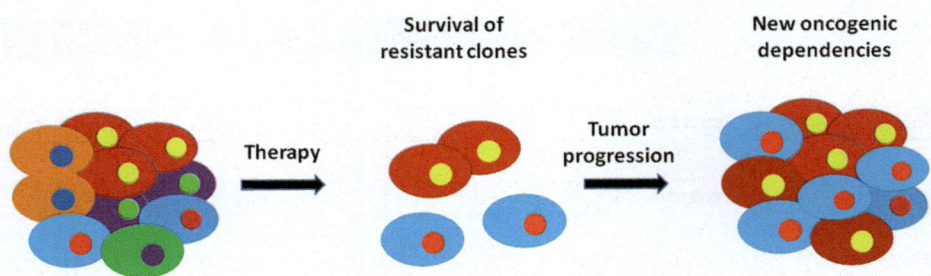

Survival of
resistant clones

New oncogenic
dependencies

Therapy

Tumor
progression

Fig. 3.3 Intra-tumor heterogeneity and resistance. Heterogeneity of tumor cells may alter the therapeutic response to specific therapies, because a small fraction of tumor clones becomes insensitive to therapy and survives, resulting in disease relapse and tumor progression

Melanoma is the most aggressive and serious form of skin cancer accounting for the sixth most common cause of cancer-related deaths [72]. It is a poorly differentiated high-grade malignant tumor of melanocytes (cells producing melanin pigments) whose incidence has shown a gradual increase in recent years leading to an unfavorable prognosis in the presence of advanced metastatic disease, with a low 5-year survival rate [73]. Cutaneous melanoma can be divided into four major subtypes: nodular melanoma, superficial spreading, lentigo maligna, and acral lentiginous [74]. The complex interaction between genetic and environmental factors has been shown to determine the neoplastic transformation of epidermal melanocytes resulting in cancer development [75]. Recent epidemiological, clinical, and genetic studies showed that melanomas are phenotypically and genetically heterogeneous tumors harboring different genetic alterations. The key genetic alterations involved in melanoma pathogenesis concern three main oncogenes: BRAF, NRAS, and c-KIT [76]. Acral or mucosal melanomas as well as those arising in areas of chronic skin damage usually harbor both wild-type *NRAS* and *BRAF*, but show alterations in *c-KIT* and, frequently, a greater copy number of genes downstream of the RAS/BRAF signaling pathway, such as cyclin D1 (*CCND1*) and cyclin-dependent kinase 4 (*CDK4*) [77]. The mitogen-activated protein kinase (MAPK) signaling pathway has been shown to be mainly involved in melanoma onset and progression. Alterations in the RAS/RAF/MEK/ERK signaling cascade may occur at different levels, leading

to an aberrant cell proliferation and apoptosis [78]. NRAS resulted be the most frequently mutated isoform in melanoma, since NRAS mutations, associated with nodular lesions and increased sun exposure, were identified in 33% of primary and 26% of metastatic melanomas [79, 80]. The substitutions of glutamine at position 61 by a lysine or an arginine (Q61K and Q61R) are the most commonly detected *NRAS* mutations [81]. *BRAF* mutations are most commonly harbored by melanomas located in areas without sun exposure-induced chronic damage and have been shown to occur early during tumor progression stages, inducing cell proliferation and, subsequently, senescence [82, 83]. Generally, *BRAF* mutations are more commonly present in younger patients and with a higher number of nevi. Increased exposure to UV radiations during youth is correlated with *BRAF* mutations, whereas high rates of sun exposure throughout the course of life are associated with *NRAS* mutations [84]. Approximately 40–60% of advanced cutaneous melanomas harbors activating *BRAF* mutations, exhibiting some clinical characteristics correlated with a poorer prognosis [85, 86]. However, significant improvements in overall survival of patients with metastatic melanoma have been recently achieved by targeting mutated BRAF [77, 87]. The most frequently detected *BRAF* mutation in 80–90% of melanoma cases is the substitution of glutamic acid for valine at amino acid 600 (V600E), whereas about 16% of the remaining activating mutations consist of an alternate substitution (lysine for valine) at the V600 locus (V600K), detected at slightly higher levels in melanomas of older patients [88, 89]. The *BRAF* V600E mutation promotes proliferation and malignant transformation via constitutive activation of BRAF, regardless of the upstream activation by extracellular stimuli and RAS. However, the melanoma progression is driven by other factors which cooperate with BRAF. Data from cohort studies strongly indicated that *NRAS* and *BRAF* mutations are almost always mutually exclusive in melanoma, suggesting that probably the simultaneous presence of both mutations does not provide benefit for tumor growth and survival and occurrence of each mutation may be specifically correlated with some subtypes of melanoma [90–92]. However, during these years, some rare exception has been reported [93]. In the last years, some studies postulated that *NRAS* and *BRAF* mutations may be simultaneously detected in the same tumor specimens, suggesting that these mutations are not mutually exclusive in melanoma, but exhibit intra-tumor heterogeneity. In this regard, Sensi et al. [94] have observed, using high-sensitivity sequencing methods, that *NRAS* Q61R and *BRAF* V600E mutations are mutually exclusive at the single-cell level, but may be simultaneously present in the same human melanoma, since a small cell subpopulation of the same tumor mass may harbor one of two mutations. Moreover, *NRAS*^{Q61R}-mutated clones showed a higher proliferative ability both in vitro and in vivo compared to *BRAF*^{V600E}-mutated clones [94]. In the same year, using in vitro assays, the same group of authors showed that the simultaneous expression of *NRAS* Q61R and *BRAF* V600E in the same human melanoma cell may induce senescence and enhance the susceptibility to cell-mediated cytotoxicity by both HLA class I antigen-restricted and nonspecific T cells, suggesting a relationship not only epistatic but also of synthetic lethality between *NRAS* and *BRAF*, resulting in a selection against double mutant cells [95]. Recently, Chiappetta et al. [96] reported that, when *NRAS* and *BRAF* mutations coexist in the same sample of nodular melanoma, these show different mutation frequencies: one is a low-frequency mutation and the other is a high-frequency mutation. These recent findings could

lead to limit the clinical use of BRAF inhibitors in melanomas that contain different *BRAF*- and *NRAS*-mutated cell subpopulations, as the cancer cell growth and survival are regulated in a manner heterogeneous within the same tumor. Therefore, in the light of these observations, it is crucial to develop and use more sensitive and specific technical approaches, in order to select the subgroups of patients which are more likely to respond to BRAF inhibitors, based on the frequency by which both mutations occur within the same melanoma. In addition, the molecular mechanisms responsible for the occurrence of two mutations in the same tumor should be further studied.

The identification of cancer driver genes, such as epidermal growth factor receptor gene (*EGFR*), allowed to implement promising approaches of personalized medicine in NSCLC patients [97, 98].

EGFR activation induces the dimerization of receptor, favoring, in turn, an intracellular protein-tyrosine kinase activity that leads to auto-phosphorylation and activation of downstream signaling pathways, such as angiogenesis, proliferation, and apoptosis [99]. The selective inhibition of EGFR signaling by TKIs, including gefitinib and erlotinib, occurs through targeting of ATP-binding site and inactivation of the tyrosine kinase domain [100, 101]. The intra-tumor heterogeneity seems to play a key role also in NSCLC treatment, since NSCLC patients with *EGFR*-activating mutations exhibit different responses to tyrosine kinase inhibitors (TKIs). Indeed, clinical data showed that most of patients harboring EGFR mutations exhibits high response rates to TKIs, whereas a small group of them gives rise to mixed responses [102, 103]. Tumors may be intrinsically insensitive to treatment with EGFR TKIs prior to therapy (intrinsic or primary resistance) or, after being initially sensitive to therapy, may develop a resistance acquired after TKI treatment (acquired or secondary resistance). Acquired resistance not only makes tumors resistant to originally used drugs but may also cause cross-resistance to other drugs with different mechanisms of action. The intra-tumor heterogeneity, that implicates differences

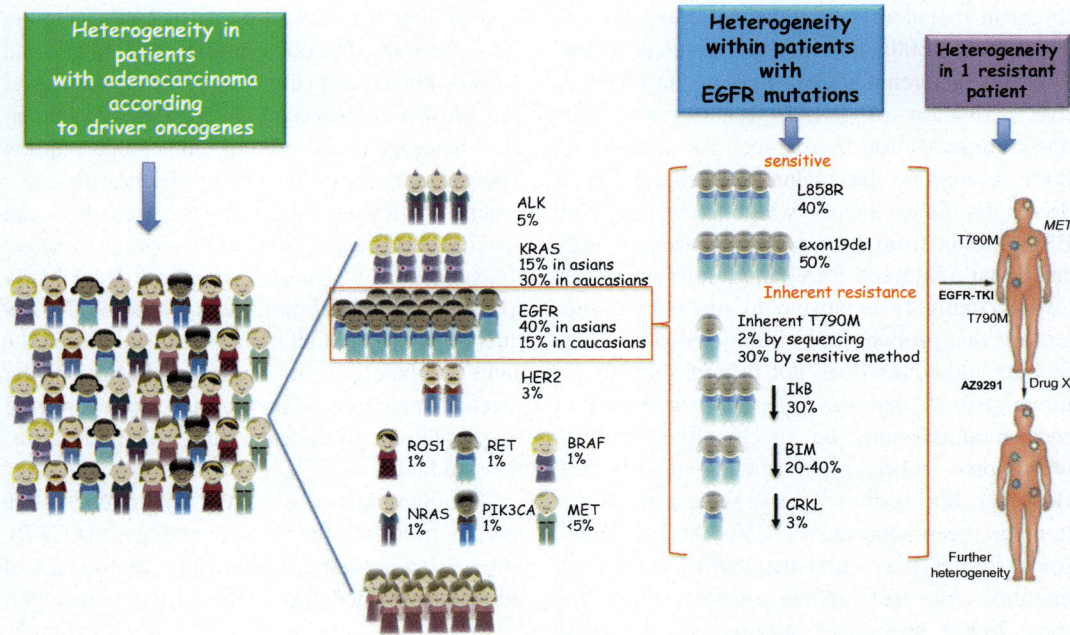

Fig. 3.4 The efficacy of target therapy in NSCLC is affected by tumor heterogeneity

in the mutational status, extent of amplification, and expression levels of EGFR, reduces effectiveness of targeted therapy in NSCLC [104, 105]. The sequential therapy, that involves the consecutive use of different drugs after the failure of that previously used, may represent an interesting clinical option to overcome the resistance induced by selection of a therapy-resistant subclone [106]. An example of sequential therapy is represented by the treatment of EGFR-mutated NSCLC patients (with mutation EGFR L585R or EGFR exon 19 deletion) with first-generation EGFRIs (gefitinib or erlotinib). After the initial response, subsequently, the occurrence of a resistance mutation (EGFR T790M) causes tumor progression [107]. Nevertheless, cells harboring this resistance-conferring mutation have been shown to be responsive to the third-generation EGFRIs, rociletinib and AZD9291 [108, 109]. However, a subclone harboring a EGFR T790M variant may become resistant to therapy with AZD9291 or rociletinib generating another

selection mechanism, resulting in the reappearance of subclones negative for EGFR T790M and EGFR C797S mutant cells or resistant subclones positive for EGFR T790M [110, 111] (Fig. 3.4).

Conclusions and Futures Perspective

Knowing the evolutionary history of a tumor in the space and time is a crucial factor for developing screening methods able to early detect disease when genetic variability is low and tumor is evolving. The correlations observed between tumor diversity and clinical outcome make it necessary the development of more sensitive and specific clinical approaches in order to better characterize and measure tumor heterogeneity and early identify the subclonal events within tumor [15]. The combination therapy may help us to overcome tumor resistance caused by intratumor heterogeneity, enhancing the efficacy of targeted agents and chemotherapy and improving survival rates in cancer patients.

In recent years, with the advent of new cancer genomic sequencing technologies, significant advances in the detection of single-nucleotide variants were made [112, 113]. In particular, NGS technologies are providing new methods of genome sequencing at high speed and greater resolution power, leading to identification of tumor-specific genetic changes belonging to different clonal populations within a given tumor. Despite encouraging results obtained from several studies, however, there are still some technical restrictions that may limit the potential application of these technologies in clinical practice, including issues concerning sequencing methods requiring DNA pre-amplification, and selection criteria of individual cell subclones within a tumor.

Additional molecular investigations on single cancer cells are needed in order to increase our knowledge about genetic variability of individual cells present in several tumors and responsible for the complex question concerning cancer clonal evolution during all stages of tumorigenesis.

References

1. Ramos P, Bentires-Alj M. Mechanism-based cancer therapy: resistance to therapy, therapy for resistance. Oncogene. 2015;34(28):3617–26. doi:10.1038/onc.2014.314, onc2014314 [pii].
2. Vogelstein B, Papadopoulos N, Velculescu VE, Zhou S, Diaz Jr LA, Kinzler KW. Cancer genome landscapes. Science. 2013;339(6127):1546–58. doi:10.1126/science.1235122, 339/6127/1546 [pii].
3. Vignot S, Frampton GM, Soria JC, Yelensky R, Commo F, Brambilla C, et al. Next-generation sequencing reveals high concordance of recurrent somatic alterations between primary tumor and metastases from patients with non-small-cell lung cancer. J Clin Oncol. 2013;31(17):2167–72. doi:10.1200/JCO.2012.47.7737, JCO.2012.47.7737 [pii].
4. Turajlic S, Furney SJ, Lambros MB, Mitsopoulos C, Kozarewa I, Geyer FC, et al. Whole genome sequencing of matched primary and metastatic acral melanomas. Genome Res. 2012;22(2):196–207. doi:10.1101/gr.125591.111, gr.125591.111 [pii].
5. Anderson K, Lutz C, van Delft FW, Bateman CM, Guo Y, Colman SM, et al. Genetic variegation of
6. Vignot S, Besse B, Andre F, Spano JP, Soria JC. Discrepancies between primary tumor and metastasis: a literature review on clinically established biomarkers. Crit Rev Oncol Hematol. 2012;84(3):301–13. doi:10.1016/j.critrevonc.2012.05.002, S1040-8428(12)00115-1 [pii].
7. Fanale D, Corsini L, Rizzo S, Russo A. Gene signatures in CRC and liver metastasis. 2012;27–33. doi:10.1007/978-1-61779-358-5_3.
8. Campbell PJ, Yachida S, Mudie LJ, Stephens PJ, Pleasance ED, Stebbings LA, et al. The patterns and dynamics of genomic instability in metastatic pancreatic cancer. Nature. 2010;467(7319):1109–13. doi:10.1038/nature09460, nature09460 [pii].
9. Yachida S, Jones S, Bozic I, Antal T, Leary R, Fu B, et al. Distant metastasis occurs late during the genetic evolution of pancreatic cancer. Nature. 2010;467(7319):1114–7. doi:10.1038/nature09515, nature09515 [pii].
10. Fidler IJ, Kripke ML. Genomic analysis of primary tumors does not address the prevalence of metastatic cells in the population. Nat Genet. 2003;34(1):23; author reply 5. doi:10.1038/ng0503-23a, ng0503-23a [pii].
11. Koh KH, Rhee H, Kang HJ, Yang E, You KT, Lee H, et al. Differential Gene expression profiles of metastases in paired primary and metastatic colorectal carcinomas. Oncology. 2008;75(1–2):92–101. doi:10.1159/000155211.
12. Nguyen DX, Massagué J. Genetic determinants of cancer metastasis. Nat Rev Genet. 2007;8(5):341–52. doi:10.1038/nrg2101.
13. Ramaswamy S, Ross KN, Lander ES, Golub TR. A molecular signature of metastasis in primary solid tumors. Nat Genet. 2003;33(1):49–54. doi:10.1038/ng1060, ng1060 [pii].
14. Navin N, Krasnitz A, Rodgers L, Cook K, Meth J, Kendall J, et al. Inferring tumor progression from genomic heterogeneity. Genome Res. 2010;20(1):68–80. doi:10.1101/gr.099622.109, gr.099622.109 [pii].
15. Gerlinger M, Rowan AJ, Horswell S, Larkin J, Endesfelder D, Gronroos E, et al. Intratumor heterogeneity and branched evolution revealed by multiregion sequencing. N Engl J Med. 2012;366(10):883–92. doi:10.1056/NEJMoa1113205.
16. Swanton C. Intratumor heterogeneity: evolution through space and time. Cancer Res. 2012;72(19):4875–82. doi:10.1158/0008-5472.CAN-12-2217, 0008-5472.CAN-12-2217 [pii].
17. Klein CA. Selection and adaptation during metastatic cancer progression. Nature. 2013;501(7467):365–72. doi:10.1038/nature12628.
18. Bedard PL, Hansen AR, Ratain MJ, Siu LL. Tumour heterogeneity in the clinic. Nature. 2013;501(7467):355–64. doi:10.1038/nature12627.

19. Janku F. Tumor heterogeneity in the clinic: is it a real problem? Ther Adv Med Oncol. 2014;6(2):43–51. doi:10.1177/1758834013517414, 10.1177_1758834013517414 [pii].

20. Crowley E, Di Nicolantonio F, Loupakis F, Bardelli A. Liquid biopsy: monitoring cancer-genetics in the blood. Nat Rev Clin Oncol. 2013;10(8):472–84. doi:10.1038/nrclinonc.2013.110, nrclinonc.2013.110 [pii].

21. Passiglia F, Cicero G, Castiglia M, Bazan V. Biomarkers as prognostic, predictive, and surrogate endpoints. 2015:31–41. doi:10.1007/978–1–4939-2047-1_4.

22. Weinstein IB. Disorders in cell circuitry during multistage carcinogenesis: the role of homeostasis. Carcinogenesis. 2000;21(5):857–64.

23. Caruso S, Fanale D, Bazan V. Oncogene addiction in solid tumors. 2015:3–7. doi:10.1007/978–1–4939-2047-1_2.

24. Garcia SB, Novelli M, Wright NA. The clonal origin and clonal evolution of epithelial tumours. Int J Exp Pathol. 2000;81(2):89–116. iep142 [pii].

25. Navin N, Kendall J, Troge J, Andrews P, Rodgers L, McIndoo J et al. Tumour evolution inferred by single-cell sequencing. Nature. 2011;472(7341):90–4. doi:10.1038/nature09807.

26. Gatenby RA, Vincent TL. An evolutionary model of carcinogenesis. Cancer Res. 2003;63(19):6212–20.

27. Nowell PC. The clonal evolution of tumor cell populations. Science. 1976;194(4260):23–8.

28. Pandis N, Heim S, Bardi G, Idvall I, Mandahl N, Mitelman F. Chromosome analysis of 20 breast carcinomas: cytogenetic multiclonality and karyotypic-pathologic correlations. Genes Chromosomes Cancer. 1993;6(1):51–7.

29. Heim S, Teixeira MR, Dietrich CU, Pandis N. Cytogenetic polyclonality in tumors of the breast. Cancer Genet Cytogenet. 1997;95(1):16–9. S0165460896003226 [pii].

30. Pandis N, Teixeira MR, Adeyinka A, Rizou H, Bardi G, Mertens F, et al. Cytogenetic comparison of primary tumors and lymph node metastases in breast cancer patients. Genes Chromosomes Cancer. 1998;22(2):122–9. doi:10.1002/(SICI)1098-2264(199806)22:2<122::AID-GCC6>3.0.CO;2-Z [pii].

31. Teixeira MR, Pandis N, Heim S. Cytogenetic clues to breast carcinogenesis. Genes Chromosomes Cancer. 2002;33(1):1–16. doi:10.1002/gcc.1206 [pii].

32. Adeyinka A, Mertens F, Bondeson L, Garne JP, Borg A, Baldetorp B, et al. Cytogenetic heterogeneity and clonal evolution in synchronous bilateral breast carcinomas and their lymph node metastases from a male patient without any detectable BRCA2 germline mutation. Cancer Genet Cytogenet. 2000;118(1):42–7. S0165-4608(99)00150-8 [pii].

33. Hoglund M, Sall T, Heim S, Mitelman F, Mandahl N, Fadl-Elmula I. Identification of cytogenetic subgroups and karyotypic pathways in transitional cell carcinoma. Cancer Res. 2001;61(22):8241–6.

34. Teixeira MR, Heim S. Cytogenetic analysis of tumor clonality. Adv Cancer Res. 2011;112:127–49. doi:10.1016/B978-0-12-387688-1.00005-3, B978-0-12-387688-1.00005-3 [pii].

35. Heim S, Mandahl N, Mitelman F. Genetic convergence and divergence in tumor progression. Cancer Res. 1988;48(21):5911–6.

36. Adeyinka A, Kytola S, Mertens F, Pandis N, Larsson C. Spectral karyotyping and chromosome banding studies of primary breast carcinomas and their lymph node metastases. Int J Mol Med. 2000;5(3):235–40.

37. Murugaesu N, Chew SK, Swanton C. Adapting clinical paradigms to the challenges of cancer clonal evolution. Am J Pathol. 2013;182(6):1962–71. doi:10.1016/j.ajpath.2013.02.026, S0002-9440(13)00205-8 [pii].

38. Merlo LM, Pepper JW, Reid BJ, Maley CC. Cancer as an evolutionary and ecological process. Nat Rev Cancer. 2006;6(12):924–35. doi:10.1038/nrc2013, nrc2013 [pii].

39. Ding L, Raphael BJ, Chen F, Wendl MC. Advances for studying clonal evolution in cancer. Cancer Lett. 2013;340(2):212–9. doi:10.1016/j.canlet.2012.12.028.

40. Gerlinger M, McGranahan N, Dewhurst SM, Burrell RA, Tomlinson I, Swanton C. Cancer: evolution within a lifetime. Annu Rev Genet. 2014;48:215–36. doi:10.1146/annurev-genet-120213-092314.

41. de Bruin EC, McGranahan N, Mitter R, Salm M, Wedge DC, Yates L, et al. Spatial and temporal diversity in genomic instability processes defines lung cancer evolution. Science. 2014;346(6206):251–6. doi:10.1126/science.1253462, 346/6206/251 [pii].

42. Gerlinger M, Horswell S, Larkin J, Rowan AJ, Salm MP, Varela I, et al. Genomic architecture and evolution of clear cell renal cell carcinomas defined by multiregion sequencing. Nat Genet 2014;46(3):225–33. doi:10.1038/ng.2891.

43. Marusyk A, Tabassum DP, Altrock PM, Almendro V, Michor F, Polyak K. Non-cell-autonomous driving of tumour growth supports sub-clonal heterogeneity. Nature. 2014;514(7520):54–8. doi:10.1038/nature13556.

44. McGranahan N, Swanton C. Biological and therapeutic impact of intratumor heterogeneity in cancer evolution. Cancer Cell. 2015;27(1):15–26. doi:10.1016/j.ccell.2014.12.001.

45. Greenman CD, Pleasance ED, Newman S, Yang F, Fu B, Nik-Zainal S, et al. Estimation of rearrangement phylogeny for cancer genomes. Genome Res. 2012;22(2):346–61. doi:10.1101/gr.118414.110, gr.118414.110 [pii].

46. Paweletz CP, Sacher AG, Raymond CK, Alden RS, O'Connell A, Mach SL, et al. Bias-corrected targeted next-generation sequencing for rapid, multiplexed detection of actionable alterations in cell-free DNA from advanced lung cancer patients. Clin Cancer Res. 2016;22(4):915–22. doi:10.1158/1078-0432. CCR-15-1627-T, 1078-0432.CCR-15-1627-T [pii].

47. Aparicio S, Mardis E. Tumor heterogeneity: next-generation sequencing enhances the view from the pathologist's microscope. Genome Biol. 2014;15(9):463. doi:10.1186/s13059-014-0463-6, s13059-014-0463-6 [pii].

48. Russnes HG, Navin N, Hicks J, Borresen-Dale AL. Insight into the heterogeneity of breast cancer through next-generation sequencing. J Clin Invest. 2011;121(10):3810–8. doi:10.1172/JCI57088, 57088 [pii].

49. Jiang Y, Qiu Y, Minn AJ, Zhang NR. Assessing intratumor heterogeneity and tracking longitudinal and spatial clonal evolutionary history by next-generation sequencing. Proc Natl Acad Sci. 2016;113(37):E5528-E37. doi:10.1073/pnas.1522203113.

50. Guan YF, Li GR, Wang RJ, Yi YT, Yang L, Jiang D, et al. Application of next-generation sequencing in clinical oncology to advance personalized treatment of cancer. Chin J Cancer. 2012;31(10):463–70. doi:10.5732/cjc.012.10216, cjc.012.10216 [pii].

51. Ma QC, Ennis CA, Aparicio S. Opening Pandora's box – the new biology of driver mutations and clonal evolution in cancer as revealed by next generation sequencing. Curr Opin Genet Dev. 2012;22(1):3–9. doi:10.1016/j.gde.2012.01.008, S0959-437X(12)00009-3 [pii].

52. Medvedev P, Stanciu M, Brudno M. Computational methods for discovering structural variation with next-generation sequencing. Nat Methods. 2009;6(11 Suppl):S13–20. doi:10.1038/nmeth.1374, nmeth.1374 [pii].

53. Chan KCA, Jiang P, Zheng YWL, Liao GJW, Sun H, Wong J, et al. Cancer genome scanning in plasma: detection of tumor-associated copy number aberrations, single-nucleotide variants, and Tumoral heterogeneity by massively parallel sequencing. Clin Chem. 2012;59(1):211–24. doi:10.1373/clinchem.2012.196014.

54. Meyerson M, Gabriel S, Getz G. Advances in understanding cancer genomes through second-generation sequencing. Nat Rev Genet. 2010;11(10):685–96. doi:10.1038/nrg2841, nrg2841 [pii].

55. Martelotto LG, Ng CK, Piscuoglio S, Weigelt B, Reis-Filho JS. Breast cancer intra-tumor heterogeneity. Breast Cancer Res. 2014;16(3):210. doi:10.1186/bcr3658, 10.1186/bcr3658 [pii].

56. Brown TM, Fee E. Rudolf Carl Virchow: medical scientist, social reformer, role model. Am J Public Health. 2006;96(12):2104–5. doi:10.2105/AJPH.2005.078436, AJPH.2005.078436 [pii].

57. Apostoli AJ, Ailles L. Clonal evolution and tumor-initiating cells: new dimensions in cancer patient treatment. Crit Rev Clin Lab Sci. 2016;53(1):40–51. doi:10.3109/10408363.2015.1083944.

58. Gay L, Baker A-M, Graham TA. Tumour cell heterogeneity. F1000Research. 2016;5:238. doi:10.12688/f1000research.7210.1.

59. Heppner GH. Tumor heterogeneity. Cancer Res. 1984;44(6):2259–65.

60. Navin NE, Hicks J. Tracing the tumor lineage. Mol Oncol. 2010;4(3):267–83. doi:10.1016/j.molonc.2010.04.010, S1574-7891(10)00032-3 [pii].

61. Greaves M, Maley CC. Clonal evolution in cancer. Nature. 2012;481(7381):306–13. doi:10.1038/nature10762, nature10762 [pii].

62. Meacham CE, Morrison SJ. Tumour heterogeneity and cancer cell plasticity. Nature. 2013;501(7467):328–37. doi:10.1038/nature12624, nature12624 [pii].

63. Marusyk A, Polyak K. Tumor heterogeneity: causes and consequences. Biochim Biophys Acta. 2010;1805(1):105–17. doi:10.1016/j.bbcan.2009.11.002, S0304-419X(09)00074-2 [pii].

64. Melo FDSE, Vermeulen L, Fessler E, Medema JP. Cancer heterogeneity – a multifaceted view. EMBO Rep. 2013;14(8):686–95. doi:10.1038/embor.2013.92.

65. Turner NC, Reis-Filho JS. Genetic heterogeneity and cancer drug resistance. Lancet Oncol. 2012;13(4):e178–85. doi:10.1016/S1470-2045(11)70335-7, S1470-2045(11)70335-7 [pii].

66. Cao F. Differential response to EGFR- and VEGF-targeted therapies in patient-derived tumor tissue xenograft models of colon carcinoma and related metastases. Int J Oncol. 2012; doi:10.3892/ijo.2012.1469.

67. McGranahan N, Favero F, de Bruin EC, Birkbak NJ, Szallasi Z, Swanton C. Clonal status of actionable driver events and the timing of mutational processes in cancer evolution. Sci Transl Med. 2015;7(283):283ra54. doi:10.1126/scitranslmed.aaa1408, 7/283/283ra54 [pii].

68. Morris LG, Riaz N, Desrichard A, Senbabaoglu Y, Hakimi AA, Makarov V et al. Pan-cancer analysis of intratumor heterogeneity as a prognostic determinant of survival. Oncotarget. 2016;7(9):10051–63. doi:10.18632/oncotarget.7067, 7067 [pii].

69. Jamal-Hanjani M, Quezada SA, Larkin J, Swanton C. Translational implications of tumor heterogeneity. Clin Cancer Res. 2015;21(6):1258–66. doi:10.1158/1078-0432.CCR-14-1429, 21/6/1258 [pii].

70. Jamal-Hanjani M, Thanopoulou E, Peggs KS, Quezada SA, Swanton C. Tumour heterogeneity and immune-modulation. Curr Opin Pharmacol. 2013;13(4):497–503. doi:10.1016/j.coph.2013.04.006, S1471-4892(13)00055-6 [pii].

71. Ramos P, Bentires-Alj M. Mechanism-based cancer therapy: resistance to therapy, therapy for resistance. Oncogene. 2014; doi:10.1038/onc.2014.314.

72. Siegel RL, Miller KD, Jemal A. Cancer statistics, 2015. CA Cancer J Clin. 2015; doi:10.3322/caac.21254.

73. Massey PR, Prasad V, Figg WD, Fojo T. Multiplying therapies and reducing toxicity in metastatic melanoma. Cancer Biol Ther. 2015; doi:10.1080/15384047.2015.1046650.

74. Tas F, Keskin S, Karadeniz A, Dagoglu N, Sen F, Kilic L, et al. Noncutaneous melanoma have distinct features from each other and cutaneous melanoma.

Oncology. 2011;81(5–6):353–8. doi:10.1159/000334863, 000334863 [pii].

75. Oba-Shinjo SM, Correa M, Ricca TI, Molognoni F, Pinhal MA, Neves IA, et al. Melanocyte transformation associated with substrate adhesion impediment. Neoplasia. 2006; doi:10.1593/neo.05781.

76. Curtin JA, Fridlyand J, Kageshita T, Patel HN, Busam KJ, Kutzner H, et al. Distinct sets of genetic alterations in melanoma. N Engl J Med. 2005;353(20):2135–47. doi:10.1056/NEJMoa050092, 353/20/2135 [pii].

77. Kunz M. Oncogenes in melanoma: an update. Eur J Cell Biol. 2014;93(1–2):1–10. doi:10.1016/j.ejcb.2013.12.002, S0171-9335(13)00097-6 [pii].

78. Wang AX, Qi XY. Targeting RAS/RAF/MEK/ERK signaling in metastatic melanoma. IUBMB Life. 2013; doi:10.1002/iub.1193.

79. Jafari M, Papp T, Kirchner S, Diener U, Henschler D, Burg G, et al. Analysis of ras mutations in human melanocytic lesions: activation of the ras gene seems to be associated with the nodular type of human malignant melanoma. J Cancer Res Clin Oncol. 1995;121(1):23–30.

80. van Elsas A, Zerp SF, van der Flier S, Kruse KM, Aarnoudse C, Hayward NK, et al. Relevance of ultraviolet-induced N-ras oncogene point mutations in development of primary human cutaneous melanoma. Am J Pathol. 1996;149(3):883–93.

81. Ellerhorst JA, Greene VR, Ekmekcioglu S, Warneke CL, Johnson MM, Cooke CP, et al. Clinical correlates of NRAS and BRAF mutations in primary human melanoma. Clin Cancer Res. 2011;17(2):229–35. doi:10.1158/1078-0432.CCR-10-2276, 1078-0432.CCR-10-2276 [pii].

82. Pollock PM, Harper UL, Hansen KS, Yudt LM, Stark M, Robbins CM, et al. High frequency of BRAF mutations in nevi. Nat Genet. 2003;33(1):19–20. doi:10.1038/ng1054, ng1054 [pii].

83. Yeh I, von Deimling A, Bastian BC. Clonal BRAF mutations in melanocytic nevi and initiating role of BRAF in melanocytic neoplasia. J Natl Cancer Inst. 2013;105(12):917–9. doi:10.1093/jnci/djt119, djt119 [pii].

84. Bertolotto C. Melanoma: from melanocyte to genetic alterations and clinical options. Scientifica (Cairo). 2013;2013:635203. doi:10.1155/2013/635203.

85. Davies H, Bignell GR, Cox C, Stephens P, Edkins S, Clegg S, et al. Mutations of the BRAF gene in human cancer. Nature. 2002;417(6892):949–54. doi:10.1038/nature00766, nature00766 [pii].

86. Long GV, Menzies AM, Nagrial AM, Haydu LE, Hamilton AL, Mann GJ, et al. Prognostic and clinicopathologic associations of oncogenic BRAF in metastatic melanoma. J Clin Oncol. 2011;29(10):1239–46. doi:10.1200/JCO.2010.32.4327, JCO.2010.32.4327 [pii].

87. Wellbrock C, Hurlstone A. BRAF as therapeutic target in melanoma. Biochem Pharmacol. 2010;80(5):561–7. doi:10.1016/j.bcp.2010.03.019, S0006-2952(10)00207-8 [pii].

88. Thomas NE. BRAF somatic mutations in malignant melanoma and melanocytic naevi. Melanoma Res. 2006;16(2):97–103. doi:10.1097/01.cmr.0000215035.38436.87, 00008390-200604000-00001 [pii].

89. Madureira P, de Mello RA. BRAF and MEK gene rearrangements in melanoma: implications for targeted therapy. Mol Diagn Ther. 2014; doi:10.1007/s40291-013-0081-0.

90. Omholt K, Platz A, Kanter L, Ringborg U, Hansson J. NRAS and BRAF mutations arise early during melanoma pathogenesis and are preserved throughout tumor progression. Clin Cancer Res. 2003;9(17):6483–8.

91. Edlundh-Rose E, Egyhazi S, Omholt K, Mansson-Brahme E, Platz A, Hansson J, et al. NRAS and BRAF mutations in melanoma tumours in relation to clinical characteristics: a study based on mutation screening by pyrosequencing. Melanoma Res. 2006;16(6):471–8. doi:10.1097/01.cmr.0000232300.22032.86, 00008390-200612000-00001 [pii].

92. Platz A, Egyhazi S, Ringborg U, Hansson J. Human cutaneous melanoma; a review of NRAS and BRAF mutation frequencies in relation to histogenetic subclass and body site. Mol Oncol. 2008;1(4):395–405. doi:10.1016/j.molonc.2007.12.003, S1574-7891(07)00104-4 [pii].

93. Jovanovic B, Egyhazi S, Eskandarpour M, Ghiorzo P, Palmer JM, Bianchi Scarra G, et al. Coexisting NRAS and BRAF mutations in primary familial melanomas with specific CDKN2A germline alterations. J Invest Dermatol. 2010;130(2):618–20. doi:10.1038/jid.2009.287, S0022-202X(15)34686-8 [pii].

94. Sensi M, Nicolini G, Petti C, Bersani I, Lozupone F, Molla A, et al. Mutually exclusive NRASQ61R and BRAFV600E mutations at the single-cell level in the same human melanoma. Oncogene. 2006;25(24):3357–64. doi:10.1038/sj.onc.1209379, 1209379 [pii].

95. Petti C, Molla A, Vegetti C, Ferrone S, Anichini A, Sensi M. Coexpression of NRASQ61R and BRAFV600E in human melanoma cells activates senescence and increases susceptibility to cell-mediated cytotoxicity. Cancer Res. 2006;66(13):6503–11. doi:10.1158/0008-5472.CAN-05-4671, 66/13/6503 [pii].

96. Chiappetta C, Proietti I, Soccodato V, Puggioni C, Zaralli R, Pacini L, et al. BRAF and NRAS mutations are heterogeneous and not mutually exclusive in nodular melanoma. Appl Immunohistochem Mol Morphol. 2015; doi:10.1097/PAI.0000000000000071.

97. Mok TS, Wu Y-L, Thongprasert S, Yang C-H, Chu D-T, Saijo N, et al. Gefitinib or carboplatin–paclitaxel in pulmonary adenocarcinoma. N Engl J Med. 2009; doi:10.1056/NEJMoa0810699.

98. Rosell R, Moran T, Queralt C, Porta R, Cardenal F, Camps C, et al. Screening for epidermal growth factor receptor mutations in lung cancer. N Engl J Med. 2009; doi:10.1056/NEJMoa0904554.

99. Seshacharyulu P, Ponnusamy MP, Haridas D, Jain M, Ganti AK, Batra SK. Targeting the EGFR signaling pathway in cancer therapy. Expert Opin Ther Targets. 2012; doi:10.1517/14728222.2011.648617.

100. Cohen MH, Williams GA, Sridhara R, Chen G, McGuinn Jr WD, Morse D, et al. United States Food and Drug Administration drug approval summary: gefitinib (ZD1839; Iressa) tablets. Clin Cancer Res. 2004;10(4):1212–8.

101. Cohen MH, Johnson JR, Chen YF, Sridhara R, Pazdur R. FDA drug approval summary: erlotinib (Tarceva) tablets. Oncologist. 2005;10(7):461–6. doi:10.1634/theoncologist.10-7-461, 10/7/461 [pii].

102. Chen ZY, Zhong WZ, Zhang XC, Su J, Yang XN, Chen ZH, et al. EGFR mutation heterogeneity and the mixed response to EGFR tyrosine kinase inhibitors of lung adenocarcinomas. Oncologist. 2012;17(7):978–85. doi:10.1634/theoncologist.2011-0385, theoncologist.2011-0385 [pii].

103. Ryoo BY, Na, II, Yang SH, Koh JS, Kim CH, Lee JC. Synchronous multiple primary lung cancers with different response to gefitinib. Lung Cancer. 2006;53(2):245–8. doi:10.1016/j.lungcan.2006.05.010, S0169-5002(06)00235-2 [pii].

104. Fanale D, Castiglia M, Bazan V, Russo A. Involvement of non-coding RNAs in chemo- and radioresistance of colorectal cancer. 2016;937:207–228. doi:10.1007/978-3-319-42059-2_11.

105. Majem M, Remon J. Tumor heterogeneity: evolution through space and time in EGFR mutant non small cell lung cancer patients. Transl Lung Cancer Res. 2013;2(3):226–37. doi:10.3978/j.issn.2218-6751.2013.03.09, tlcr-02-03-226 [pii].

106. Venkatesan S, Swanton C. Tumor evolutionary principles: how intratumor heterogeneity influences cancer treatment and outcome. Am Soc Clin Oncol Educ Book. 2016;35:e141–9. doi:10.14694/EDBK_158930, 158930 [pii].

107. Pao W, Miller VA, Politi KA, Riely GJ, Somwar R, Zakowski MF, et al. Acquired resistance of lung adenocarcinomas to gefitinib or erlotinib is associated with a second mutation in the EGFR kinase domain. PLoS Med. 2005;2(3):e73. doi:10.1371/journal.pmed.0020073, 05-PLME-RA-0027R1 [pii].

108. Walter AO, Sjin RT, Haringsma HJ, Ohashi K, Sun J, Lee K, et al. Discovery of a mutant-selective covalent inhibitor of EGFR that overcomes T790M-mediated resistance in NSCLC. Cancer Discov. 2013;3(12):1404–15. doi:10.1158/2159-8290.CD-13-0314, 2159-8290.CD-13-0314 [pii].

109. Cross DA, Ashton SE, Ghiorghiu S, Eberlein C, Nebhan CA, Spitzler PJ, et al. AZD9291, an irreversible EGFR TKI, overcomes T790M-mediated resistance to EGFR inhibitors in lung cancer. Cancer Discov. 2014;4(9):1046–61. doi:10.1158/2159-8290.CD-14-0337, 2159-8290.CD-14-0337 [pii].

110. Thress KS, Paweletz CP, Felip E, Cho BC, Stetson D, Dougherty B, et al. Acquired EGFR C797S mutation mediates resistance to AZD9291 in non–small cell lung cancer harboring EGFR T790M. Nat Med. 2015;21(6):560–2. doi:10.1038/nm.3854.

111. Piotrowska Z, Niederst MJ, Karlovich CA, Wakelee HA, Neal JW, Mino-Kenudson M, et al. Heterogeneity underlies the emergence of EGFRT790 wild-type clones following treatment of T790M-positive cancers with a third-generation EGFR inhibitor. Cancer Discov. 2015;5(7):713–22. doi:10.1158/2159-8290.CD-15-0399, 2159-8290.CD-15-0399 [pii].

112. Koboldt DC, Zhang Q, Larson DE, Shen D, McLellan MD, Lin L, et al. VarScan 2: somatic mutation and copy number alteration discovery in cancer by exome sequencing. Genome Res 2012;22(3):568–76. doi:10.1101/gr.129684.111, gr.129684.111 [pii].

113. Larson DE, Harris CC, Chen K, Koboldt DC, Abbott TE, Dooling DJ, et al. SomaticSniper: identification of somatic point mutations in whole genome sequencing data. Bioinformatics. 2012;28(3):311–7. doi:10.1093/bioinformatics/btr665, btr665 [pii].

Tissue Versus Liquid Biopsy: Opposite or Complementary?

4

Walter Arancio, Beatrice Belmonte,
Marta Castiglia, Arianna Di Napoli,
and Claudio Tripodo

The main pillar of cancer diagnosis has been classically represented by the cyto-/histopathological analysis of cells and tissues. The detection of morphological features of cellular atypia (e.g., altered nuclear/cytoplasmic area ratio; nuclear dysmorphism) and disarranged hierarchical architecture of the tissue (i.e., dysplasia) are funding elements in the diagnosis of malignancies, yet the pieces of information conveyed by these features are often insufficient for the precise identification of a specific cancer histotype, and sometimes they prove faulty [1–6].

Ancillary techniques, prototypically immuno-cyto-/histochemistry, have substantially pushed forward the sensitivity and specificity of cell-/tissue-based histopathological diagnosis especially in settings in which morphological clues are of limited significance, such as tumors of

W. Arancio • B. Belmonte • C. Tripodo (✉)
Tumor Immunology Unit, Human Pathology Section,
Department ProSaMI (Dipartimento per la
Promozione della Salute e Materno Infantile
"G. D'Alessandro"), Palermo University School of
Medicine, Via del vespro 129, 90127 Palermo, Italy
e-mail: claudio.tripodo@unipa.it

M. Castiglia
Department of Surgical, Oncological and Oral
Sciences, Section of Medical Oncology, University of
Palermo, Via del Vespro 129, 90127 Palermo, Italy

A. Di Napoli
Department of Clinical and Molecular Medicine,
Sant'Andrea Hospital, Sapienza University,
Rome, Italy

hematopoietic and mesenchymal tissues. Through the detection of protein epitopes either specifically expressed (e.g., ALK-1 in anaplastic large T-cell lymphoma) [7] or downregulated (e.g., Bap-1 in malignant mesothelioma) [8] by cells, the differentiation between reactive or premalignant modifications of the tissue and malignant transformation can be achieved.

In situ immunological detection of epitopes has changed the very essence of pathology moving its role from diagnosis and prognostication (essentially based on pathological staging) to refined risk stratification and prediction of treatment success. In this setting notable examples are the detection of CD20 expression by B-cell lymphoid clones prompting anti-CD20 immunotherapy [9] and the semiquantitative grading of HER2 expression on ductal breast adenocarcinoma cells driving the adoption of anti-HER strategies [10].

Notably, in specific settings, the information that can be inferred from cell- or tissue-based immunodetection analyses encompasses genetics. Indeed, the expression and localization of a specific protein can be correlated to peculiar genetic events such as translocations as in the case of MYC and BCL2 expression by malignant B cells in high-grade B-cell lymphomas [11] (Fig. 4.1), duplications/amplifications (e.g., HER2 overexpression in breast adenocarcinoma) [12–14], or mutations (e.g., nuclear vs. membrane expression of beta-catenin in *APC*-mutated colon adenocarcinoma [15–19] or nuclear vs.

© Springer International Publishing AG 2017
A. Giordano et al. (eds.), *Liquid Biopsy in Cancer Patients*, Current Clinical Pathology,
DOI 10.1007/978-3-319-55661-1_4

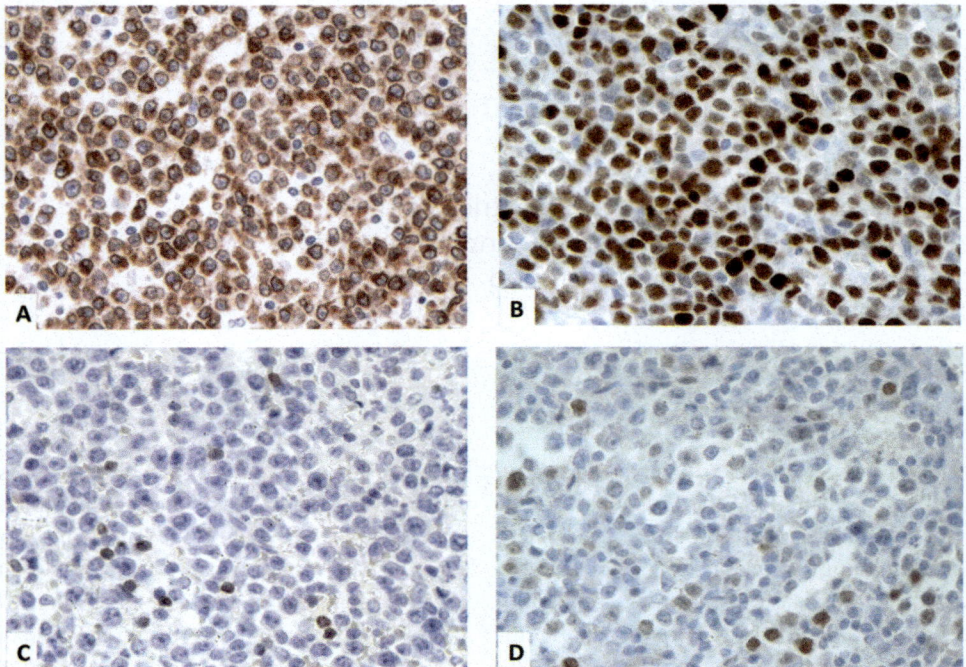

Fig. 4.1 Immunohistochemical expression of BCL2 and MYC protein in a high-grade B-cell lymphoma (HGBL) with *MYC* (**a**) and *BCL2* (**b**) rearrangements compared to a diffuse large B-cell lymphoma (DLBCL nos) lacking *BCL2* (**c**) and *MYC* (**d**) rearrangements (original magnification ×400)

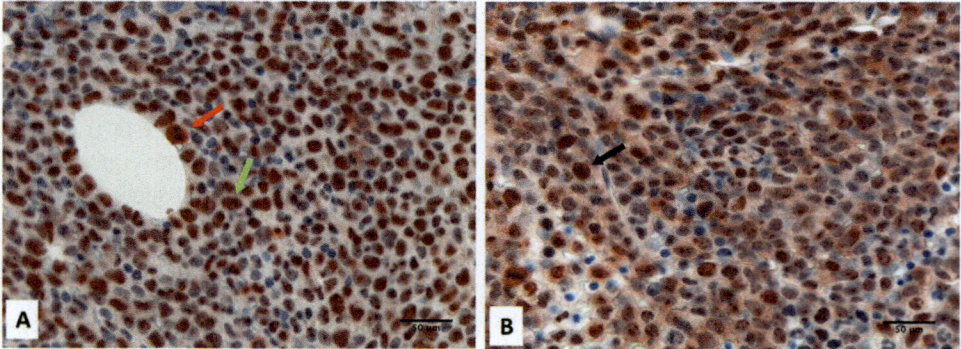

Fig. 4.2 Representative microphotographs of differential expression of NPM in acute myeloid leukemia. While samples with wild-type NPM show nuclear staining (**a**, *green arrow*) or cytoplasmic staining during mitosis (**a**, *red arrow*), samples with specific NPM mutations show only cytoplasmic expression during all the phases of the cell cycle (**b**, *black arrow*)

cytoplasmic expression of NPM) (Fig. 4.2). Besides detecting altered intensities/localizations of target proteins, immunocyto-/histochemical techniques can allow the specific identification of peptides resulting from the translation of mutated transcripts. This is made possible when the mutational event leads to the synthesis of a protein with a different epitopic profile from that of the wild-type form, which can be identified by the adoption of a specific antibody against the mutation-associated epitope (e.g., anti-EGFR with exon 19 deletion) [20].

Integrating the role of immunogenetics are methods based on the hybridization of probes complementary to specific genomic DNA, mRNA, or miRNA sequences. These techniques, either relying on fluorescence microscopy (e.g., fluorescent in situ hybridization for major genetic events, such as amplifications, translocations, and/or deletions) or bright-field microscopy (e.g., chromogenic in situ hybridization for transcript detection), provide a more direct insight into genetic/molecular features of malignant cells/tissues without fully losing the topographic information. However, the association between genetic/molecular information and tissue morphology/topography is an invaluable, yet still poorly understood, resource.

On these bases, cell- and tissue-based ancillary techniques have progressively gained their consolidated role as gold standard diagnostic tools in cancer, extending their influence over disease prognostication and prediction of treatment outcome.

Along with the expanding comprehension of the genetic complexity of cancer, the concepts of clonal heterogeneity and clonal evolution have emerged as determinants of cancer pathobiology [21–23]. The notion that malignancies are composed by a complex mosaic of subclones sharing funding genetic lesions but differentially enriched in additional events shaping their capability to adapt to the coevolving cancer microenvironment and resist treatment has claimed for an unprecedented level of integration between clinical, pathological, and molecular data [24–27]. In this context, the novel focus on tumor-derived cells, DNA and RNA circulating in the periphery characterizing the "liquid biopsy" (LB) approach, is delineating the new frontiers of cancer theragnostics.

The aim of liquid biopsy is to detect and analyze biological material originated within and from the tumor [28, 29]. This technique is very ductile, allowing to collect information about the pathological state of the patient without being burdened by the risk of comorbidities associated with traditional biopsy techniques that sometimes are hardly performed, especially in compromised oncological patients.

The information acquired through LB can be either diagnostic, prognostic, or predictive as it can be used for the early detection of a specific malignancy, for monitoring its progression, its response to therapy, the arousal of resistant clones, or its relapse following complete remission [30]. Notably, LB can be also easily adopted for population screening efforts and preventive medicine [31–34] .

LB relies on biological fluids that can be informative about the disease under investigation. Several reports suggest that cancers are usually very active in releasing cancer-derived molecules or cells into the peripheral blood or other biological fluids. Indeed, blood and its derivatives/components (serum, plasma, platelets, microvesicles/exosomes, and circulating cells) are the samples of election [29] for LB, but analyses on other fluids have been reported, such as the liquor for molecular diagnosis and mutation tracking of central nervous system malignancies [35] or the saliva [32, 36] and urine [37, 38] for the analysis of contiguous or distant tumors. Of note, the saliva and urine are becoming increasingly adopted as LB substrates owing to their noninvasive way of collection and capability of magnifying specific markers [39].

In details, LB relies on very different entities as source of information: circulating cells derived from cancer, cancer-cell-derived cell-free DNA [40, 41], RNA molecules [42–45], tumor-educated platelets [46, 47], and even immune cells, such as T-cells, which repertoire diversification provides an insight into the response to immunological therapies [48].

Circulating tumor cells (CTCs) are very informative, but their use has been somehow limited by their relative paucity in the bloodstream and by the intrinsic difficulties in their selection from the high background noise of the normal circulating cells. CTCs detach from the tumor foci and can be found in both the blood and lymphatic circulation, either as single cells or in the form of cell clusters/aggregates (microemboli) [49]. Nevertheless, the identification of tumor-specific or tumor-enriched membrane-bound epitopes has allowed sorting this specific population from blood samples and using them to profile and characterize the tumor.

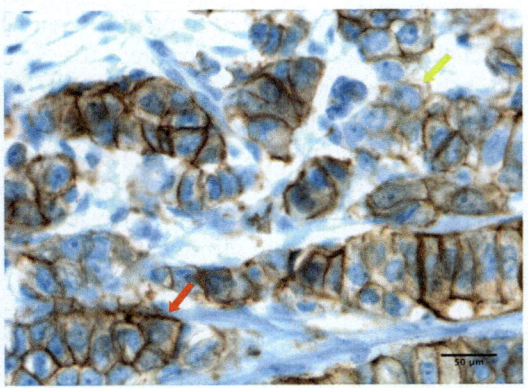

Fig. 4.3 Representative microphotograph showing heterogeneity membrane expression of Her2-neu in mammary neoplastic cells. In particular the distribution of Her2-neu is different even in the same tumoral area, with complete membrane positivity (*red arrow*) or negative expression (*yellow arrow*)

A prototypical example is that of epithelial cell adhesion molecule (EpCAM), which has been used for the positive selection of CTCs of colorectal cancer patients to identify tumor-specific transcripts [50]. In this regard, a note of caution should come from the analyses of tumor tissues, from which a dramatic heterogeneity in the topographic distribution of most surface tumor cell markers emerged (Fig. 4.3).

Alternatively, label-independent techniques rely on sorting CTCs through peculiar physical characteristics, especially size [51].

Isolated CTCs can be analyzed by high sensitivity molecular approaches, such as modified real-time PCR [52–54], digital PCR (dPCR), droplet digital PCR (ddPCR), and next-generation sequencing (NGS). One notable example is represented by the study of *ALK*-gene rearrangements on CTCs from patients with lung adenocarcinomas [55]. CTCs can also be cultivated in vitro [56] or used to generate patient-derived xenografts [57, 58].

Among the different LB specimens, CTCs have the greatest informative potential being representative of the entire cellular program of the malignancy and are therefore mainly used in specialized applications such as functional studies [58, 59] aimed at identifying new therapeutic targets.

Circulating free DNA (cfDNA) has become the standard source for liquid biopsies. DNA is a very stable molecule, and cancer-derived cfDNA (also known as circulating tumor DNA, ctDNA) can be highly enriched in plasma, accounting for up to 10% of the total cfDNA [60]. Such enrichment stems from passive mechanisms of release by dying cancer cells, including those undergoing apoptosis or necrosis or phagocytosis by macrophages, but also from active mechanisms of release from vital cancer cells, which still remain unclear. Of note, the 150–180 bp length, typical of nucleosome spacing, has been reported to be particularly enriched in cancer-derived cfDNA [61], which might open a prospect on this form of circulating DNA as a biomarker of cancer-bearing patients.

The quantification and characterization of cfDNA through LB has been associated with several biological features of the tumor, such as stage, tumor burden, vascularization [60], and the response to the therapy [62].

cfDNA has proven particularly useful in detecting and quantifying clinically relevant mutations (e.g., in *EGFR*, *KRAS*, and *BRAF* mutations) from which inferring the tumoral burden change over time or the relapse of the underlying cancer [63–65]. Moreover, it has been successfully adopted to monitor and eventually overcome the arousal of therapy-resistant clones due to selective pressures, as in the case of the detection and quantification of the *EGFR* T790M mutation that confers resistance to tyrosine kinase pharmacological inhibition used routinely in the treatment of NSCLC patients [66, 67]. Other remarkable examples come from the setting of diffuse large B-cell lymphomas, where cfDNA genotyping allowed quick, noninvasive, and accurate identification of mutations that were missed in the "traditional" tissue biopsy probably due to spatial tumor heterogeneity, where tissue analysis just allows the identification of mutations represented in the biopsied foci [41].

Overall, the possibility to monitor the malignancy as a whole, comprising primary and "metastatic" lesions, indeed represents one major advance of LB over traditional approaches.

The analysis of cfDNA has propelled the development of several advanced PCR techniques able to detect and quantify mutations with very low burden, aiming at very high sensitivity and specificity rates [68]. NGS technology has been also applied using ultradeep sequencing approaches. Nevertheless, NGS application on LB is extremely challenging, requiring a careful validation of the whole pipeline, from the specimen collection to the bioinformatic analysis [69–71].

Circulating tumor-derived RNAs have been reported to be used in LB, but the intrinsic instability of RNA molecules has so far hampered this approach. Gene fusion-derived transcripts, tumor-specific transcript, and splice variants can be detected by the analysis of these molecules, but successful examples are still rare and somehow far from the routine clinical use [72, 73]. For this reason, a great effort has been done in identifying specialized entities naturally enriched in RNAs such as exosomes and platelets [47, 74].

Exosomes are small stable vesicles that are actively released from the cell of origin and carry a plethora of biological molecules, encompassing DNA, RNAs, miRNAs, and proteins.

Even if difficult to purify in comparison with other biological entities, exosomes have been reported as useful sources of information in LB, especially for the analyses of the carried miRNAs in the diagnosis and prognostication of several forms of cancer [75–77]. Interestingly it has been recently reported that exosomes could be a good source to evaluate the androgen receptor splice variant 7 (*AR*-V7), which is associated with resistance to hormonal therapy in castration-resistant prostate cancer (CRPC). Moreover it was showed that using this approach, it could be possible to predict hormonal therapy resistance, earning an important clinical impact [78].

Platelets have been clearly demonstrated to be actively enriched in RNAs derived from cancer cells, becoming so-called tumor-educated platelets (TEPs). In contrast to exosomes, TEPs are very easy to harvest from blood by centrifugation, and the RNAs extracted from them have been proven to be a good source for tumor-derived transcript analyses [47].

The need for finding good sources of RNAs to be analyzed through LB is not trivial. RNA molecules have been found to sustain several layers of regulation that are subverted during the cancer transformation. Long noncoding RNAs (lncRNAs) are key regulators of transcription, and some of them have been reported to be specifically deregulated in cancer, as in the case of metastasis-associated lung adenocarcinoma transcript 1 (*MALAT1*) [79]. MicroRNAs have a central role in the regulation of the transcriptional output of the cell, and their roles in tumorigenesis and as tumor-associated markers or even as therapeutic targets are consolidated [80]. Circular RNAs represent a rather novel yet interesting class of ncRNAs with regulatory functions, which are emerging as key players in cancer [81]. Circular RNAs appear to be of particular interest in LB applications because, lacking free ends, they are conspicuously more stable in comparison with linear RNAs.

The emerging applications of LB aim at gaining more complex pieces of information about the underlying tumor, extending beyond genotyping. Examples of this novel approaches include studies about the differential DNA-releasing capability from different subclones in advanced lung cancer [82] or the assessment of intratumoral DNA methylation and epigenetic heterogeneity directly desumed from LB [83, 84].

In brief, the LB allows to monitor the onset and development of the tumor through a noninvasive approach to swiftly tailor the therapy on the patient with an efficient and economically affordable approach.

On the other hand, in comparison with traditional tissue-based biopsy, LB does not allow (yet) the specification of tumor histotype and the characterization of elements relevant for the pathological staging, such as the local invasion of relevant structures (e.g., neural invasion in melanoma), relying on circulating cells or biological molecules released from the tumor, and it may require dedicated techniques and expertise of molecular and cellular biology (Fig. 4.4).

Considering that we are still at the dawn of this approach and that LB has been quickly adopted in the clinical practice in many cancer

Tissue Biopsy vs. Liquid Biopsy

Tissue Biopsy	Liquid Biopsy
• Allows histological diagnosis and staging	• Does not allow tumor histotype specification and staging
• Often difficult and invasive	• Non-invasive procedure
• Not always representative for the entire variety of malignant clones: TUMOR HETEROGENEITY	• Representative of the different localization of the malignant clones: TUMOR HETEROGENEITY
• Multiple sampling are not always feasible	• Easily repeatable and highly reproducible
• Single snapshot over time and space	• Real-time monitoring of disease (MRD and PD)
• Still the gold standard for tumor characterization	• Lack of standardization, still used mainly in translational research

Fig. 4.4 Direct comparison between tissue and liquid biopsy (LB). LB allows the monitoring of the onset and development of the tumor through a noninvasive approach to swiftly tailor the therapy on the patient with an efficient and economically affordable approach. On the other hand, in comparison with traditional tissue-based biopsy, LB does not allow (yet) the specification of tumor histotype and the characterization of local invasion of relevant structures (e.g., neural invasion in melanoma). Tissue biopsy represents still the gold standard for tumor molecular characterization, but it is sometimes hampered by tumor heterogeneity; LB may thus be fundamental to overcome this issue and complement tissue biopsy for a better clinical management of different types of solid tumors

settings, it is highly probable that it will soon become a widespread approach complementary to tissue-based analyses and profoundly influencing population-based screening, early diagnosis, monitoring of the oncological patient, and clinical follow-up after remission.

References

1. Torous VF, Schnitt SJ, Collins LC. Benign breast lesions that mimic malignancy. Pathology. 2017;49:181–96.
2. Underwood JC. More than meets the eye: the changing face of histopathology. Histopathology. 2017;70:4–9.
3. Cheah AL, Billings SD, Rowe JJ. Mesenchymal tumours of the breast and their mimics: a review with approach to diagnosis. Pathology. 2016;48:406–24.
4. Rastogi V, Puri N, Arora S, et al. Artefacts: a diagnostic dilemma – a review. J Clin Diagn Res. 2013;7:2408–13.
5. Gayathri B, Kalyani R, Harendra KM, Krishna PK. Fine needle aspiration cytology of Hashimoto's thyroiditis – a diagnostic pitfall with review of literature. J Cytol. 2011;28:210–3.
6. Magro G, Longo FR, Angelico G, et al. Immunohistochemistry as potential diagnostic pitfall in the most common solid tumors of children and adolescents. Acta Histochem. 2015;117:397–414.
7. Pileri SA, Pulford K, Mori S, et al. Frequent expression of the NPM-ALK chimeric fusion protein in anaplastic large-cell lymphoma, lympho-histiocytic type. Am J Pathol. 1997;150:1207–11.
8. Cigognetti M, Lonardi S, Fisogni S, et al. BAP1 (BRCA1-associated protein 1) is a highly specific marker for differentiating mesothelioma from reactive mesothelial proliferations. Mod Pathol. 2015;28:1043–57.
9. Witkowska M, Smolewski P. Development of anti-CD20 antigen-targeting therapies for B-cell Lymphoproliferative malignancies – the state of the art. Curr Drug Targets. 2016;17:1072–82.
10. Browne BC, O'Brien N, Duffy MJ, et al. HER-2 signaling and inhibition in breast cancer. Curr Cancer Drug Targets. 2009;9:419–38.
11. Dalla-Favera R, Bregni M, Erikson J, et al. Human c-myc onc gene is located on the region of chromosome 8 that is translocated in Burkitt lymphoma cells. Proc Natl Acad Sci U S A. 1982;79:7824–7.
12. Torrisi R, Rotmensz N, Bagnardi V, et al. HER2 status in early breast cancer: relevance of cell staining patterns, gene amplification and polysomy 17. Eur J Cancer. 2007;43:2339–44.
13. Stoss OC, Scheel A, Nagelmeier I, et al. Impact of updated HER2 testing guidelines in breast cancer – re-evaluation of HERA trial fluorescence in situ hybridization data. Mod Pathol. 2015;28:1528–34.

14. Viale G. The current state of breast cancer classification. Ann Oncol. 2012;23(Suppl 10):x207–10.
15. Barker N, Morin PJ, Clevers H. The Yin-Yang of TCF/beta-catenin signaling. Adv Cancer Res. 2000;77:1–24.
16. Senda T, Iizuka-Kogo A, Onouchi T, Shimomura A. Adenomatous polyposis coli (APC) plays multiple roles in the intestinal and colorectal epithelia. Med Mol Morphol. 2007;40:68–81.
17. Phelps RA, Broadbent TJ, Stafforini DM, Jones DA. New perspectives on APC control of cell fate and proliferation in colorectal cancer. Cell Cycle. 2009;8:2549–56.
18. Tucker EL, Pignatelli M. Catenins and their associated proteins in colorectal cancer. Histol Histopathol. 2000;15:251–60.
19. Herter P, Kuhnen C, Müller KM, et al. Intracellular distribution of beta-catenin in colorectal adenomas, carcinomas and Peutz-Jeghers polyps. J Cancer Res Clin Oncol. 1999;125:297–304.
20. Allo G, Bandarchi B, Yanagawa N, et al. Epidermal growth factor receptor mutation-specific immunohistochemical antibodies in lung adenocarcinoma. Histopathology. 2014;64:826–39.
21. Li S, Mason CE, Melnick A. Genetic and epigenetic heterogeneity in acute myeloid leukemia. Curr Opin Genet Dev. 2016;36:100–6.
22. Izzo F, Landau DA. Genetic and epigenetic determinants of B-cell lymphoma evolution. Curr Opin Hematol. 2016;23:392–401.
23. Zhang M, Rosen JM. Developmental insights into breast cancer intratumoral heterogeneity. Trends Cancer. 2015;1:242–51.
24. Cheng X, Chen H. Tumor heterogeneity and resistance to EGFR-targeted therapy in advanced nonsmall cell lung cancer: challenges and perspectives. Onco Targets Ther. 2014;7:1689–704.
25. Roesch A. Tumor heterogeneity and plasticity as elusive drivers for resistance to MAPK pathway inhibition in melanoma. Oncogene. 2015;34:2951–7.
26. Burrell RA, Swanton C. Tumour heterogeneity and the evolution of polyclonal drug resistance. Mol Oncol. 2014;8:1095–111.
27. Brioli A, Melchor L, Cavo M, Morgan GJ. The impact of intra-clonal heterogeneity on the treatment of multiple myeloma. Br J Haematol. 2014;165:441–54.
28. Crowley E, Di Nicolantonio F, Loupakis F, Bardelli A. Liquid biopsy: monitoring cancer-genetics in the blood. Nat Rev Clin Oncol. 2013;10:472–84.
29. Huang WL, Chen YL, Yang SC, et al. Liquid biopsy genotyping in lung cancer: ready for clinical utility? Oncotarget. 2017. doi: 10.18632/oncotarget.14613. [Epub ahead of print].
30. Rolfo C, Castiglia M, Hong D, et al. Liquid biopsies in lung cancer: the new ambrosia of researchers. Biochim Biophys Acta. 1846;2014:539–46.
31. Hofman P. Liquid biopsy for early detection of lung cancer. Curr Opin Oncol. 2017;29:73–8.
32. Kaczor-Urbanowicz KE, Martín Carreras-Presas C, Kaczor T, et al. Emerging technologies for salivaomics in cancer detection. J Cell Mol Med. 2016. doi: 10.1111/jcmm.13007. [Epub ahead of print] Review.
33. Kalniņa Z, Meistere I, Kikuste I, et al. Emerging blood-based biomarkers for detection of gastric cancer. World J Gastroenterol. 2015;21:11636–53.
34. Tóth K, Barták BK, Tulassay Z, Molnár B. Circulating cell-free nucleic acids as biomarkers in colorectal cancer screening and diagnosis. Expert Rev Mol Diagn. 2016;16:239–52.
35. Marchiò C, Mariani S, Bertero L, et al. Liquoral liquid biopsy in neoplastic meningitis enables molecular diagnosis and mutation tracking: a proof of concept. Neuro-Oncology. 2016;pii: now244. [Epub ahead of print].
36. Kaczor-Urbanowicz KE, Martin Carreras-Presas C, Aro K, et al. Saliva diagnostics – Current views and directions. Exp Biol Med (Maywood). 2017;242(5):459–72. doi:10.1177/1535370216681550.
37. Li G, Zhao A, Péoch M, et al. Detection of urinary cell-free miR-210 as a potential tool of liquid biopsy for clear cell renal cell carcinoma. Urol Oncol. 2017; pii: S1078–1439(16):30414–8. doi: 10.1016/j.urolonc.2016.12.007.
38. Salvi S, Martignano F, Molinari C, et al. The potential use of urine cell free DNA as a marker for cancer. Expert Rev Mol Diagn. 2016;16(12):1283–90.
39. Christensen E, Birkenkamp-Demtröder K, Nordentoft I, et al. Liquid biopsy analysis of FGFR3 and PIK3CA hotspot mutations for disease surveillance in bladder cancer. Eur Urol. 2017;pii: S0302–2838(16):30920–4. doi: 10.1016/j.eururo.2016.12.016.
40. Bedin C, Enzo MV, Del Bianco P, et al. Diagnostic and prognostic role of cell-free DNA testing for colorectal cancer patients. Int J Cancer. 2017;140(8):1888–98. doi:10.1002/ijc.30565.
41. Rossi D, Diop F, Spaccarotella E, et al. Diffuse large B-cell lymphoma genotyping on the liquid biopsy. Blood. 2017;pii: blood-2016-05-719641. doi: 10.1182/blood-2016-05-719641.
42. Lombo TB, Ganguly A, Tagle DA. Diagnostic potential of extracellular RNA from biofluids. Expert Rev Mol Diagn. 2016;16:1135–8.
43. Suraj S, Dhar C, Srivastava S. Circulating nucleic acids: an analysis of their occurrence in malignancies. Biomed Rep. 2017;6:8–14.
44. Konishi H, Ichikawa D, Arita T, Otsuji E. Microarray technology and its applications for detecting plasma microRNA biomarkers in digestive tract cancers. Methods Mol Biol. 2016;1368:99–109.
45. Sestini S, Boeri M, Marchiano A, et al. Circulating microRNA signature as liquid-biopsy to monitor lung cancer in low-dose computed tomography screening. Oncotarget. 2015;6:32868–77.
46. Joosse SA, Pantel K. Tumor-educated platelets as liquid biopsy in cancer patients. Cancer Cell. 2015;28:552–4.
47. Best MG, Sol N, Kooi I, et al. RNA-Seq of tumor-educated platelets enables blood-based pan-cancer, multiclass, and molecular pathway cancer diagnostics. Cancer Cell. 2015;28:666–76.

48. Akyüz N, Brandt A, Stein A, et al. T-cell diversifica-
    tion reflects antigen selection in the blood of patients
    on immune checkpoint inhibition and may be
    exploited as liquid biopsy biomarker. Int J Cancer.
    2016. doi: 10.1002/ijc.30549. [Epub ahead of print].
49. Pantel K, Speicher MR. The biology of circulating
    tumor cells. Oncogene. 2016;35:1216–24.
50. Vojtechova G, Benesova L, Belsanova B, et al.
    Monitoring of circulating tumor cells by a combina-
    tion of Immunomagnetic enrichment and RT-PCR in
    colorectal cancer patients undergoing surgery. Adv
    Clin Exp Med. 2016;25:1273–9.
51. Hofman V, Long E, Ilie M, et al. Morphological anal-
    ysis of circulating tumour cells in patients undergoing
    surgery for non-small cell lung carcinoma using the
    isolation by size of epithelial tumour cell (ISET)
    method. Cytopathology. 2012;23:30–8.
52. Douillard JY, Ostoros G, Cobo M, et al. Gefitinib treat-
    ment in EGFR mutated caucasian NSCLC: circulating-
    free tumor DNA as a surrogate for determination of
    EGFR status. J Thorac Oncol. 2014;9:1345–53.
53. Kimura H, Fujiwara Y, Sone T, et al. High sensitivity
    detection of epidermal growth factor receptor muta-
    tions in the pleural effusion of non-small cell lung
    cancer patients. Cancer Sci. 2006;97:642–8.
54. Mok T, Wu YL, Lee JS, et al. Detection and dynamic
    changes of EGFR mutations from circulating tumor
    DNA as a predictor of survival outcomes in NSCLC
    patients treated with first-line intercalated erlotinib
    and chemotherapy. Clin Cancer Res. 2015;21:
    3196–203.
55. Ilie M, Long E, Butori C, et al. ALK-gene rearrange-
    ment: a comparative analysis on circulating tumour
    cells and tumour tissue from patients with lung adeno-
    carcinoma. Ann Oncol. 2012;23:2907–13.
56. Bobek V, Kacprzak G, Rzechonek A, Kolostova K.
    Detection and cultivation of circulating tumor cells in
    malignant pleural mesothelioma. Anticancer Res.
    2014;34:2565–9.
57. Lowes LE, Goodale D, Xia Y, et al. Epithelial-to-
    mesenchymal transition leads to disease-stage differ-
    ences in circulating tumor cell detection and
    metastasis in pre-clinical models of prostate cancer.
    Oncotarget. 2016;7:76125–39.
58. Pantel K, Alix-Panabières C. Functional studies on
    viable circulating tumor cells. Clin Chem.
    2016;62:328–34.
59. Alix-Panabières C, Bartkowiak K, Pantel K.
    Functional studies on circulating and disseminated
    tumor cells in carcinoma patients. Mol Oncol.
    2016;10:443–9.
60. Diehl F, Schmidt K, Choti MA, et al. Circulating
    mutant DNA to assess tumor dynamics. Nat Med.
    2008;14:985–90.
61. Heitzer E, Ulz P, Geigl JB. Circulating tumor DNA as
    a liquid biopsy for cancer. Clin Chem.
    2015;61:112–23.
62. Sirera R, Bremnes RM, Cabrera A, et al. Circulating
    DNA is a useful prognostic factor in patients with

advanced non-small cell lung cancer. J Thorac Oncol.
    2011;6:286–90.
63. Gonzalez-Cao M, Mayo-de-Las-Casas C, Molina-
    Vila MA, et al. BRAF mutation analysis in circulating
    free tumor DNA of melanoma patients treated with
    BRAF inhibitors. Melanoma Res. 2015;25:486–95.
64. Karachaliou N, Mayo-de las Casas C, Queralt C, et al.
    Association of EGFR L858R mutation in circulating
    free DNA with survival in the EURTAC trial. JAMA
    Oncol. 2015;1:149–57.
65. Sorensen BS, Wu L, Wei W, et al. Monitoring of epi-
    dermal growth factor receptor tyrosine kinase inhibi-
    tor-sensitizing and resistance mutations in the plasma
    DNA of patients with advanced non-small cell lung
    cancer during treatment with erlotinib. Cancer.
    2014;120:3896–901.
66. Wang W, Song Z, Zhang Y. A comparison of ddPCR
    and ARMS for detecting EGFR T790M status in
    ctDNA from advanced NSCLC patients with acquired
    EGFR-TKI resistance. Cancer Med. 2017;6:154–62.
67. Wang Z, Chen R, Wang S, et al. Quantification and
    dynamic monitoring of EGFR T790M in plasma cell-
    free DNA by digital PCR for prognosis of EGFR-TKI
    treatment in advanced NSCLC. PLoS One.
    2014;9:e110780.
68. Molina-Vila MA, Mayo-de-Las-Casas C, Giménez-
    Capitán A, et al. Liquid biopsy in non-small cell lung
    cancer. Front Med (Lausanne). 2016;3:69.
69. Malapelle U, Pisapia P, Rocco D, et al. Next genera-
    tion sequencing techniques in liquid biopsy: focus on
    non-small cell lung cancer patients. Transl Lung
    Cancer Res. 2016;5:505–10.
70. Yee SS, Lieberman DB, Blanchard T, et al. A novel
    approach for next-generation sequencing of circulat-
    ing tumor cells. Mol Genet Genomic Med.
    2016;4:395–406.
71. Rachiglio AM, Abate RE, Sacco A, et al. Limits and
    potential of targeted sequencing analysis of liquid
    biopsy in patients with lung and colon carcinoma.
    Oncotarget. 2016;7:66595–605.
72. Nilsson RJ, Karachaliou N, Berenguer J, et al.
    Rearranged EML4-ALK fusion transcripts sequester
    in circulating blood platelets and enable blood-based
    crizotinib response monitoring in non-small-cell lung
    cancer. Oncotarget. 2016;7:1066–75.
73. Dong WW, Li HM, Qing XR, et al. Identification and
    characterization of human testis derived circular
    RNAs and their existence in seminal plasma. Sci Rep.
    2016;6:39080.
74. Record M, Carayon K, Poirot M, Silvente-Poirot S.
    Exosomes as new vesicular lipid transporters involved
    in cell-cell communication and various pathophysi-
    ologies. Biochim Biophys Acta. 2014;1841:108–20.
75. Rosell R, Wei J, Taron M. Circulating MicroRNA
    signatures of tumor-derived exosomes for early diag-
    nosis of non-small-cell lung cancer. Clin Lung Cancer.
    2009;10:8–9.
76. Cazzoli R, Buttitta F, Di Nicola M, et al. microRNAs
    derived from circulating exosomes as noninvasive

biomarkers for screening and diagnosing lung cancer. J Thorac Oncol. 2013;8:1156–62.

77. Giallombardo M, Chacártegui Borrás J, Castiglia M, et al. Exosomal miRNA analysis in non-small cell lung cancer (NSCLC) Patients' plasma through qPCR: a feasible liquid biopsy tool. J Vis Exp. 2016;(111). doi: 10.3791/53900.

78. Del Re M, Biasco E, Crucitta S, et al. The detection of androgen receptor splice variant 7 in plasma-derived Exosomal RNA strongly predicts resistance to hormonal therapy in metastatic prostate cancer patients. Eur Urol. 2017;71(4):680–7. doi:10.1016/j.eururo.2016.08.012.

79. Liu J, Peng WX, Mo YY, Luo D. MALAT1-mediated tumorigenesis. Front Biosci (Landmark Ed). 2017;22:66–80.

80. Ji W, Sun B, Su C. Targeting MicroRNAs in cancer Gene therapy. Genes (Basel). 2017;8:e21.

81. Dong Y, He D, Peng Z, et al. Circular RNAs in cancer: an emerging key player. J Hematol Oncol. 2017;10:2.

82. Mao X, Zhang Z, Zheng X, et al. Capture-based targeted ultradeep sequencing in paired tissue and plasma samples demonstrates differential subclonal ctDNA-releasing capability in advanced lung cancer. J Thorac Oncol. 2016;pii: S1556-0864(16)33575-4. doi: 10.1016/j.jtho.2016.11.2235.

83. Pisanic TR, Athamanolap P, Poh W, et al. DREAMing: a simple and ultrasensitive method for assessing intratumor epigenetic heterogeneity directly from liquid biopsies. Nucleic Acids Res. 2015;43:e154.

84. Lissa D, Robles AI. Methylation analyses in liquid biopsy. Transl Lung Cancer Res. 2016;5:492–504.

Technical Aspects for the Evaluation of Circulating Tumor Cells (CTCs)

A.B. Di Stefano, M. Castiglia, M. Ciaccio, and Viviana Bazan

Nowadays, the circulating tumor cells (CTCs) are valid prognostic markers useful for disease progression monitoring in many different tumors: prostate, breast, colorectal, and lung cancers [1]. Moreover, the number of CTCs is correlated with tumor size and stages, and consequently the decrease of CTCs is correlated with the efficacy of the therapeutic treatment.

Today, there are many approaches for the isolation and detection of CTCs. The isolation techniques aim at the enrichment of CTCs from whole blood samples. Normally they are concentrated in a range between 1 and 10 CTCs per ml of blood, with a million of leukocytes and a billion of erythrocytes that have to be removed for a better yield of CTCs. CTC selection can be achieved by exploiting both their biological and physical properties, such as the presence of typical membrane markers or the cells size [2].

In this chapter, we will introduce the current available strategies that can be used for CTC enrichment and analysis. The techniques that take advantage from CTC *biological characteristics* for isolation are mainly immunomagnetic methods. These approaches couple isolation and detection phases; the isolation phase is based on the identification of specific markers expressed on cell surface, while the detection phase exploits several methods such as immunofluorescence, flow cytometry, or reverse transcription polymerase chain reaction (RT-PCR). We will now briefly discuss these methods:

- *CellSearch assay (Veridex)* is a simple method that evaluates the expression of both membrane epithelial cell adhesion molecule (EpCAM) and the cytoplasmic epithelial cytokeratin (8, 18, and 19) markers on CTCs. With this platform, CD45+ leucocytes are negatively selected and excluded from the analysis, whereas the nuclei of CTCs are evaluated using DAPI stains [3]. These immunostainings are revealed through fluorescence imaging with microscopy or with CellTracks system. With this system marked cells are detected and enumerated through flow cytometry. Instead, ImageStream system is the upgrade technology developed by Amnis Corporation that integrates together with

A.B. Di Stefano • M. Castiglia
Department of Surgical, Oncogical and Oral Sciences, Section of Medical Oncology, University of Palermo, Via del Vespro 127, Palermo 90127, Italy

M. Ciaccio
Section of Clinical Biochemistry and Clinical Molecular Medicine, Department of Biopathology and Medical Biotechnology, University of Palermo – U.O.C. Laboratory Medicine – CoreLab, Policlinico University Hospital, Palermo, Italy

V. Bazan (✉)
Department of Experimental Biomedicine and Clinical Neurosciences, University of Palermo, Palermo, Italy
e-mail: viviana.bazan@usa.net

immunomagnetic isolation and also the fluorescence microscopy and flow cytometry analysis. However, the CellSearch technology remains the only FDA-approved method for CTC analysis in clinical practice [4].

- *Adna test* is a novel PCR-based assay. In particular, CTCs are first isolated through an immunomagnetic assay with antibody-linked Dynabeads against epithelial specific markers, such as EPCAM and, for breast tumors, also MUC-1. After the extraction of mRNAs, a quantitative real-time PCR is performed on EPCAM$^+$ CTC cells against the specific cancer markers, allowing gene expression analysis of CTCs [5].

- *Aptamers* are small synthetic single-stranded nucleic acids that bind specific target with high affinity. Aptamers can be specifically designed to bind CTCs, and they have been reported to be a valid alternative to antibodies because of their high specificity and tissue penetration rate. They are normally spotted in a microfluidic device and used for the isolation of CTCs from whole blood [2].

- *GILUPI* is a new easy CellCollector® device that can be used for ex vivo and in vivo CTC isolation. It is composed of a stainless steel wire of 16 cm coated with anti-EpCAM antibodies that can be placed for 30 min directly in the vein. It can be used on different tumors, but recently, it was demonstrated that the GILUPI CellCollector® is capable to capture EpCAM$^+$ cells in the blood of prostate cancer patients [6].

In parallel to the aforementioned technologies, several other methods based on CTCs' *physical characteristics* have been developed, and we will now discuss them. These methods are able to distinguish CTCs from other cells by size evaluation. CTCs measure 7–18 μm in diameter and are larger than leukocytes, and for this reasons it is possible to separate them using specific filters and chemical materials or through centrifugation. Differently than biological isolation methods, these techniques are not based on immunomagnetic procedure, thus yielding a greater number of isolated cells. Nevertheless

this may not always be an advantage as it might happen that also other cells could be recovered and considered as CTCs. To avoid this inconvenience, it is fundamental to characterize CTCs after the isolation phase. Indeed, the detection of CTCs is afterward obtained through immunocytochemistry or RT-PCR methods. The principle physical methods used for CTCs recovering are:

- *ISET* (isolation by size of epithelial tumor cells) is a method of blood filtration that isolates and enriches CTCs, in a marker-independent manner. Recently, Laget et al. have reported that by using an ISET device, it is possible to isolate CTCs both fixed in a slide for a microscopic or molecular analysis and as a cell suspension that might be used for in vivo and in vitro analysis (such as culturing and subsequent molecular and proteomic analysis). In the same paper, they compared the exome mutational profile through NGS between fixed and viable cancer cells, even at single cell, and before or after ISET system, reporting no differences between experimental conditions [7].

- *Density-gradient centrifugation* is a method that allows the isolation of CTCs and the exclusion of blood cell. OncoQuick or Ficoll techniques separate the polymorphonuclear cells, platelets, and erythrocytes, from CTCs and mononuclear cells using a density gradient. *OncoQuick* method divides the cells through a porous filter that separates CTC and mononuclear cells from other blood cells in the interphase. The remaining blood cells are deposited as a pellet on the bottom of the tube. With the **Ficoll** method, the separation occurs through a branched polysaccharide. This matrix is able to separate CTCs from other blood cells through the aid of specific centrifugation steps. Many studies have demonstrated that the OncoQuick system is better because it can isolate CTCs from greater blood volume, and it can reduce the white blood cell, improving downstream analysis [2].

- *Dielectrophoresis* method is based on the evidence that cells in suspension are characterized by a specific conductivity. It is therefore possible to separate cells by applying to the suspension a specific electric field. The Dep forces exerted on the particles can discriminate, using changed dielectric properties, different cells, even between normal or cancer cells. The main differences are due in terms of cell membrane, size or correlation of origin site, blood, or solid tumors [8]. Nowadays, the DEPArray is used to identify stem cells, leukocytes, platelets, cancer cells, and also viable CTCs [9].

In the last few years, liquid biopsy has emerged as an important noninvasive practice alternative to tissue biopsy. This simple technique allows the detection and monitor of specific elements such as CTCs, ctDNA, and exosomes that can provide important information about tumor progression. Many techniques of CTC isolation, enrichment, and detection (Fig. 5.1) were described technically on this chapter, but they have some limitations that can lead to underestimation of the CTC population.

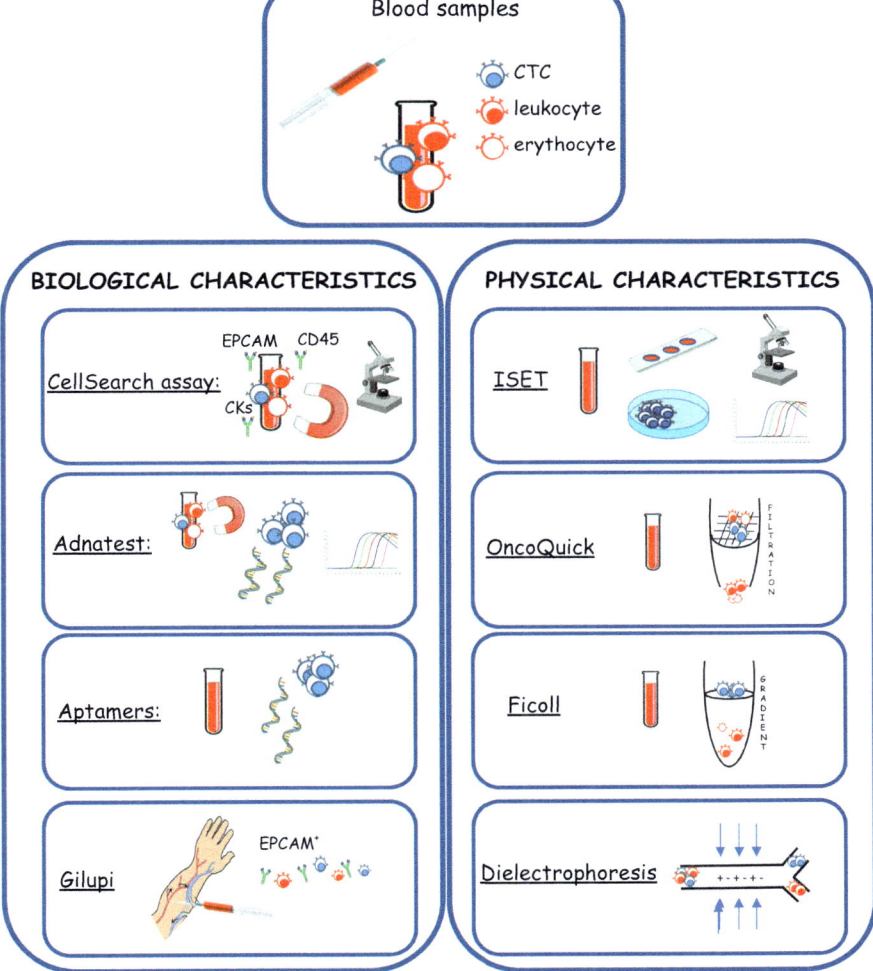

Fig. 5.1 In this figure are summarized the techniques discussed in the chapter that are available for CTC isolation. On the *left*, there are the techniques based on CTC biological characteristics and on the *right* the ones based on CTC physical characteristics

The number of CTC from blood samples is very limited, and their isolation only through biological or physical characteristics could lead to a substantial loss of CTCs. Cell size and membrane marker expression may not be enough for a perfect isolation of CTCs, whereas genetic analysis can perfectly complete the analysis. Actually, the only system approved in clinical practice is the CellSearch system; nevertheless, it has still some limitations. Indeed during epithelial-to-mesenchymal transition (EMT), tumor cells loose EpCAM expression leading to an underestimation of CTCs.

In conclusion, it is necessary to improve the current technologies, exploiting the combination between genetic and proteomic analyses, for a better assessment of the CTCs, in patient clinical management.

References

1. Rolfo C, Castiglia M, Hong D, et al. Liquid biopsies in lung cancer: the new ambrosia of researchers. Biochim Biophys Acta. 2014;1846(2):539–46.
2. Yang D, Wang L, Tian X. Application of circulating tumor cells scope technique on circulating tumor cell research. Mol Cell Ther. 2014;2:8.
3. Allard WJ, Matera J, Miller MC, et al. Tumor cells circulate in the peripheral blood of all major carcinomas but not in healthy subjects or patients with non-malignant diseases. Clin Cancer Res. 2004;10(20): 6897–904.
4. Yu M, Stott S, Toner M, Maheswaran S, Haber DA. Circulating tumor cells: approaches to isolation and characterization. J Cell Biol. 2011;192(3): 373–82.
5. Andreopoulou E, Yang LY, Rangel KM, et al. Comparison of assay methods for detection of circulating tumor cells in metastatic breast cancer: AdnaGen AdnaTest BreastCancer select/detect™ versus Veridex CellSearch™ system. Int J Cancer. 2012;130(7):1590–7.
6. Theil G, Fischer K, Weber E, et al. The use of a new CellCollector to isolate circulating tumor cells from the blood of patients with different stages of prostate cancer and clinical outcomes – a proof-of-concept study. PLoS One. 2016;11(8):e0158354.
7. Laget S, Broncy L, Hormigos K, et al. Technical insights into highly sensitive isolation and molecular characterization of fixed and live circulating tumor cells for early detection of tumor invasion. PLoS One. 2017;12(1):e0169427.
8. Gascoyne PR, Shim S. Isolation of circulating tumor cells by dielectrophoresis. Cancers (Basel). 2014;6(1):545–79.
9. Gascoyne PR, Shim S, Noshari J, Becker FF, Stemke-Hale K. Correlations between the dielectric properties and exterior morphology of cells revealed by dielectrophoretic field-flow fractionation. Electrophoresis. 2013;34(7):1042–50.

Technical Aspects for the Evaluation of Circulating Nucleic Acids (CNAs): Circulating Tumor DNA (ctDNA) and Circulating MicroRNAs

M. Castiglia, A. Perez, M.J. Serrano, M. Ciaccio, V. Bazan, and Antonio Russo

M. Castiglia and A. Perez contributed equally to this work.

M. Castiglia • A. Perez
Department of Surgical, Oncological and Oral Sciences, Section of Medical Oncology, University of Palermo, Via del Vespro 129, 90127 Palermo, Italy

M.J. Serrano
GENYO, Centre for Genomics and Oncological Research (Pfizer/University of Granada/ Andalusian Regional Government),
PTS Granada Av. de la Ilustración, 114-18016 Granada, Spain

M. Ciaccio
Section of Clinical Biochemistry and Clinical Molecular Medicine, Department of Biopathology and Medical Biotechnology, University of Palermo – U.O.C. Laboratory Medicine – CoreLab, Policlinico University Hospital, Palermo, Italy

V. Bazan • A. Russo, MD, PhD (✉)
Department of Surgical, Oncological and Oral Sciences, Section of Medical Oncology, University of Palermo, Via del Vespro 129, 90127 Palermo, Italy

Institute for Cancer Research and Molecular Medicineand Center of Biotechnology, College of Science and Biotechnology, Philadelphia, PA, USA
e-mail: antonio.russo@usa.net

Circulating nucleic acids (CNAs), for example, circulating tumor DNA (ctDNA) and circulating microRNA (miRNA), represent promising biomarkers in several diseases including cancer. They can be isolated from many body fluids, such as blood, saliva, and urine. Also ascites, cerebrospinal fluids, and pleural effusion may be considered as a source of CNAs, but with several and intrinsic limitations. Therefore, blood withdrawal represents one of the best sources for CNAs due to the very simple and minimally invasive way of sampling. Moreover, it can be repeated at different time points, giving the opportunity for a real-time monitoring of the disease.

CNAs are spread from both cancer and normal cells, but in cancer patients their concentrations are greater [1, 2]. Nevertheless, the mechanisms underlying their release are not fully understood. Some evidences show that CNAs can be released through a passive mechanism; indeed, infiltrating phagocytes clear apoptotic or necrotic cells under normal physiologic circumstances. This does not happen efficiently within the tumoral mass, leading to the accumulation of cellular debris and its inevitable release into the circulation. Another possible way of CNAs release could be through extracellular vesicles, such as exosomes. In this case, CNAs are packed inside exosome and actively secreted by cells. This seems to be more realistic for miRNAs, whereas for DNA there are still conflicting data.

Circulating Tumor DNA (ctDNA)

Circulating cell-free DNA (cfDNA) is highly fragmented, and therefore it represents a challenging analyte. It has been shown that the length of cfDNA strands is often between 200 and 180 base pairs, suggesting that apoptosis likely produces the majority of cfDNA in circulation [3]. Circulating tumor DNA (ctDNA) is part of the cfDNA deriving from the tumor mass. The easiest way to identify the ctDNA is to investigate the presence of somatic driver mutations, which, by definition, can be exclusively found on tumor. Nevertheless, several methods have shown that the fraction of ctDNA varies greatly, between 0.01% and more than 90% [3]. Moreover, different tumor types do not release the same amount of ctDNA, and, even in patients with the same disease, the concentration of ctDNA may vary consistently [4].

Several pre-analytical variables, such as blood collection and handling, ctDNA extraction protocols, and storage temperature may affect the quantity and quality of ctDNA fragments in a sample [5–8]. As previously mentioned, blood represents the most used source for ctDNA. Nevertheless, there is a big question: serum or plasma?

In the majority of clinical trails, EDTA containing tubes are used for blood collection (4–9 [9]). Using these tubes clotting is inhibited, and thus it is possible to recover plasma that represent the matrix of choice for ctDNA extraction. Actually also serum can be used as a matrix to isolate ctDNA; indeed, it has been reported that the amount of ctDNA in serum can be 2–24 times higher than in plasma. This can be a consequence of the clotting process that causes white blood cells (WBCs) breaking, finally leading to the release of wild-type DNA. This contamination causes a further dilution of the tumor-specific DNA, making it even more difficult to detect. However, it has been reported that in some cases it might be advantageous to analyze both serum and plasma, as this increases the chances to detect the specific mutation [10].

Another important pre-analytical aspect is the time that elapses between the withdrawal and its processing for plasma recovery. Indeed, the more the time passes, the more is the risk of WBCs lysis, leading again to ctDNA contamination with wild-type background DNA. Moreover ctDNA is associated with a high turnover (15 min half-life), and therefore after blood collection, it is recommended to proceed with plasma preparation by centrifugation within 1 h [11]. Plasma can be stored for a long period at −20 °C or immediately processed for ctDNA extraction.

ctDNA extraction can be performed through different kits; recently, Sorber L et al. [12] have compared the isolation efficiency of the most used kit, the QIAamp circulating nucleic acid kit (QIA), with four other cfDNA isolation kits: the PME free-circulating DNA Extraction Kit (PME), the Maxwell RSC ccfDNA Plasma Kit (RSC), the EpiQuick Circulating Cell-Free DNA Isolation Kit (EQ), and two consecutive versions of the NEXTprep-Mag cfDNA Isolation Kit ($NpM_{V1/2}$). A total of ten samples were used, and five of them harbored KRAS mutations. In the study, the detection of KRAS mutation and total cell-free DNA concentration were performed with droplet digital PCR, whereas real-time PCR was used to evaluate cfDNA integrity. They showed that QIA and the RSC kits displayed similar isolation efficiencies, whereas the yield generated by the PME and NpM_{V2} kits was significantly lower [12]. Interestingly, Sonnenberg et al. developed an electrokinetic technique that allowed rapid isolation of cfDNA directly from blood [13, 14].

Following extraction, another important issue is the quantification method. There is no standardization of the quantification method, which can lead to different results. The most commonly used techniques include spectrophotometric methods, fluorescent dyes, or quantitative PCR-based methods [15]. The identification of a reliable and efficient method for cfDNA quantification is fundamental for the clinical evaluation of ctDNA as a liquid biopsy in order to obtain consistent data, comparable between laboratories.

Plasma DNA investigation can be achieved through two different analytical approaches: a targeted approach and an untargeted approach (Fig. 6.1). The targeted approach relies on the possibility to analyze known genetic mutations that occurs in hotspot region of specific genes with implications for therapy decisions; this is the case, for example, of KRAS, EGFR, and BRAF genes in lung, colon, and melanoma tumors, respectively. Among these methods, we can include real-time PCR; digital PCR (dPCR);

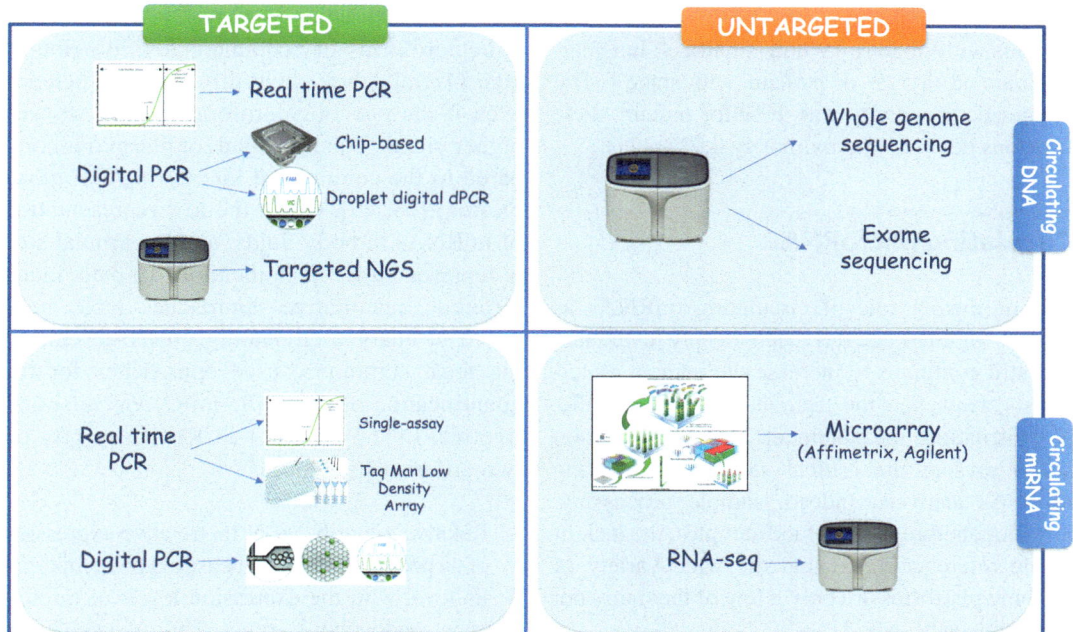

Fig. 6.1 Targeted and untargeted approaches for circulating DNA and circulating miRNAs evaluation

droplet digital PCR (ddPCR); beads, emulsions, amplification, and magnetics (BEAMing); and targeted next-generation sequencing (NGS).

In the untargeted approach, it is possible to investigate ctDNA without the knowledge of any specific mutations present in the primary tumor. This can be achieved through whole genome sequencing using NGS platforms. Nevertheless, this analysis is quite expensive and sometimes difficult to interpret; thus, it can be used for biomarkers discovery in the context of disease monitoring, detection of molecular resistance, and identification of new therapeutic targets. Despite whole genome sequencing, a more cost-effective method in the exome sequencing, which does not require prior knowledge of the genetic landscape of the tumor.

As previously mentioned, the main targeted approaches are real-time PCR, dPCR, ddPCR, BEAMing [16], and targeted NGS. Real-time PCR represents the oldest technique, but its sensitivity has been dramatically improved thanks to the introduction of the ARMS technology (amplification refractory mutation system) [17, 18]. Nevertheless, the power of this technique in

detecting mutant allele at a very low frequency is limited, and therefore other more sophisticated methods have been developed. Through the dPCR approach, the DNA sample is partitioned into thousands of single PCR reactions, improving detection power [19]. In ddPCR, the partitioning is obtained through an emulsion PCR, each generated droplets ideally represent a PCR reactor. At the end of the analysis, software allows to identify a positive or a negative signal indicating the presence or absence of a target sequence. Therefore, a mutated ctDNA can be detected in a wide background of wild-type sequences. The dPCR platforms now available are various, each of them with a more or less different workflow, but they all share a very high sensitivity [20].

NGS is emerging as a very interesting technique because it has revolutionized our approach to molecular testing, indeed we can analyze *multiple genes and multiple patients at a time* with a consistent reduction in time and money. Of great interest, there is the paper of Newman et al. that has developed cancer personalized profiling by deep sequencing (CAPP-Seq) [21]. CAPP-Seq method is able to detect ctDNA in 100% of patients with stage II–IV non–small-cell lung carcinoma and in 50% of patients with stage I. The diagnostic specificity was 96% for mutant allele fractions down to approximately 0.02% [21].

Circulating MicroRNA

The promising role of circulating miRNAs as disease biomarkers has been deeply evaluated and still continues to increase the interest of scientists. However, the technical aspects of miRNAs isolation, measurement, and quantification still represent the critical steps of circulating miRNAs analysis. Indeed, sample processing, isolation, hemolysis in blood samples, the lack of stable reference gene, and the wide variety of genome platforms are only a few of the many not negligible aspects [22].

In circulating miRNAs analysis, the first and pivotal step is to identify a feasible source of nucleic acids. As reported in the study of Weber et al., the most common source of circulating miRNAs are plasma, serum, urine, and saliva but also microvesicles and exosomes [23]. Even if the exosomal miRNAs can probably provide more information, their isolation is complex [24]. The isolation of circulating miRNAs from plasma or serum is easier despite the high content of blood components in these body fluids. Furthermore, plasma and serum specimens often show a different spectrum of miRNAs also within the same individuals. Serum seems to be better source for miRNA isolation because the yield of miRNA is greater than the one obtained from plasma; this is probably due to the contamination of RNAs deriving from platelets during the clotting process [25]. Also in plasma, the levels of miRNA could be influenced by hemolysis as recently reported by Kirschner et al. In fact, miR-16 and miR-451 plasma levels are highly increased as usually they are in blood cells [26, 27]. Generally, the concentration of miRNAs in body fluids is very low. Therefore, the isolation and enrichment of miRNAs is an extremely delicate and important procedure. Nowadays, for the RNAs isolation we can rely

on manual extraction methods such as the phenol/chloroform or commercially distributed kits. Overall, they show differential efficiency even if the phenol/chloroform method showed higher yields (400 ng/500 uL of plasma) if compared to the commercial kits (50 ng/200 uL of plasma) [28, 29]. Given the low representation of miRNAs in body fluids, another crucial step is represented by quantification. To date, many different quantitative approaches have been tested to analyze circulating miRNAs. One of the most commonly used approaches for the quantification of a specific miRNA is quantitative real-time PCR (qRT-PCR). It can rely on two different strategies:

1. Relative quantification: the relative expression of a specific miRNA is measured by comparing its level with the expression levels of a reference endogenous gene. Unfortunately, the debate on the most reliable endogenous miRNA is still open. Indeed, some groups speculate on the high reliability of miR-16, which expression levels are highly stable in different tissues, while some others demonstrated inconsistent expression of miR-16 in plasma and serum [30, 31]. However, a combination of several genes among all those selected seems to be the best approach to follow [32].

2. Absolute quantification: this method relies on the generation of a standard curve. The results of absolute quantification are often indicated as copies per uL of plasma or serum. In the last years, the introduction of digital technologies (dPCR, ddPCR) has deeply increased the sensibility of the standard PCR approaches. Indeed, without the aid of a standard curve, PCR-positive and PCR-negative reactions are counted and then the result is converted as number of copies of the specific target.

Regarding the expression profile of circulating miRNAs, the most commonly used platform is TaqMan Low Density Array (TLDA, ThermoFisher) based on qRT-PCR. This high-sensitive platform allows analyzing up to 754 miRNAs at the same time. Generally, the 382-well format is the most developed for its reduced costs, high throughput, and simple workflow. Moreover, its high sensibility allows the use of a low input of RNA (1-500 ng) [33, 34]. Another platform used for miRNAs profile is Microarray technology. Microarray is based on the hybridization of nucleic acids on different supports and for its less sensitivity, generally requires a higher RNA input (100 ng-1ug) that probably represents the major limitation of this application. Moreover, it can often be difficult to discriminate mature from immature miRNAs forms due to background and cross-hybridization issues [35, 36]. The recent introduction of deep sequencing miRNAs (miRNA-seq), a NGS approach, allowed not only to assess miRNA expression levels but also to identify unknown miRNAs. The major limitation of using routinely NGS is strictly correlated to its high costs as well as time consuming. Moreover, it generally requires big amount of input RNA even if there are attempts to work with less starting material (5 ng). Nowadays, the most popular NGS technology used for circulating miRNAs analysis is Solexa sequencing by Illumina [37, 38]. Recently, a novel technology combining serial analysis of gene expression (SAGE) with NGS technology has been developed. The so-called digital gene expression (DGE) allows to simultaneously study novel potential miRNAs and analyze their expression level [22]. In conclusion, the choice of the proper platform to analyze circulating miRNAs strictly depends on the aim and conditions of the study.

References

1. Delgado PO, Alves BC, Gehrke FS, et al. Characterization of cell-free circulating DNA in plasma in patients with prostate cancer. Tumour Biol. 2013;34:983–6.
2. Hashad D, Sorour A, Ghazal A, Talaat I. Free circulating tumor DNA as a diagnostic marker for breast cancer. J Clin Lab Anal. 2012;26:467–72.
3. Diaz LA Jr, Bardelli A. Liquid biopsies: genotyping circulating tumor DNA. J Clin Oncol. 2014;32(6):579–86. doi:10.1200/JCO.2012.45.2011. Epub 2014 Jan 21.
4. Bettegowda C, Sausen M, Leary RJ, et al. Detection of circulating tumor DNA in early- and late-stage human malignancies. Sci Transl Med. 2014;6:224ra224.
5. Umetani N, Kim J, Hiramatsu S, et al. Increased integrity of free circulating DNA in sera of patients with colorectal or periampullary cancer: direct quantitative PCR for ALU repeats. Clin Chem. 2006;52:1062–9.
6. Chan KC, Yeung SW, Lui WB, et al. Effects of pre-analytical factors on the molecular size of cell-free DNA in blood. Clin Chem. 2005;51:781–4.
7. Swinkels DW, Wiegerinck E, Steegers EA, de Kok JB. Effects of blood-processing protocols on cell-free DNA quantification in plasma. Clin Chem. 2003;49:525–6.
8. Chiu RW, Poon LL, Lau TK, et al. Effects of blood-processing protocols on fetal and total DNA quantification in maternal plasma. Clin Chem. 2001;47:1607–13.
9. Malapelle U, Pisapia P, Rocco D, Smeraglio R, di Spirito M, Bellevicine C, Troncone G. Next generation sequencing techniques in liquid biopsy: focus on non-small cell lung cancer patients. Transl Lung Cancer Res 2016;5(5):505–510.
10. Karachaliou N, Mayo-de las Casas C, Queralt C, et al. Association of EGFR L858R mutation in circulating free DNA with survival in the EURTAC trial. JAMA Oncol. 2015;1:149–57.
11. Malapelle U, Pisapia P, Rocco D, et al. Next generation sequencing techniques in liquid biopsy: focus on non-small cell lung cancer patients. Transl Lung Cancer Res. 2016;5:505–10.
12. Sorber L, Zwaenepoel K, Deschoolmeester V, et al. A comparison of cell-free DNA isolation kits: isolation and quantification of cell-free DNA in plasma. J Mol Diagn. 2017;19:162–8.
13. Sonnenberg A, Marciniak JY, Rassenti L, et al. Rapid electrokinetic isolation of cancer-related circulating cell-free DNA directly from blood. Clin Chem. 2014;60:500–9.
14. Sonnenberg A, Marciniak JY, Skowronski EA, et al. Dielectrophoretic isolation and detection of cancer-related circulating cell-free DNA biomarkers from blood and plasma. Electrophoresis. 2014;35:1828–36.
15. Devonshire AS, Whale AS, Gutteridge A, et al. Towards standardisation of cell-free DNA measurement in plasma: controls for extraction efficiency, fragment size bias and quantification. Anal Bioanal Chem. 2014;406:6499–512.
16. Bidard FC, Madic J, Mariani P, et al. Detection rate and prognostic value of circulating tumor cells and circulating tumor DNA in metastatic uveal melanoma. Int J Cancer. 2014;134:1207–13.
17. Spindler KL, Pallisgaard N, Vogelius I, Jakobsen A. Quantitative cell-free DNA, KRAS, and BRAF mutations in plasma from patients with metastatic colorectal cancer during treatment with cetuximab and irinotecan. Clin Cancer Res. 2012;18:1177–85.
18. Spindler KL, Pallisgaard N, Andersen RF, Jakobsen A. Changes in mutational status during third-line treatment for metastatic colorectal cancer – results of consecutive measurement of cell free DNA, KRAS and BRAF in the plasma. Int J Cancer. 2014;135:2215–22.

19. Taly V, Pekin D, Benhaim L, et al. Multiplex pico-droplet digital PCR to detect KRAS mutations in circulating DNA from the plasma of colorectal cancer patients. Clin Chem. 2013;59:1722–31.

20. Sorber L, Zwaenepoel K, Deschoolmeester V, et al. Circulating cell-free nucleic acids and platelets as a liquid biopsy in the provision of personalized therapy for lung cancer patients. Lung Cancer. 2016;107:100.

21. Newman AM, Bratman SV, To J, et al. An ultrasensitive method for quantitating circulating tumor DNA with broad patient coverage. Nat Med. 2014;20:548–54.

22. Hruštincová A, Votavová H, Dostálová MM. Circulating MicroRNAs: methodological aspects in detection of these biomarkers. Folia Biol (Praha). 2015;61:203–18.

23. Weber JA, Baxter DH, Zhang S, et al. The microRNA spectrum in 12 body fluids. Clin Chem. 2010;56:1733–41.

24. Hunter MP, Ismail N, Zhang X, et al. Detection of microRNA expression in human peripheral blood microvesicles. PLoS One. 2008;3:e3694.

25. Fang C, Zhu DX, Dong HJ, et al. Serum microRNAs are promising novel biomarkers for diffuse large B cell lymphoma. Ann Hematol. 2012;91:553–9.

26. Kirschner MB, Kao SC, Edelman JJ, et al. Haemolysis during sample preparation alters microRNA content of plasma. PLoS One. 2011;6:e24145.

27. Cheng HH, Yi HS, Kim Y, et al. Plasma processing conditions substantially influence circulating microRNA biomarker levels. PLoS One. 2013;8:e64795.

28. Monleau M, Bonnel S, Gostan T, et al. Comparison of different extraction techniques to profile microRNAs from human sera and peripheral blood mononuclear cells. BMC Genomics. 2014;15:395.

29. Kroh EM, Parkin RK, Mitchell PS, Tewari M. Analysis of circulating microRNA biomarkers in plasma and serum using quantitative reverse transcription-PCR (qRT-PCR). Methods. 2010;50:298–301.

30. Xiang M, Zeng Y, Yang R, et al. U6 is not a suitable endogenous control for the quantification of circulating microRNAs. Biochem Biophys Res Commun. 2014;454:210–4.

31. Filková M, Aradi B, Senolt L, et al. Association of circulating miR-223 and miR-16 with disease activity in patients with early rheumatoid arthritis. Ann Rheum Dis. 2014;73:1898–904.

32. Chen X, Liang H, Guan D, et al. A combination of let-7d, let-7g and let-7i serves as a stable reference for normalization of serum microRNAs. PLoS One. 2013;8:e79652.

33. Ge Q, Zhou Y, Lu J, Bai Y, Xie X, Lu Z. miRNA in plasma exosome is stable under different storage conditions. Molecules. 2014;19(2):1568–75.

34. Zearo S, Kim E, Zhu Y, Zhao JT, Sidhu SB, Robinson BG, Soon PSh. MicroRNA-484 is more highly expressed in serum of early breast cancer patients compared to healthy volunteers. BMC Cancer 2014;14:200.

35. Steudemann C, Bauersachs S, Weber K, Wess G. Detection and comparison of microRNA expression in the serum of Doberman Pinschers with dilated cardiomyopathy and healthy controls. BMC Vet Res. 2013;9:12.

36. Blenkiron C, Askelund KJ, Shanbhag ST, et al. MicroRNAs in mesenteric lymph and plasma during acute pancreatitis. Ann Surg. 2014;260:341–7.

37. Creighton CJ, Reid JG, Gunaratne PH. Expression profiling of microRNAs by deep sequencing. Brief Bioinform. 2009;10:490–7.

38. Wang Z, Gerstein M, Snyder M. RNA-Seq: a revolutionary tool for transcriptomics. Nat Rev Genet. 2009;10:57–63.

Technical Aspects for the Evaluation of Exosomes and Their Content

Simona Fontana, Marco Giallombardo, and Riccardo Alessandro

Introduction and Exosome as Biomarkers in Liquid Biopsies

In addition to circulating tumor cells (CTCs) and circulating free tumor nucleic acids (cfNA) including DNA, miRNAs, mRNA, and long noncoding RNA, liquid biopsy is a precious source of exosomes, small vesicles that, as a growing body of evidence suggests, may be used as biomarkers for the diagnosis and prognosis of malignant tumors.

Exosomes are nanometer-sized vesicles (40–100 nm diameter) of endocytic origin released by all living cells, including tumor cells [1].

Initially, exosomes were described as "garbage bags" through which cells eliminated unnecessary molecular components [2]. Today, numerous remarkable findings clearly highlighted that exosomes are not only cell "cleaners" but are pivotal mediators of intercellular signaling that act independently but synergistically with soluble growth factors [3]. They function as cell-free messengers and play a relevant role in the cell-cell communication, strongly depending on the nature of the transported molecules (proteins, mRNAs, miRNAs, and lipids). Exosomes are largely released in biological fluids, such as plasma, urine, cerebrospinal fluid, epididymal fluid, amniotic fluid, malignant and pleural effusions, saliva, bronchoalveolar lavage fluid, synovial fluid, and breast milk, indicating their role as cellular shuttles across distant body compartments [1, 4, 5]. Tumor cells actively shed exosomes (tumor-derived exosomes – TDEs) into their surrounding microenvironment, and growing evidence indicates that these vesicles have pleiotropic functions in the modulation of tumor progression, promoting immune escape, tumor invasion, neovascularization, metastasis, and drug resistance [1]. In plasma of cancer patients, total exosomes were found to be significantly more abundant than in healthy donors' plasma, especially in patients with advanced cancers [6]. Not only total exosome fraction is enriched in plasma of cancer patients but also the specific content of TDEs might vary depending on the type of tumor, disease stage, and therapeutic treatment. Over the past few years, a significant body of literature has demonstrated that TDEs carry tumor-specific RNAs and proteins that are widely considered very attractive targets for diagnostic application. Thus, one of the most intriguing biomedical utility of exosomes is their potential application as biomarkers in clinical diagnostics. Moreover, compared with free biomarkers detected in conventional biofluids such as serum or urine, exosomal biomarkers display higher specificity and sensitivity due to their

S. Fontana (✉) • M. Giallombardo • R. Alessandro
Department of Biopathology and Medical
Biotecnologies, University of Palermo,
via Divisi, 83 – 9133, Palermo, Italy
e-mail: simona.fontana@unipa.it; markgiallo@gmail.com; riccardo.alessandro@unipa.it

© Springer International Publishing AG 2017
A. Giordano et al. (eds.), *Liquid Biopsy in Cancer Patients*, Current Clinical Pathology,
DOI 10.1007/978-3-319-55661-1_7

outstanding stability. At the light of their potential application in the clinical practice, many efforts have been recently done to improve the technical aspects of exosome isolation in order to have pure exosome samples and to make exosomal diagnostics more cost-efficient.

Isolation Methods

Mass spectrometry-based proteomic and amplified, ultrahigh sensitivity RNA technologies have clearly displayed that exosomes contain a complex set of macromolecules, including proteins and RNAs, that can be transferred to target cells mediating intercellular interactions between neighboring cells. The specific molecular composition of TDEs, besides to elicit interest for its biological meaning as regulator of tumor progression, has a strong attractive power for its potential diagnostic utility.

Even if exosomes represent a recognized stable source of putative biomarkers in body fluids, several issues concerning the isolation methods make still questionable their suitability for diagnostic use in the clinical practice.

There are two crucial points that must be controlled to achieve a good quality in exosome sample preparations: (1) the appropriate collection/storage of the body fluid samples and (2) the purity of the isolated exosomes.

Since no strictly defined conditions for storing/isolating exosomes are reported, different laboratories use high variable protocols. For example, there are studies demonstrating that the use of different anticoagulants in blood samples can affect exosome yields. The use of human plasma versus serum for exosome isolation has been a subject of much discussion because of the possibility of exosome losses from sera due to clotting. However, it was recently reported that plasma or serum can be considered as equally good sources of circulating exosomes in terms of recovery, purity, morphology, and biological function [7]. Other critical aspects that can affect exosome recovery from body fluid samples are (a) the processing timing after collection and (b) the freezing/thawing cycles with particular atten-

tion to the thawing conditions. Indeed, it has been reported that body fluid samples thawed on ice showed a lower exosome recovery compared to the ones thawed at room temperature or 37 °C, indicating that the thawing conditions play a more crucial role in EV recovery than multiple freezing-thawing cycles. Although several groups agree that multiple freezing-thawing cycles of a sample affect exosome characteristics/concentration, some suggest that repeating these cycles for up to ten times has no influence on the size and composition of EVs to any significant degree. The common idea is that, when possible, the starting sample should be handled rapidly after collection, avoiding extensive waiting periods between further processing stages (i.e., centrifugation steps). In blood/plasma samples, all the necessary precautions (i.e., processing temperature, upright sample position for transport, no agitation) should be undertaken to avoid platelet activation and thus potential platelet-derived EV generation. Moreover, once isolated, EV aliquots should be prepared and stored at −70 to −80 °C until use [8].

For an effective use of exosomes as source of biomarker discovery, pure exosome samples are required. One of the major issues in purifying exosomes from body fluids is the co-isolation of contaminating non-exosomal material (such as other types of extracellular vesicles, lipoproteins, or RNA/protein complexes) or the loss of exosomal materials due to damaged membrane integrity that can both generate significant artifacts in the downstream *omics* analyses. To date, a reference approach for isolating exosomes from biological fluids is lacking; thus different laboratories carry out different protocols for exosome purification. The failure of standardized parameters leads to qualitative/quantitative variability and discrepancies in acquired data that represent the real drawback for using exosomal proteins as reliable diagnostic, prognostic, and therapeutic biomarkers.

The main methodologies used for exosome purification/isolation that could serve as the backbone for potential new variants are four: (1) differential centrifugation/ultracentrifugation with/without a sucrose gradient/cushion; (2) size

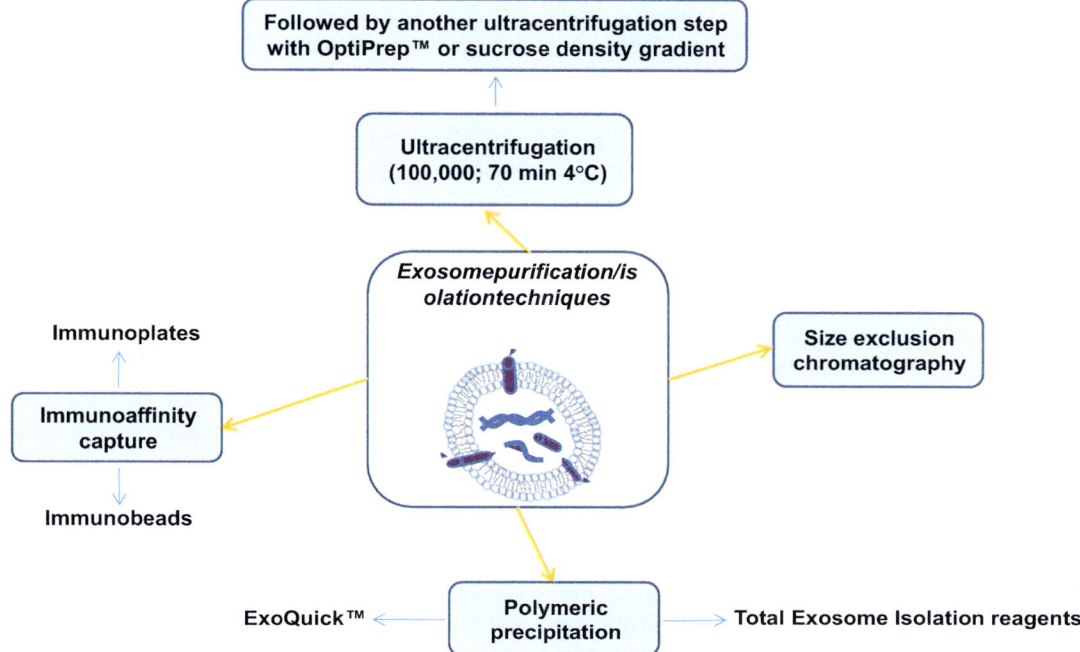

Fig. 7.1 Overview of the different exosome purification/isolation techniques

exclusion chromatography (SEC); (3) immunoaffinity capture; and (4) polymeric precipitation (Fig. 7.1). Each of these methodologies shows pros and cons.

Differential ultracentrifugation is the current gold standard for exosome isolation. In its classical form, initially proposed by Raposo's group [9], it consists of sequential centrifugation steps carried out at 4 °C with increasing centrifugal forces allowing to remove unwanted components from the samples in order to obtain exosome enrichment. The three first centrifugations enable to sequentially remove intact cells (300 g for 10 min), dead cells and apoptotic bodies (2000 g for 10 min), and cell debris and microvesicles (10,000 g for 30 min). After each centrifugation, the obtained pellet is being discarded while the supernatant is subjected to the next centrifugation step. After the 10,000 × g spin, the supernatant is finally ultracentrifuged at 100,000 × g for 90 min, and exosome pellet is obtained. The Raposo's protocol is focused on the purification of exosomes from conditioned cell culture media; thus there has been an increasing need to adapt

the method for other types of samples as body fluids. For example, Théry et al. proposed to dilute the samples with an equal volume of PBS before further processing due to the viscosity of the respective fluids [10]. Moreover, due to the complexity of the viscous fluid samples, the time and centrifugation speeds have been increased/adapted, and serial filtration through 0.45 and 0.2 mm filters is used before exosome pelleting [10]. Since some argue that during EV isolation by centrifugation aggregates of large proteins and/or proteins that were nonspecifically associated with EVs are also being sedimented, it has been proposed to add to differential UC a density-gradient-based step using sucrose or iodixanol (OptiPrep™) that supposedly eliminates this contamination allowing to obtain an exosome population with a greater purity [10].

The ultracentrifugation approach has several weaknesses: (I) it is highly labor-intensive and time-consuming (up to 2 days per preparation, for a protocol with density gradients); (II) no more than six samples at a time can be processed; (III) a large amount of starting material is needed;

and (IV) exosome yields are typically low. However to date, sequential centrifugations, when combined with density-gradient ultracentrifugation, can produce highly pure exosome preparations. As demonstrated by the analysis of *omics* data, the OptiPrep density-gradient centrifugation outperforms other methods as those based on precipitation [11]. However, the suitability of the density-gradient method in a clinical setting is questionable, due to difficulties in upscaling and automating this procedure.

Size-exclusion chromatography (SEC) is a method where a solution of molecules is separated based on the component's size, not molecular weight. This method is usually preceded by a low-speed centrifugation step that allows to remove larger components from the sample (cells, cellular debris, organelles, etc.) that is then filtered (0.8 and 0.2 μm pore size filter) to preconcentrate the vesicles. SEC is performed using heteroporous beads made of a neutral, crosslinked polymeric support, packed into a column. These beads consist of numerous pores or tunnels of varying sizes separation. Thus, particles in a sample, depending on their size, will move through the filtration column at different rates: larger particles will elute more rapidly, while the smaller ones more slowly, due to their ability to penetrate the stationary phase (gel) of the column. In theory, the obtained eluted fraction at a certain time should contain a population of particles of the same size. After the loading of filtered sample on the column, the collected fractions are ultracentrifuged (100,000 × g, 1 h and longer) to pellet down the exosomes that will be resuspended in PBS and used in downstream assays [12]. To avoid deformation and eventual rupture into smaller exosome particles, SEC is performed by gravity or with the application of the smallest possible force. Moreover, the selection of the appropriate gel type is crucial to the recovery of exosomes, rather than proteins or lipoproteins. Additionally, the short isolation time and relatively low cost are also beneficial [12].

Another promising alternative for isolating exosomes involves the use of immobilized antibodies recognizing specific exosomal antigens, such as CD63, CD81, CD82, CD9, Alix, annexin,

EpCAM, and Rab5, that can be used by themselves or in combination. These antibodies can be covalently attached to a variety of supports, including magnetic beads, chromatograph matrices, plates, and microfluidic devices [10, 13]. Devices containing antibodies against CD63, CD81, or CD9 for exosome capture and characterization are already commercialized by HansaBioMed (www.hansabiomed.eu) and Life Technologies (www.lifetechnologies.com/exosomes) [14]. Similarly, Aethlon Medical (www.aethlonmedical.com) has proposed an affinity capture strategy based on the use of a patented lectin that targets mannose residues exposed on exosomes [14]. Although these methodologies are very interesting and promising, it remains to be confirmed how well they work and if (a) they can be considered specific for exosomes, since a number of cells contain mannose on their surface and circulating cancer cells can expose EpCAM antigen, and (b) they ensure the capture of all exosome types. Anyway, it is definitely worth investigating.

The appeal of polymeric precipitation method for recovering exosomes is related to its relativerapidity, ability to high EV recoveries, and no request of laborious ultracentrifugation. The method is based on use of a polymer solution, such as polyethylene glycol (PEG), routinely used for precipitating viruses [15]. Several commercial products using the polymeric precipitation have been developed, such as ExoQuick from System Biosciences exosomes (www.systembio.com) and five Total Exosome Isolation reagents from Life Technologies (www.lifetechnologies.com/exosomes), enabling fast recovery of exosomes from various sample types. When these reagents are added to sample (conditioned media, plasma, urine, saliva, milk, cerebrospinal fluid, ascitic fluid, and amniotic fluid), they work by binding water molecules and inducing the precipitation of less-soluble components such as exosomes. Finally, the exosomes can be collected by low-speed centrifugation [14]. The major drawbacks of polymer-based precipitation concern the co-isolation of nonvesicular contaminants, including lipoproteins and the presence in isolated exosomes of the polymer material that may not be compatible with downstream *omics* analyses.

To make real the applicability of exosomes in liquid biopsy, it is clear that it is mandatory to develop specific and reliable methods to work with well-defined preparations, and to this end it is urgent to reach a consensus regarding the procedures for exosome isolation and characterization by integrating the observations coming from different research groups.

Content Characterization

Exosomal miRNAs

It has been demonstrated that exosomes contain several nucleic acids, such as microRNAs (miRNAs), that can be shuttled to other cells keeping their biological activity [16, 17]. MicroRNAs are small noncoding (18–25 nucleotides) RNA molecules with a length between 18 and 25 nucleotides [18]. They have biological functions as single-strand molecules, targeting the 3′-UTR of the target mRNA and leading to posttranscriptional regulations in several biological processes, such as cell growth, adhesion, motility, apoptosis, angiogenesis, and differentiation, among others [18–23].

Several reasons led researchers to study the exosomal miRNA content, especially of tumor-derived exosomes isolated from different body fluids; in this context, it was recently demonstrated that this content could mirror the parental tissue condition, reflecting the pathological status in several cancer diseases, like was reported in lung adenocarcinoma [24]. This feature might be exploitable then as novel liquid biopsy signature, giving the opportunity to validate a new class of noninvasive diagnostic and prognostic biomarkers.

Nowadays, 2838 miRNAs have been described in exosomes released from different cytotypes (www.exocarta.org), and several new high-throughput technologies have been exploited in order to accelerate these analysis.

Microarray, microRNA ready-to-use PCR cards/panels, and next-generation RNA sequencing (NGS RNA-seq) are the high-throughput technologies mostly used to get comprehensive microRNA expression profiles in cancer and healthy tissues as well as in exosomes [24–27].

Microarray is a powerful tool for monitoring the expression of thousands of miRNAs (with already known or unknown functions) in a single experiment. This technology was applied to analyze miRNAs into exosomes isolated from plasma/serum of patients affected by several types of cancer. The obtained data allowed to define specific exosomal miRNA panel with diagnostic potential for both NSCLC (miR-17-3p, miR-21, miR-106a, miR-146, miR-155, miR-191, miR-192, miR-203, miR-205, miR-210, miR-212, miR-214) [24] and ovarian cancer (miR-21, miR-141, miR-200a, miR-200b, miR-200c, miR-203, miR-205, miR-214) [27]. Similarly, in esophageal squamous cell carcinoma, microarray analysis allowed to select one serum exosomal miRNA (miR-1246) with strong diagnostic and prognostic value [28].

The microRNA ready to use PCR cards/panels are really sensitive high-throughput expression profiling method useful also in case of minimal amounts of starting template. Briefly, these PCR 96–384-well cards/panels contain primers in each well in the plate per well giving the opportunity to detect in one experiment a really large amount of miRNAs. Promising results, obtained by comparing the miRNA profiles of circulating exosomes of patients affected by lung carcinoma and control subjects, have allowed to select plasma exosomal miRNA panels detecting, in the lung, the presence/absence of residual tumor mass after tumor removal (miR-205, miR-19a, miR-19b, miR-30b, miR-20a) [29] or able to discriminate lung adenocarcinoma from granuloma tissue (miR-151a-5p, miR-30a-3p, miR-200b-5p, miR-629, miR-100, miR-154-3p) [30].

Recently, a new technique called RNA sequencing (RNA-seq) is intended to replace microarray technology. RNA-seq, also known as whole transcriptome shotgun sequencing (WTSS), is a specific next-generation sequencing (NGS) technology able to get, in the same experiment, quantitative and qualitative values of selected RNA populations in a sample. This profiling method was applied to analyze prostate cancer circulating exosomes allowing to select two exosomal miRNAs (miR-1290 and miR-375) as potential prognostic biomarkers for castration-resistant prostate cancer patients [26].

Nevertheless, among the individual miRNA analysis methods, quantitative real-time PCR (both with TaqMan® or SYBR® Green chemistry) is still the most used for exosomal miRNA analysis and also used in order to validate data obtained from high-throughput technologies. Several exosomal analyses, carried out through qPCR, have provided interesting results for the detection of circulating tumor biomarkers. For example, in lung and breast cancer, exosomal miRNAs with diagnostic, prognostic, and predictive value have been identified [30, 31].

A recently developed type of high sensitive individual assay PCR technology, the droplet digital polymerase chain reaction (ddPCR), offers the opportunity to detect a very low copy number of miRNAs and then to perform easily miRNA analysis in clinical samples [32]. Briefly, ddPCR is a PCR method based on water-oil emulsion droplet technology where the sample is fractionated into a large number of droplets (around 20,000) and the PCR amplification is performed in each individual droplet, leading to really high sensitivity [32]. Though this technique was possible to detect in serum exosomes released by liver cancer cells, very low quantity of mir-29 is usually undetectable through classic qPCR [32].

All these methods, applied to miRNAs analysis of exosomes released into different biofluids in cancer patients, open the door to the opportunity to highlight and select new potential classes of noninvasive diagnostic, prognostic, and drug resistance biomarkers in a liquid biopsy scenario.

Exosomal Proteins

In general, the available published data on TDE proteomics clearly shows that proteins identified in these nanovesicles (both released by tumor cell lines and isolated from body fluids) can be sorted into two groups: one group represents a conserved set of proteins irrespective of exosome origin; the second one is formed by proteins specifically related to the producer host cell, showing that TDEs have a unique cell-specific protein composition.

Within the group of common proteins, those most frequently identified belong to the following classes: membrane adhesion proteins (integrins); components of the ESCRT machinery (Alix, TSG101, vacuolar protein sorting-associated protein 28 homolog (vps-28), vacuolar protein sorting-associated protein 4B (vps-4B), ubiquitin-like modifier-activating enzyme, and ubiquitin); membrane transport/trafficking (annexins, Rab protein family); cytoskeletal components (actin, cytokeratins, ezrin, tubulin, and myosin); lysosomal markers (lysosome membrane protein 2, cathepsin D, CD63, LAMP-1/2); antigen presentation proteins (HLA class I and II/peptide complexes); metabolic enzymes (GAPDH, pyruvate, enolase alpha); heat shock proteins (Hsc70, Hsp70, Hsp90); kinases (LYN, MINK1, and MAP4K4); tetraspanins (CD9, CD81, CD82, tetraspanin-8); proteases (ADAM10, DPEP1, ST14); transporters (ATP7A, ATP7B, MRP2, SLC1A4, SLC16A1, CLIC1); and receptors (CD46, CD55, NOTCH1) [1]. All these proteins are cataloged in the ExoCarta website (http://www.exocarta.org/), a primary resource for high-quality exosomal datasets accessible also from Vesiclepedia (http://www.microvesicles.org), a manually curated compendium that contains molecular data identified in all classes of EVs, including apoptotic bodies, exosomes, large dense-core vesicles, microparticles, and shedding microvesicles [33, 34].

As more proteome studies are performed, it is becoming ever more apparent that beyond the set of conserved proteins, TDEs contain proteins that are not found in the exosomes from both non-tumor cells and/or body fluids of healthy individuals. All of the proteomic data that has been obtained so far demonstrates that TDEs express a discrete set of proteins specifically related to the tumor phenotype and involved in cell proliferation, antigen presentation, signal transduction, migration, invasion, and angiogenesis, supporting the hypothesis that exosomes may play a crucial role in modulating tumor progression and preparing the metastatic niche [1]. This suggests that the potential role of exosomal profiles as biomarkers is not only diagnostic but also prognostic and predictive of the therapeutic response. Several data acquired in the last years strongly support the effective clinical impact of exosomes that as multimolecular aggregates also offer the unique opportunity to identify combination of different biomarkers.

Recently, by using mass spectrometry analyses, a cell surface proteoglycan, glypican-1 (GPC1), was found specifically enriched on cancer cell-derived exosomes. GPC1-positive circulating exosomes (GPC1 (+) crExos) were detected in the serum of patients with pancreatic cancer with absolute specificity and sensitivity, allowing to discriminate healthy subjects and patients with a benign pancreatic disease from patients with pancreatic cancer [35].

A specific protein signature comprised of TYRP2, VLA-4, HSP70, an HSP90 isoform, and MET was also identified in circulating exosomes from subjects with advanced melanoma. It was found that the co-expression of TYRP2 and MET in exosomes, as well as increased protein amount per exosome, predicted disease progression, and their use as indicator of metastatic disease and tumor burden, was proposed [36]. In another interesting paper, the role of exosomal survivin as a diagnostic and/or prognostic marker in early breast cancer patients was proposed. The authors found that the levels of this protein (and of its splice variant) were significantly higher in all serum samples of women affected by breast cancer compared to controls. Moreover, the variable expression of survivin-2B level correlated with cancer stages [37]. Exosomes have been suggested as promising biomarkers also in NSCLC. It was reported that the markers CD151, CD171, and tetraspanin-8 identified in plasma exosomes were strong separators of patients with cancer of all histological subtypes versus patients without cancer [38]. Interestingly, in addition to plasma/serum, other biofluids, such as urine, may represent valuable sources of exosomal biomarkers.

Higher levels of leucine-rich α-2-glycoprotein (LRG1) were found, for example, in urinary exosomes, such as in lung tissue, of NSCLC patients, suggesting that LRG1 may be a candidate biomarker for noninvasive diagnosis of NSCLC [39].

The potential use of urinary exosomes was overall reported for the diagnosis and clinical management of urogenital cancers, such as bladder and prostate cancers. It was demonstrated that exosomes isolated from both high-grade bladder cancer cells and urine of patients with high-grade bladder cancer (HiG-BlCa) contain the bioactive protein EDIL3 promoting angiogenesis and migration of bladder cancer cells and endothelial cells. This protein was also found significantly enriched in exosomes purified from the urine of patients with HiG-BlCa in comparison to urine exosomes of healthy controls [40]. Besides the use as biomarkers, the identification of this molecule and of its associated oncogenic pathways could lead to novel therapeutic targets and treatment strategies.

A comparative study of protein profiling by mass spectrometry-based proteomics highlighted the expression of ITGA3 and ITGB1 (proteins involved in migration/invasion processes) on exosomes released by prostate cancer cell lines (LNCaP and PC3T). Afterward, these proteins were found more abundant in urine exosomes of metastatic patients compared to benign prostatic hyperplasia or prostate cancer (PCa), suggesting the potential use of urine exosomes for identification of patients with metastatic PCa in a noninvasive manner [41]. In another study, 15 control and 16 prostate cancer samples of urinary exosomes were analyzed, and 246 proteins were found differentially expressed in the two groups. By applying specific criteria to create a focus list, the authors highlighted 17 proteins that at 100% specificity displayed individual sensitivities above 60%. Among them, there were TM256, showing the highest sensitivity (94%), LAMTOR1 and ADIRF (81% sensitivity), VATL, several Rab class members, and proteasomal proteins. Moreover, several well-known prostate cancer biomarkers including PSA, FOLH1/PMSA, TGM4, and TMPRSS were also found to

Table 7.1 Potential tumor biomarkers found in exosomes isolated from body fluids of patients with various cancers

Biofluid	Exo-protein/tumor biomarker[a]	Tumor type	Reference
Plasma/serum	Glypican-1	Pancreatic cancer	[35]
	TYRP2, VLA-4, HSP70, an HSP90 isoform and MET	Melanoma	[36]
	Survivin	Breast cancer	[37]
	CD151, CD171, and tetraspanin-8	Non-small cell lung cancer (NSCLC)	[38]
	Claudin-4	Ovarian cancer	[43]
	Caveolin-1, CD63	Melanoma	[44]
	EGFR	Lung cancer	[45]
	EGFRVIII mutated	Glioblastoma	[46]
	Galectin-9	Nasopharyngeal cancer	[47]
	MIF	Pancreatic cancer	[48]
	TGF-β and MAGE 3/6	Ovarian cancer	[49]
	TGF-β	Acute myeloid leukemia (AML)	[50]
Urine	LRG-1	NSCLC	[39]
	EDIL-3/Del1	High-grade bladder cancer	[40]
	ITGA3 and ITGB1	Metastatic prostate cancer	[41]
	MMP-9, CAIX, DKK4, CP, PODXL	Renal cell carcinoma	[51]
	TACSTD2	Bladder cancer	[52]
	TM256, LAMTOR1, ADIRF VATL, several Rab class members, and proteasomal proteins	Prostate cancer	[42]

[a]Proteins found in exosomes isolated from biofluids and described as potential tumor biomarkers

be enriched in urinary exosomes from prostate cancer patients compared to controls. Even if, compared to some of the novel candidates, these known prostate cancer marker proteins showed lower degree of specificity and/or sensitivity, their presence in urinary exosomes gives further credibility to the novel proteins identified [42]. A summary of proteins found in exosomes obtained from body fluids of patients with cancer is reported in Table 7.1. Studies on exosomes in body fluids of cancer patients have provided promising indications about their effective use in clinical settings and merit further advance in order to develop new and valid noninvasive cancer diagnostic and prognostic tools needed for enhancing positive outcomes in cancer.

References

1. Fontana S, et al. Contribution of proteomics to understanding the role of tumor-derived exosomes in cancer progression: state of the art and new perspectives. Proteomics. 2013;13(10–11):1581–94.

2. Pan BT, Johnstone RM. Fate of the transferrin receptor during maturation of sheep reticulocytes in vitro: selective externalization of the receptor. Cell. 1983;33(3):967–78.
3. Ludwig AK, Giebel B. Exosomes: small vesicles participating in intercellular communication. Int J Biochem Cell Biol. 2012;44(1):11–5.
4. Properzi F, Logozzi M, Fais S. Exosomes: the future of biomarkers in medicine. Biomark Med. 2013;7(5): 769–78.
5. Lin J, et al. Exosomes: novel biomarkers for clinical diagnosis. ScientificWorldJournal. 2015;2015:657086.
6. Whiteside TL. The potential of tumor-derived exosomes for noninvasive cancer monitoring. Expert Rev Mol Diagn. 2015;15(10):1293–310.
7. Muller L, et al. Isolation of biologically-active exosomes from human plasma. J Immunol Methods. 2014;411:55–65.
8. Szatanek R, et al. Isolation of extracellular vesicles: determining the correct approach (review). Int J Mol Med. 2015;36(1):11–7.
9. Raposo G, et al. B lymphocytes secrete antigen-presenting vesicles. J Exp Med. 1996;183(3):1161–72.
10. Thery C, et al. Isolation and characterization of exosomes from cell culture supernatants and biological fluids. Curr Protoc Cell Biol. 2006. Chapter 3:Unit 3 22.
11. Van Deun J, et al. The impact of disparate isolation methods for extracellular vesicles on downstream RNA profiling. J Extracell Vesicles 2014;3:24858. http://dx.doi.org/10.3402/jev.v3.24858.

12. Taylor DD, Shah S. Methods of isolating extracellular vesicles impact down-stream analyses of their cargoes. Methods. 2015;87:3–10.

13. Chen C, et al. Microfluidic isolation and transcriptome analysis of serum microvesicles. Lab Chip. 2010;10(4):505–11.

14. Zeringer E, et al. Strategies for isolation of exosomes. Cold Spring Harb Protoc. 2015;2015(4):319–23.

15. Gooding Jr GV, Hebert TT. A simple technique for purification of tobacco mosaic virus in large quantities. Phytopathology. 1967;57(11):1285.

16. Zhang J, et al. Exosome and exosomal microRNA: trafficking, sorting, and function. Genomics Proteomics Bioinformatics. 2015;13(1):17–24.

17. Valadi H, et al. Exosome-mediated transfer of mRNAs and microRNAs is a novel mechanism of genetic exchange between cells. Nat Cell Biol. 2007;9(6):654–9.

18. Bartel DP. MicroRNAs: genomics, biogenesis, mechanism, and function. Cell. 2004;116(2):281–97.

19. Corrado C, et al. Exosomes as intercellular signaling organelles involved in health and disease: basic science and clinical applications. Int J Mol Sci. 2013;14(3):5338–66.

20. Corrado C, et al. Chronic myelogenous leukaemia exosomes modulate bone marrow microenvironment through activation of epidermal growth factor receptor. J Cell Mol Med. 2016;20:1829–39.

21. Lv MM, et al. Exosomes mediate drug resistance transfer in MCF-7 breast cancer cells and a probable mechanism is delivery of P-glycoprotein. Tumour Biol. 2014;35(11):10773–9.

22. Melo SA, et al. Cancer exosomes perform cell-independent microRNA biogenesis and promote tumorigenesis. Cancer Cell. 2014;26(5):707–21.

23. Taverna S, et al. Role of exosomes released by chronic myelogenous leukemia cells in angiogenesis. Int J Cancer. 2012;130(9):2033–43.

24. Rabinowits G, et al. Exosomal microRNA: a diagnostic marker for lung cancer. Clin Lung Cancer. 2009;10(1):42–6.

25. Liang RQ, et al. An oligonucleotide microarray for microRNA expression analysis based on labeling RNA with quantum dot and nanogold probe. Nucleic Acids Res. 2005;33(2):e17.

26. Huang X, et al. Exosomal miR-1290 and miR-375 as prognostic markers in castration-resistant prostate cancer. Eur Urol. 2015;67(1):33–41.

27. Taylor DD, Gercel-Taylor C. MicroRNA signatures of tumor-derived exosomes as diagnostic biomarkers of ovarian cancer. Gynecol Oncol. 2008;110(1):13–21.

28. Takeshita N, et al. Serum microRNA expression profile: miR-1246 as a novel diagnostic and prognostic biomarker for oesophageal squamous cell carcinoma. Br J Cancer. 2013;108(3):644–52.

29. Aushev VN, et al. Comparisons of microRNA patterns in plasma before and after tumor removal reveal new biomarkers of lung squamous cell carcinoma. PLoS One. 2013;8(10):e78649.

30. Cazzoli R, et al. microRNAs derived from circulating exosomes as noninvasive biomarkers for screening and diagnosing lung cancer. J Thorac Oncol. 2013;8(9):1156–62.

31. Eichelser C, et al. Increased serum levels of circulating exosomal microRNA-373 in receptor-negative breast cancer patients. Oncotarget. 2014;5(20):9650–63.

32. Takahashi K, et al. Analysis of extracellular RNA by digital PCR. Front Oncol. 2014;4:129.

33. Kalra H, et al. Vesiclepedia: a compendium for extracellular vesicles with continuous community annotation. PLoS Biol. 2012;10(12):e1001450.

34. Simpson RJ, Kalra H, Mathivanan S. ExoCarta as a resource for exosomal research. J Extracell Vesicles. 2012;1:18374. http://dx.doi.org/10.3402/jev.v1i0.18374 .

35. Melo SA, et al. Glypican-1 identifies cancer exosomes and detects early pancreatic cancer. Nature. 2015;523(7559):177–82.

36. Peinado H, et al. Melanoma exosomes educate bone marrow progenitor cells toward a pro-metastatic phenotype through MET. Nat Med. 2012;18(6):883–91.

37. Khan S, et al. Early diagnostic value of survivin and its alternative splice variants in breast cancer. BMC Cancer. 2014;14:176.

38. Sandfeld-Paulsen B, et al. Exosomal proteins as diagnostic biomarkers in lung cancer. J Thorac Oncol. 2016;11:1701–10.

39. Li Y, et al. Proteomic identification of exosomal LRG1: a potential urinary biomarker for detecting NSCLC. Electrophoresis. 2011;32(15):1976–83.

40. Beckham CJ, et al. Bladder cancer exosomes contain EDIL-3/Del1 and facilitate cancer progression. J Urol. 2014;192(2):583–92.

41. Bijnsdorp IV, et al. Exosomal ITGA3 interferes with non-cancerous prostate cell functions and is increased in urine exosomes of metastatic prostate cancer patients. J Extracell Vesicles. 2013;2:22097. http://dx.doi.org/10.3402/jev.v2i0.22097

42. Overbye A, et al. Identification of prostate cancer biomarkers in urinary exosomes. Oncotarget. 2015;6(30):30357–76.

43. Li J, et al. Claudin-containing exosomes in the peripheral circulation of women with ovarian cancer. BMC Cancer. 2009;9:244.

44. Logozzi M, et al. High levels of exosomes expressing CD63 and caveolin-1 in plasma of melanoma patients. PLoS One. 2009;4(4):e5219.

45. Yamashita T, et al. Epidermal growth factor receptor localized to exosome membranes as a possible biomarker for lung cancer diagnosis. Pharmazie. 2013;68(12):969–73.

46. Graner MW, et al. Proteomic and immunologic analyses of brain tumor exosomes. FASEB J. 2009;23(5):1541–57.

47. Klibi J, et al. Blood diffusion and Th1-suppressive effects of galectin-9-containing exosomes released by Epstein-Barr virus-infected nasopharyngeal carcinoma cells. Blood. 2009;113(9):1957–66.

48. Costa-Silva B, et al. Pancreatic cancer exosomes initiate pre-metastatic niche formation in the liver. Nat Cell Biol. 2015;17(6):816–26.

49. Szajnik M, et al. Exosomes in plasma of patients with ovarian carcinoma: potential biomarkers of tumor progression and response to therapy. Gynecol Obstet (Sunnyvale). 2013;Suppl 4:3.

50. Hong CS, et al. Plasma exosomes as markers of therapeutic response in patients with acute myeloid leukemia. Front Immunol. 2014;5:160.

51. Raimondo F, et al. Differential protein profiling of renal cell carcinoma urinary exosomes. Mol BioSyst. 2013;9(6):1220–33.

52. Chen CL, et al. Comparative and targeted proteomic analyses of urinary microparticles from bladder cancer and hernia patients. J Proteome Res. 2012;11(12): 5611–29.

Actionable Molecular Targets in Cancer Liquid Biopsy

8

Pierluigi Scalia, Stephen J. Williams,
Antonio Russo, and Antonio Giordano

The possibility to detect nucleic acid sequences in the bloodstream deriving from an underlying tumor process has disclosed a unique opportunity in medical oncology. Whether the nucleic acid material is leaked in the blood at any step of cancer development (circulating tumor DNA or ctDNA) or it is obtained from isolated circulating tumor cells (CTCs), the detection and analysis of the meaningful sequence defects harbored in instrumental molecular targets (which we call liquid biopsy) constitutes an invaluable tool toward leading the current oncology practice toward a less invasive and fully personalized diagnostic-therapeutic workflow. In spite of the current technical limitations that liquid biopsy still bears in terms of enrichment and/or isolation of the target test material (CTCs, ctDNA, etc.) from the bloodstream (widely discussed in the other chapters), current advancements in nanotechnologies as well as in pathway-driven biology knowledge of the cancer process now allow medical science to adopt universal pre-analytical and analytic methodologies. The key aspect that currently concerns the medical oncology field still remains what molecular targets should be pursued in the clinical practice (sequential monotherapies versus smart combinations) at the light of the experience accumulating on the mechanisms of acquired resistance to molecular monotherapies (even the most effective ones). While the previous chapters provide cancer-specific perspective on the use of liquid biopsy, in this chapter we summarize the general evidences toward the use of individual and combined molecular targets in liquid biopsy focusing on the experimental work conducted in the last few years toward validating this tool in parallel with the target validation data obtained by cancer genome wide studies. Even though the chapter is not meant to provide an exhaustive source for the constantly growing validated molecular targets in liquid biopsy testing (covered by other authors and through the references herein), it aims to provide an overview of the currently tested molecular targets shown to be linked to the evolution of the disease while focusing on the diagnostic and/or therapeutic monitoring value of the test.

P. Scalia, MD, PhD (✉) • S.J. Williams
Sbarro Institute for Cancer Research & Molecular
Medicine, 1900 N. 12th Street, Philadelphia,
PA 19122, USA

Caltanissetta, ISOPROG, Via G Borremans 49, 93100
Caltanissetta, Italy
e-mail: pscalia@shro.org

A. Russo
Department of Surgical, Oncological and Oral
Sciences, Section of Medical Oncology, University of
Palermo, Via del Vespro 129, 90127 Palermo, Italy

A. Giordano
Sbarro Institute for Cancer Research & Molecular
Medicine, 1900 N. 12th Street, Philadelphia,
PA 19122, USA

© Springer International Publishing AG 2017
A. Giordano et al. (eds.), *Liquid Biopsy in Cancer Patients*, Current Clinical Pathology,
DOI 10.1007/978-3-319-55661-1_8

In this context, Vogelstein et al. [1] have provided a useful frame toward the simplification of cancer molecular targets by confirming that a number of 140 genes are the most commonly targeted by sequence defects in cancer and that each tumor typically harbors two to eight mutations (out of the 33–66 average somatic mutations detected per typical solid tumor) in any of these "driver" genes (genes that specifically confer a growth advantage to cancer cells), while the other mutations detected by sequencing analysis stand as passenger mutations. Passenger mutations do not provide any advantage nor do they alter the function of the resulting protein product. Furthermore, they have suggested that cancer can be viewed as a pathway-linked disease by assigning all cancer driver genes basically to 12 signaling pathways that ultimately attend one of two possible roles in the cancer cell: fate, survival, or genome maintenance. In regard to the number of somatic mutations that can be acquired and therefore can be detected in sequence testing, certain tumor types, such as melanomas and lung cancer, do contain a higher than average number of somatic mutations (~200) due to the underlying role of the potent mutagenic factors involved (such as UV light and cigarette smoking, respectively). At the higher and lower spectrum of genomic defects detectable in cancer are those bearing mismatch repair defects (carrying thousands of mutations and linked to rare syndromes) and pediatric tumors and white blood cell cancers (leukemias) displaying only a few point mutations (<10/tumor). A key consideration that carries practical relevance when analyzing the somatic mutations carrying "driver" capability is that the vast majority (~95%) are single-base substitutions (mostly missense such as EGFR T790 M or BRAF V600E), while the rest (~5%) are deletions/insertions of one or few bases. A definite intrinsic value toward the analysis of a cancer molecular target has the identification of a gain of function (oncogenic) versus loss of function (tumor suppressing) behavior when its mutational pattern is analyzed by DNA sequencing. In this regard, Vogelstein et al. have suggested

the adoption of a 20/20 rule which is that to define as oncogenes, all those driver genes carrying sequence mutations where >20% of the recorded mutations, first, are at recurrent positions and, second, are missense. On the other hand, they suggest to define a tumor suppressor gene when >20% of the recorded mutations are inactivating. Using this rule, all of the recognized cancer driver genes bearing intragenic driver mutations (also subcategorized as mut drivers) have been assigned to a specific group even when conflicting studies can be found in the literature.

In spite of the higher level of complexity present in the mutational spectrum, e.g., when considering epi-driver genes (genes that are overexpressed and confer a growth advantage to the cancer cell without a driver mutation in their coding region) or those genes affecting cancer progression in other modes rather than defects in the coding DNA sequence (such as mutations affecting promoter function or via lncRNAs), it is presently clear that perfecting our actionable knowledge of the known 140 (mut-)driver genes in order to fingerprint those three to eight key mutations harbored by each cancer carries enough clinical power to allow the adoption of the long invoked "magic bullets" combination as first therapeutic option, in order to reduce morbidity and mortality while working on the longer goal of disease eradication.

If the above considerations apply to any DNA test currently available, a specific discussion must be provided on the potential of using liquid biopsy in order to perform sequence-based testing in a cancer patient. In this case, in fact, since liquid biopsy first appeared a decade ago, a number of actual or potential technical and theoretical limitations have been a concern. In particular, it has been debated on whether embracing this approach and, even more important, under what circumstances as compared to classic tissue biopsy. First, let's remind that at present, the use of liquid biopsy regards obtaining target DNA material either via circulating tumor cells (CTCs) or via circulating tumor

DNA (ctDNA). While CTCs would appear as the most logical approach in light of the possibility to identify a definite cancer element in the bloodstream from which to extract DNA material, recent published data, discussed in this chapter, can possibly change this view of ctDNA leading to the concept that DNA obtained from CTCs and ctDNA are different entities and as such differently exploitable. Due to the still ongoing optimization of CTC retrieval from blood with abatement of the surface marker bias linked to the current enrichment techniques, we will here focus on the data obtained on ctDNA at the light of the comparative data between CTCs and ctDNA. The evidences accumulated so far on a sufficient cohort of tested subjects (see references in Table 8.1) provide the first available insight to draw some initial conclusions on the positive value of liquid biopsy in the routine cancer testing practice as a parallel and nonexclusive biopsy approach. In particular, the conclusion reported herein summarizes the results of the study conducted by Bettegowda et al. [2] on 640 patients. In this study, different sequence analysis methods were used (PCR ligation, BEAMing, and SafeSeq), and the analytical methods used displayed comparable results (linear range) in the detection of the underlying sequence defects. The sensitivity observed in sequence mutant detection from ctDNA compared to the primary tumor tested by tissue biopsy was 87.2% throughout several targets with KRAS mutational status alone between plasma and tumor showing a concordance of 95% making a strong point for the test specificity (with 99.2% all target specificity on a set of 206 patients with advanced tumor grade). Mutant fragments of ctDNA were detected in the plasma (1–5 ml) of >75% of patients with advanced tumors of the pancreas, ovaries, colon, bladder, gastroesophageal, breast, melanoma, liver, and head and neck, while the detection was <50% in patients with advanced brain, kidney, prostate, and thyroid tumors. For the localized (nonmetastatic) forms, detection rates were 73% for CRC, 57% for GI, 48% for pancreas,

and 50% for breast tumors. A comparative part of the study pairing CTC and ctDNA detection from the same patients showed that ctDNA was detected even when CTCs were not detectable using current standard methods, and, as expected, the number of ctDNA fragments reflected the tumor staging (increasing from stage 1 to stage 4). We have conveyed in Table 8.1 the current molecular targets tested in liquid biopsy in the clinical setting at centers that have adopted this approach and participated to the discussed collaborative study. Ultimately, the experience accumulated on liquid biopsy, so far, suggests that a growing range of sequence-based investigative applications both at the clinical and research level are feasible and easily standardized using this approach which has to be considered as a distinct as well as parallel tool to tissue biopsy. The distinct advantage in using ctDNA versus CTCs as observed in the first large study cited herein will need further validation without subtracting valuable applications to both methods. Finally, we invite clinical practitioners to consider liquid biopsy, at this time, not as a test per se but to an invaluable new platform under which molecular targets' panels are being conveyed for those cancers where a reliable source of pathologic tissue material cannot be obtained without unreasonable, costly, or invasive approaches (as reviewed in other chapters). We suggest that liquid biopsy might be used as a routine instrument for the disease and drug effect monitoring of all diagnosed cancer cases due to the satisfactory results in this group along with the cost/benefit advantage as compared to multiple tissue biopsies (not always feasible). A parallel, present, and future goal of liquid biopsy-based testing, through constant gain of experience and technical innovation, regards the development of molecular target panels with higher preventive-predictive value in order to add to the established personalization of molecular therapeutics and also early interventions and prediction in healthy patients bearing cancer-predisposing genomic defects.

Table 8.1 Actionable cancer targets tested in liquid biopsy analysis

Actionable target (Dx or Rx)	% (n) of mutated samples with single-base mt/insertion/deletion	Current use (Dx:Rx value)	Validation in liquid biopsy (source of liquid biopsy)	Analytic method	References
JAK2	20.9 (32,692)	Not established	Not determined	–	–
BRAF	15.5 (24288)	Rx, melanoma	(ctDNA)	ddPCR	[3]
			(ctDNA)	PCR	[4]
			(ctDNA)	ddPCR	[5]
KRAS	14.9 (23261)	Dx, multiple	(exosomes)	dPCR	[6]
			(ctDNA)	PCR	[7]
			(CTC & ctDNA)	ddPCR	[8]
			(ctDNA)	NGS	[9]
TP53	9.2 (14438)	Dx, multiple	(ctDNA)	dPCR	[10]
			(exosomes)	dPCR	[6]
			(ctDNA)	NGS	[11]
FLT3	7.4 (11520)	Rx under development	Not available	–	–
EGFR	6.8 (10628)	Rx, multiple	(ctDNA)	NGS	[12]
			(cfDNA)	Seq	[13]
			(cfDNA)	NGS	[14]
KIT	3.0 (4720)	Rx, GIST, AML	(ctDNA)	NGS	[30]
PIK3CA	2.9 (4560)	Dx, breast	(cfDNA)	NGS	[15]
			(ctDNA)	dPCR	[16]
			(CTC)	NGS	[17]
IDH1	2.9 (4509)	Not established	Not validated	–	–
CTNNB1	2.1 (3262)	Dx, multiple	No (ctDNA)	NGS	[18]
FGFR3	1.9 (2948)	Rx under evaluation	(ctDNA)	NGS	[19]
NRAS	1.8 (2738)	Dx, multiple	(ctDNA)	ddPCR	[5, 20]
APC	1.6 (2561)	Dx, colon	(ctDNA)	NGS&dPCR	[21]
			(ctDNA)	NGS&dPCR	[22]
			(ctDNA)	NGS	[23]
NPM1	1.6 (1471)	Not established			
PTEN	1.1 (1719)	Rx under evaluation	(CTC)	NGS	[24]
			(ctDNA)	NGS	[25]
VHL	0.8 (1287)	Dx, VHL syndrome	(CTC)	NGS	[26]
IDH2	0.7 (1029)	Not established	(ctDNA)	NGS	[25]
CDKN2A	0.6 (968)	Dx, multiple	(ctDNA)	MPS	[27]
			(ctDNA)	NGS	[28]
TET2	0.6 (864)	Not established	–	–	–
ABL1	0.5 (851)	Rx, CML	–	–	–
HRAS	0.5 (812)	Dx under evaluation	–	–	–
DNMT3A	0.5 (788)	Not established			–
NOTCH1	0.4 (661)	Not established	(exosomes)	NGS	[29]
			(ctDNA)	NGS	[12]
PDGFRA	0.4 (653)	Rx under evaluation, GIST	(ctDNA)	NGS	[30]
NF2	0.4 (609)	Dx, neurofibromatosis, mesothelioma	(ctDNA)	NGS	[31]
			(ctDNA)	NGS	[28]
MPL	0.3 (531)	Not established			
SF3B1	0.3 (516)	Dx under evaluation	(ctDNA)	NGS	[32]
RET	0.3 (500)	Dx under evaluation	(ctDNA)	NGS&dPCR	[22]

The actionable targets in the table originate from Vogelstein et al. (2013) (source: COSMIC open database) and represent single-base mutated driver genes (both oncogenes and tumor suppressor genes) found most frequently in cancer with a mutation hit >500/tumor. Bolded correspond to targets with clinically available therapeutics. The complete list available through the cited reference

ctDNA circulating tumor DNA, *CTC* circulating tumor cell, *NGS* next-generation sequencing, *dPCR* digital PCR, *ddPCR* droplet digital PCR, *Dx* diagnostic, *Rx* therapeutic

References

1. Vogelstein B, Papadopoulos N, Velculescu VE, Zhou S, Diaz Jr LA, Kinzler KW. Cancer genome landscapes. Science. 2013;339:1546–58.
2. Bettegowda C, Sausen M, Leary RJ, Kinde I, Wang Y, Agrawal N, Bartlett BR, Wang H, Luber B, Alani RM, Antonarakis ES, Azad NS, Bardelli A, Brem H, Cameron JL, Lee CC, Fecher LA, Gallia GL, Gibbs P, Le D, Giuntoli RL, Goggins M, Hogarty MD, Holdhoff M, Hong SM, Jiao Y, Juhl HH, Kim JJ, Siravegna G, Laheru DA, Lauricella C, Lim M, Lipson EJ, Marie SK, Netto GJ, Oliner KS, Olivi A, Olsson L, Riggins GJ, Sartore-Bianchi A, Schmidt K, Shih IM, Oba-Shinjo SM, Siena S, Theodorescu D, Tie J, Harkins TT, Veronese S, Wang TL, Weingart JD, Wolfgang CL, Wood LD, Xing D, Hruban RH, Wu J, Allen PJ, Schmidt CM, Choti MA, Velculescu VE, Kinzler KW, Vogelstein B, Papadopoulos N, Diaz Jr LA. Detection of circulating tumor DNA in early- and late-stage human malignancies. Sci Transl Med. 2014;6:224ra224.
3. Schreuer M, Meersseman G, Van Den Herrewegen S, Jansen Y, Chevolet I, Bott A, Wilgenhof S, Seremet T, Jacobs B, Buyl R, Maertens G, Neyns B. Quantitative assessment of BRAF V600 mutant circulating cell-free tumor DNA as a tool for therapeutic monitoring in metastatic melanoma patients treated with BRAF/MEK inhibitors. J Transl Med. 2016;14:95.
4. Perkins G, Yap TA, Pope L, Cassidy AM, Dukes JP, Riisnaes R, Massard C, Cassier PA, Miranda S, Clark J, Denholm KA, Thway K, Gonzalez De Castro D, Attard G, Molife LR, Kaye SB, Banerji U, de Bono JS. Multi-purpose utility of circulating plasma DNA testing in patients with advanced cancers. PLoS One. 2012;7:e47020.
5. Tsao SC, Weiss J, Hudson C, Christophi C, Cebon J, Behren A, Dobrovic A. Monitoring response to therapy in melanoma by quantifying circulating tumour DNA with droplet digital PCR for BRAF and NRAS mutations. Sci Rep. 2015;5:11198.
6. Yang S, Che SP, Kurywchak P, Tavormina JL, Gansmo LB, Correa de Sampaio P, Tachezy M, Bockhorn M, Gebauer F, Haltom AR, Melo SA, LeBleu VS, Kalluri R. Detection of mutant KRAS and TP53 DNA in circulating exosomes from healthy individuals and patients with pancreatic cancer. Cancer Biol Ther. 2017. http://dx.doi.org/10.1080/15384047.2017.1281499.
7. Sherwood JL, Corcoran C, Brown H, Sharpe AD, Musilova M, Kohlmann A. Optimised pre-analytical methods improve KRAS mutation detection in circulating tumour DNA (ctDNA) from patients with non-small cell lung cancer (NSCLC). PLoS One. 2016;11:e0150197.
8. Earl J, Garcia-Nieto S, Martinez-Avila JC, Montans J, Sanjuanbenito A, Rodriguez-Garrote M, Lisa E, Mendia E, Lobo E, Malats N, Carrato A, Guillen-Ponce C. Circulating tumor cells (Ctc) and kras mutant circulating free Dna (cfdna) detection in peripheral blood as biomarkers in patients diagnosed with exocrine pancreatic cancer. BMC Cancer. 2015;15:797.
9. Takai E, Totoki Y, Nakamura H, Kato M, Shibata T, Yachida S. Clinical utility of circulating tumor DNA for molecular assessment and precision medicine in pancreatic cancer. Adv Exp Med Biol. 2016;924: 13–7.
10. Parkinson CA, Gale D, Piskorz AM, Biggs H, Hodgkin C, Addley H, Freeman S, Moyle P, Sala E, Sayal K, Hosking K, Gounaris I, Jimenez-Linan M, Earl HM, Qian W, Rosenfeld N, Brenton JD. Exploratory analysis of TP53 mutations in circulating tumour DNA as biomarkers of treatment response for patients with relapsed high-grade serous ovarian carcinoma: a retrospective study. PLoS Med. 2016;13:e1002198.
11. Guo N, Lou F, Ma Y, Li J, Yang B, Chen W, Ye H, Zhang JB, Zhao MY, Wu WJ, Shi R, Jones L, Chen KS, Huang XF, Chen SY, Liu Y. Circulating tumor DNA detection in lung cancer patients before and after surgery. Sci Rep. 2016;6:33519.
12. Schwaederle M, Husain H, Fanta PT, Piccioni DE, Kesari S, Schwab RB, Banks KC, Lanman RB, Talasaz A, Parker BA, Kurzrock R. Detection rate of actionable mutations in diverse cancers using a biopsy-free (blood) circulating tumor cell DNA assay. Oncotarget. 2016;7:9707–17.
13. Newman AM, Lovejoy AF, Klass DM, Kurtz DM, Chabon JJ, Scherer F, Stehr H, Liu CL, Bratman SV, Say C, Zhou L, Carter JN, West RB, Sledge Jr GW, Shrager JB, Loo Jr BW, Neal JW, Wakelee HA, Diehn M, Alizadeh AA. Integrated digital error suppression for improved detection of circulating tumor DNA. Nat Biotechnol. 2016;34:547–55.
14. Janku F, Angenendt P, Tsimberidou AM, Fu S, Naing A, Falchook GS, Hong DS, Holley VR, Cabrilo G, Wheler JJ, Piha-Paul SA, Zinner RG, Bedikian AY, Overman MJ, Kee BK, Kim KB, Kopetz ES, Luthra R, Diehl F, Meric-Bernstam F, Kurzrock R. Actionable mutations in plasma cell-free DNA in patients with advanced cancers referred for experimental targeted therapies. Oncotarget. 2015;6:12809–21.
15. Kim ST, Lee WS, Lanman RB, Mortimer S, Zill OA, Kim KM, Jang KT, Kim SH, Park SH, Park JO, Park YS, Lim HY, Eltoukhy H, Kang WK, Lee WY, Kim HC, Park K, Lee J, Talasaz A. Prospective blinded study of somatic mutation detection in cell-free DNA utilizing a targeted 54-gene next generation sequencing panel in metastatic solid tumor patients. Oncotarget. 2015;6:40360–9.
16. Beaver JA, Jelovac D, Balukrishna S, Cochran RL, Croessmann S, Zabransky DJ, Wong HY, Valda Toro P, Cidado J, Blair BG, Chu D, Burns T, Higgins MJ, Stearns V, Jacobs L, Habibi M, Lange J, Hurley PJ, Lauring J, VanDenBerg DA, Kessler J, Jeter S, Samuels ML, Maar D, Cope L, Cimino-Mathews A, Argani P, Wolff AC, Park BH. Detection of cancer

DNA in plasma of patients with early-stage breast cancer. Clin Cancer Res. 2014;20:2643–50.

17. Schneck H, Blassl C, Meier-Stiegen F, Neves RP, Janni W, Fehm T, Neubauer H. Analysing the mutational status of PIK3CA in circulating tumor cells from metastatic breast cancer patients. Mol Oncol. 2013;7:976–86.

18. Liao W, Yang H, Xu H, Wang Y, Ge P, Ren J, Xu W, Lu X, Sang X, Zhong S, Zhang H, Mao Y. Noninvasive detection of tumor-associated mutations from circulating cell-free DNA in hepatocellular carcinoma patients by targeted deep sequencing. Oncotarget. 2016;7:40481–90.

19. Allen JM, Schrock AB, Erlich RL, Miller VA, Stephens PJ, Ross JS, Ou SI, Ali SM, Vafai D. Genomic profiling of circulating tumor DNA in relapsed EGFR-mutated lung adenocarcinoma reveals an acquired FGFR3-TACC3 fusion. Clin Lung Cancer. 2016 doi: http://dx.doi.org/10.1016/j.cllc.2016.12.006.

20. Bronte G, Silvestris N, Castiglia M, Galvano A, Passiglia F, Sortino G, Cicero G, Rolfo C, Peeters M, Bazan V, Fanale D, Giordano A, Russo A. New findings on primary and acquired resistance to anti-EGFR therapy in metastatic colorectal cancer: do all roads lead to RAS? Oncotarget. 2015;6:24780–96.

21. Beije N, Helmijr JC, Weerts MJ, Beaufort CM, Wiggin M, Marziali A, Verhoef C, Sleijfer S, Jansen MP, Martens JW. Somatic mutation detection using various targeted detection assays in paired samples of circulating tumor DNA, primary tumor and metastases from patients undergoing resection of colorectal liver metastases. Mol Oncol. 2016;10:1575–84.

22. Kurihara S, Ueda Y, Onitake Y, Sueda T, Ohta E, Morihara N, Hirano S, Irisuna F, Hiyama E. Circulating free DNA as non-invasive diagnostic biomarker for childhood solid tumors. J Pediatr Surg. 2015;50:2094–7.

23. Lin JK, Lin PC, Lin CH, Jiang JK, Yang SH, Liang WY, Chen WS, Chang SC. Clinical relevance of alterations in quantity and quality of plasma DNA in colorectal cancer patients: based on the mutation spectra detected in primary tumors. Ann Surg Oncol. 2014;21(Suppl 4):S680–6.

24. Jiang R, Lu YT, Ho H, Li B, Chen JF, Lin M, Li F, Wu K, Wu H, Lichterman J, Wan H, Lu CL, OuYang W, Ni M, Wang L, Li G, Lee T, Zhang X, Yang J, Rettig M, Chung LW, Yang H, Li KC, Hou Y, Tseng HR, Hou S, Xu X, Wang J, Posadas EM. A comparison of isolated circulating tumor cells and tissue biopsies using whole-genome sequencing in prostate cancer. Oncotarget. 2015;6:44781–93.

25. Rothe F, Laes JF, Lambrechts D, Smeets D, Vincent D, Maetens M, Fumagalli D, Michiels S, Drisis S, Moerman C, Detiffe JP, Larsimont D, Awada A, Piccart M, Sotiriou C, Ignatiadis M. Plasma circulating tumor DNA as an alternative to metastatic biopsies for mutational analysis in breast cancer. Ann Oncol. 2014;25:1959–65.

26. Rad FH, Ulusakarya A, Gad S, Sibony M, Juin F, Richard S, Machover D, Uzan G. Novel somatic mutations of the VHL gene in an erythropoietin-producing renal carcinoma associated with secondary polycythemia and elevated circulating endothelial progenitor cells. Am J Hematol. 2008;83:155–8.

27. De Mattos-Arruda L, Weigelt B, Cortes J, Won HH, Ng CK, Nuciforo P, Bidard FC, Aura C, Saura C, Peg V, Piscuoglio S, Oliveira M, Smolders Y, Patel P, Norton L, Tabernero J, Berger MF, Seoane J, Reis-Filho JS. Capturing intra-tumor genetic heterogeneity by de novo mutation profiling of circulating cell-free tumor DNA: a proof-of-principle. Ann Oncol. 2014;25:1729–35.

28. Sheffield BS, Tinker AV, Shen Y, Hwang H, Li-Chang HH, Pleasance E, Ch'ng C, Lum A, Lorette J, McConnell YJ, Sun S, Jones SJ, Gown AM, Huntsman DG, Schaeffer DF, Churg A, Yip S, Laskin J, Marra MA. Personalized oncogenomics: clinical experience with malignant peritoneal mesothelioma using whole genome sequencing. PLoS One. 2015; 10:e0119689.

29. San Lucas FA, Allenson K, Bernard V, Castillo J, Kim DU, Ellis K, Ehli EA, Davies GE, Petersen JL, Li D, Wolff R, Katz M, Varadhachary G, Wistuba I, Maitra A, Alvarez H. Minimally invasive genomic and transcriptomic profiling of visceral cancers by next-generation sequencing of circulating exosomes. Ann Oncol. 2016;27:635–41.

30. Kang G, Bae BN, Sohn BS, Pyo JS, Kang GH, Kim KM. Detection of KIT and PDGFRA mutations in the plasma of patients with gastrointestinal stromal tumor. Target Oncol. 2015;10:597–601.

31. Wang Y, Springer S, Zhang M, McMahon KW, Kinde I, Dobbyn L, Ptak J, Brem H, Chaichana K, Gallia GL, Gokaslan ZL, Groves ML, Jallo GI, Lim M, Olivi A, Quinones-Hinojosa A, Rigamonti D, Riggins GJ, Sciubba DM, Weingart JD, Wolinsky JP, Ye X, Oba-Shinjo SM, Marie SK, Holdhoff M, Agrawal N, Diaz Jr LA, Papadopoulos N, Kinzler KW, Vogelstein B, Bettegowda C. Detection of tumor-derived DNA in cerebrospinal fluid of patients with primary tumors of the brain and spinal cord. Proc Natl Acad Sci U S A. 2015;112:9704–9.

32. Del Giudice I, Marinelli M, Wang J, Bonina S, Messina M, Chiaretti S, Ilari C, Cafforio L, Raponi S, Mauro FR, Di Maio V, De Propris MS, Nanni M, Ciardullo C, Rossi D, Gaidano G, Guarini A, Rabadan R, Foa R. Inter- and intra-patient clonal and subclonal heterogeneity of chronic lymphocytic leukaemia: evidences from circulating and lymph nodal compartments. Br J Haematol. 2016;172:371–83.

Liquid Biopsy in Breast Cancer

9

Lorena Incorvaia, Marta Castiglia,
Alessandro Perez, Daniela Massihnia,
Stefano Caruso, Sevilay Altintas, Valentina Calò,
and Antonio Russo

Introduction

Breast cancer (BC) to date remains the most common cancer in women [1].

The increased incidence is due to wide introduction of mammography screening programs and continues to grow with the aging of the population, while the prevalence is increasing as a consequence of improvements in treatment outcomes. At the same time, mortality has decreased thanks to an efficient screening that enables disease diagnosis at a very early stage. Moreover, chemotherapy and endocrine adjuvant therapy have strongly implemented treatment in BC.

Nowadays, BC is often diagnosed at local disease stage, and, after surgery, based on individual's risk of relapse, the patients undergo adjuvant systemic treatment or/and regional irradiation to decrease the risk of recurrence. Some patients, however, will eventually develop recurrent or metastatic disease.

According to standard practice, the choice of treatment strategy includes assays for estrogen (ER) and progesterone (PgR) receptor expression levels, overexpression of human epidermal growth factor receptor 2 (Her-2), or amplification status of the correlate oncogene, but also histological grade and Ki67 to evaluate proliferation of tumor cells.

These features result in the identification of different clinical subgroups of BC:

- The "luminal" tumors, which express ER and PgR receptors and are characterized by endocrine responsiveness and further subdivided into "luminal A" and "luminal B" according to the expression levels of Ki67
- The "Her-2 positive" subgroup, which gets clinical benefit from treatment with "trastuzumab," selective monoclonal antibody that targets Her-2, used in both early and advanced disease settings
- The "triple-negative" subgroup, characterized by the absence of the tree receptors, hormonal receptors, and Her-2, with, therefore, a lower availability of therapeutic options

Lorena Incorvaia and Marta Castiglia contributed equally to this work.

L. Incorvaia • M. Castiglia • A. Perez • D. Massihnia
V. Calò • A. Russo, MD, PhD (✉)
Department of Surgical, Oncological and Oral
Sciences, Section of Medical Oncology, University
of Palermo, Via del Vespro 129, 90127 Palermo, Italy
e-mail: lorena.incorvaia@unipa.it;
martacastiglia@gmail.com; ale-like@libero.it;
danielamassi87@gmail.com;
valentinacalo74@libero.it; antonio.russo@usa.net

S. Caruso, MD, PhD (✉)
Génomique Fonctionnelle des Tumeurs Solides,
INSERM, UMR 1162, 75010 Paris, France
e-mail: steno.caruso@gmail.com

S. Altintas
Multidisciplinary Oncologic Centre Antwerp
(MOCA), Edegem, Belgium

© Springer International Publishing AG 2017
A. Giordano et al. (eds.), *Liquid Biopsy in Cancer Patients*, Current Clinical Pathology,
DOI 10.1007/978-3-319-55661-1_9

On the basis of new molecular diagnostic techniques of genomic profiling, today we know that to each clinical subgroup of BC corresponds a specific molecular subtype with distinct genomic signatures, conditioning the biologic behavior of tumors [2–4].

Current BC classification and assessment remain strongly based on clinicopathological criteria, including patient age, tumor size, lymph node invasion, histological type, and grade.

Nevertheless the established clinicopathological parameters are not sufficient anymore for risk stratification and clinical decision-making, particularly regarding adjuvant chemotherapy, since substantial over- or undertreatment may occur. ER, PgR, and Her-2 status, used for many years as only validated predictive factors to select patients for endocrine treatment and anti-Her-2 treatments, provide limited information.

Thus, novel molecular markers are under investigation to achieve a more precise prognostic and predictive evaluation of disease and a more effective "personalized treatment" in BC.

Clinicopathological information should be combined with genomic profiling to estimate recurrence risk and identify high-risk BC patients (prognostic value) and predict optimal treatment for each disease subgroup (predictive value).

Reading the Breast Cancer Genome: An Explosion of Biomarker Diversity

The recent introduction of translational analysis techniques, mainly next-generation sequencing (NGS), has led to an enormous genomic data about BC that helped the identification of several molecular alterations associated with the distinct molecular subtype of BC.

This information has revealed that BC is not a single disease but a complex and heterogeneous tumor, complicating our understanding toward molecular makeup of the tumor.

Over the tumor heterogeneity from different individuals (*intertumor heterogeneity*), even with the same clinicopathological features, there is a *spatial intra-tumor heterogeneity* due to subpopulations of tumor cells with different genomic alterations coexisting within the same tumor and a *temporal intra-tumor heterogeneity* of different cells in the same patients but at different time points, for example, between primary tumor and its metastasis (Fig. 9.1) [5–7].

This phenomenon represents one of the main barriers to precision medicine in breast cancer: the information obtained from standard tumor tissue sampling cannot be the same for the whole tumor and offer a static picture of disease. The constant molecular change of tumor cell population, spatial and temporal, requires a noninvasive approach, for real-time picture of disease. Liquid biopsy is a useful tool to follow the continuously evolving genomic landscape of breast cancer [8–10] (Fig. 9.2).

Circulating Tumor DNA (ctDNA)

Several studies have shown that ctDNA can be used in clinical practice for evaluation and decision-making in the diagnosis, treatment, and follow-up of breast cancer patients [11]. Indeed, it has been demonstrated that high levels of ctDNA correlate with tumor size, lymph node involvement, histopathological grade, and clinical staging [11, 12]. ctDNA is easier to detect in patients with metastatic breast cancer compared to patients that have a localized disease and concentrations of ctDNA increased with advanced stage of cancer [13].

Different researchers have focused on mutational analysis of genes directly involved in breast cancer both in patients with an advanced-stage disease and in patients with localized disease. Some studies have quantified the presence of tumor-specific alterations in ctDNA. In the screening and diagnosis of breast cancer, patient-specific mutations are not known before. Therefore, these studies have focused on cancer-associated alterations that are common in all types of breast cancers. Chimonidou et al. found CST6 promoter methylation in plasma ctDNA in 13–40% of breast cancer patients but none in healthy patients [14]. Accordingly, Dulaimi et al. found hypermethylation of promoters RASSF1A, APS, and DAP kinase in the serum of 70% breast cancer patients and none in serum from healthy subjects [15]. Oshiro et al. developed a digital

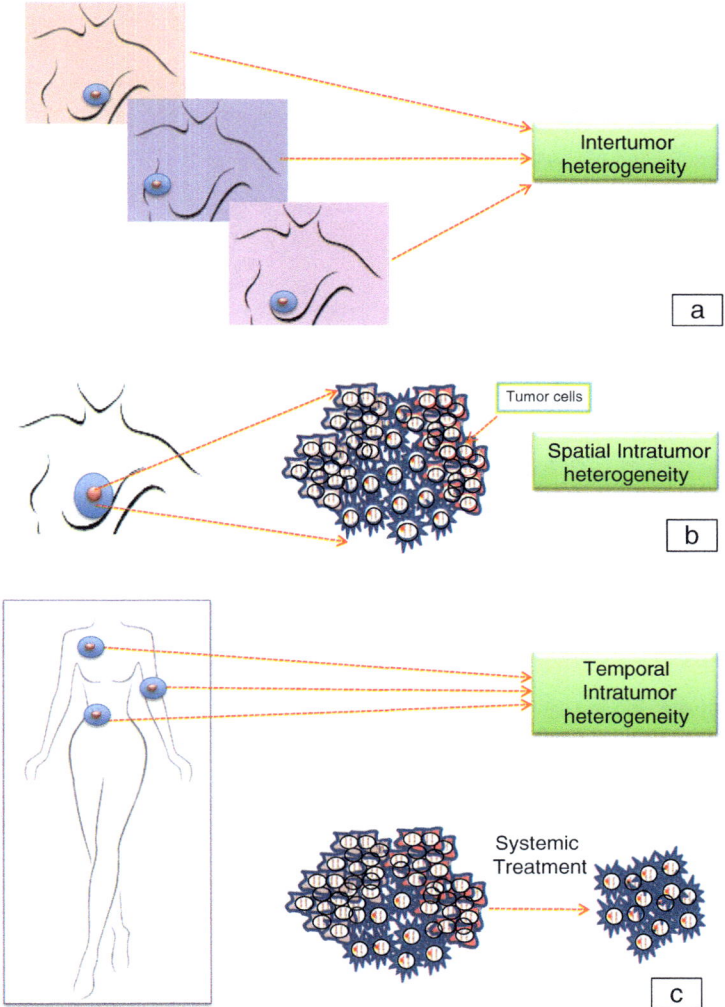

Fig. 9.1 Tumor heterogeneity in breast cancer: (**a**) intertumor heterogeneity, (**b**) spatial intra-tumor heterogeneity, and (**c**) temporal intra-tumor heterogeneity

PCR assay to evaluate three hotspot PIK3CA mutations, which is one of the main gene involved in breast cancer tumorigenesis [3]. Again by comparing healthy women with stage I–III breast cancer patients, it was shown that PIK3CA mutations in ctDNA were only detectable in the latter group [16] with a frequency of 23% (Fig. 9.3). Interestingly, Board et al. detected PIK3CA mutations in ctDNA in 80% of patients with metastatic cancer, demonstrating that advanced patients have more circulating DNA [17]. In another study, it showed that ctDNA was detectable in 86% of patients with advanced breast cancer but only 50% of patients with localized disease and at early stage [18].

Some studies have used baseline ctDNA levels to predict patients' prognosis, but results obtained are contradictory. Iqbal et al. performed a comprehensive analysis of circulating cell-free DNA in serum by the evaluation of DNA integrity index. To this end, qPCR analysis of Alu sequencing using fragments of 115 bp and 247 bp was performed in 148 BC patients at baseline, 47 patients postoperative, and 51 healthy controls. They showed that DNA integrity was significantly higher in stage IV than earlier stages, and it decreases after surgery. Moreover, DNA integrity was able to stratify patients in two groups, relapsed and disease-free patients, with higher DNA integrity in relapsed

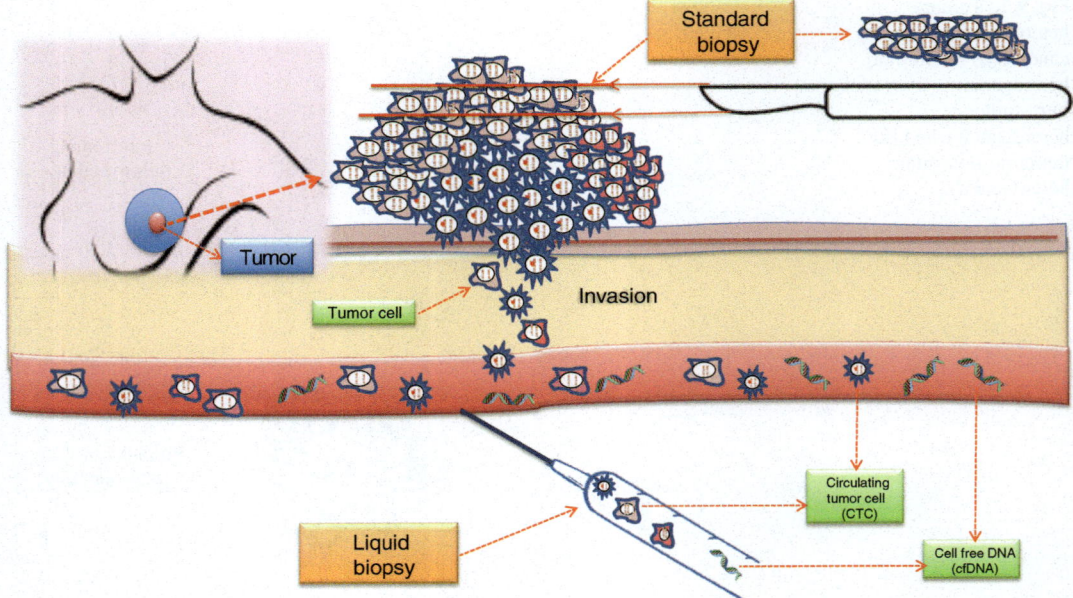

Fig. 9.2 Standard biopsy and liquid biopsy in breast cancer: the differences for a "picture" of disease

Fig. 9.3 Schematic representation of the Oshiro study design

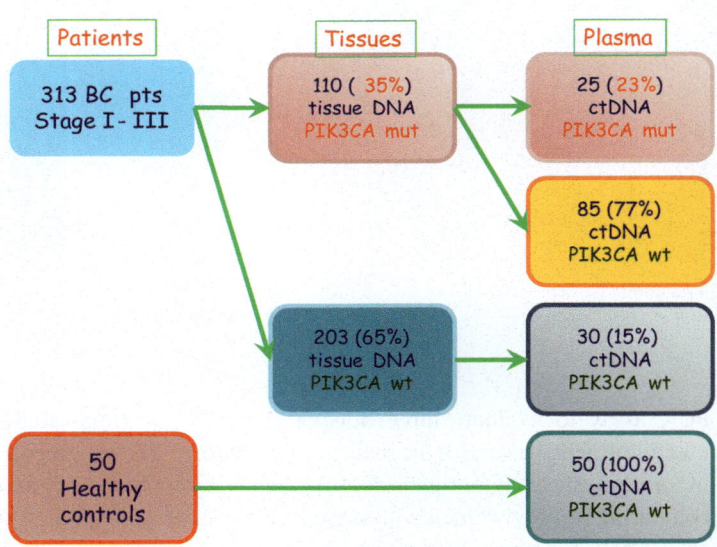

patients. Baseline serum levels of cell-free DNA and its integrity were found thus to be potential prognostic biomarkers in patients with primary breast cancer [19]. On the contrary, it was shown that OS is not associated with ctDNA levels at baseline [20]. Therefore, in contrast with CTCs that have been suggested to be strong prognostic factors, the impact of baseline ctDNA levels is still doubtful [21].

ctDNA may also be used to monitor treatment efficacy. Recent studies in breast cancer patients have found a decrease in ctDNA concentrations after surgery and chemotherapy. This prompted further studies into the use of ctDNA as a marker of treatment response [22]. Dawson et al. have compared ctDNA and CTCs for the monitoring of response to therapy in metastatic breast cancer patients. In this study, somatic mutations and structural variants were first analyzed in tumor tissue and then confirmed in plasma samples using both a microfluidic digital PCR assay and sequencing. ctDNA was detected in 29 of 30 women in 115 of 141 plasma samples collected during 2 years' time. Fluctuations in ctDNA correlate with treatment responses as also confirmed by imaging analysis. For 19 women who had progressive disease on CT imaging, 17 had growing levels of ctDNA, whereas only 7 had also CTC increase. In 10 of the 19 patients with progression, ctDNA increased an average of 5 months before the establishment of progressive disease on imaging. Increasing levels of both ctDNA and CTCs were associated with inferior OS. This group have found that ctDNA have a superior sensitivity and improved correlation with changes in tumor burden, promoting a better measure of treatment effectiveness for metastatic patients [23].

ctDNA can also be used to investigate tumor heterogeneity and clonal evolution. It is known in the literature that the metastatic cancer has different characteristics than the primary tumor [24]. Primary tumor biopsies cannot follow the evolutionary changes between metastatic lesions and primary tumor [25]. Despite these data, the current treatment decisions are often based on the molecular profile of the primary tumor without taking into consideration the heterogeneity of metastatic cancer. Moreover, many patients refuse a second tissue biopsy because the technique is very invasive and painful. Given that the ctDNA is released from all tumor components, it may provide a more complete molecular profile of changing subclone populations and better guide therapy [26]. De Mattos-Arruda et al. examined primitive tumor DNA, liver metastasis DNA, and ctDNA collected from plasma at different time points in one patient with ER+/HER2 invasive ductal lobular carcinoma with liver metastasis. They identified 16 mutations in the liver metastasis, and only 9 were also detectable in the primary tumor. Thus, ctDNA may provide a more complete picture of the mutational landscape of metastatic disease.

Based on the previously mentioned studies, it can be stated that the ctDNA could be become a valid biomarker with applications from diagnosis to prognosis but also for the monitoring of tumor evolution and therapy response, but numerous studies are still needed to go all in one direction.

Minimal Residual Disease (MRD)

Nowadays, one of the main attempts in breast cancer management is testing the feasibility of liquid biopsies to evaluate the minimal residual disease (MRD). The term MRD can be defined as the lowest levels of residual disease after a curative approach either surgical or pharmacological. In fact, evidence of MRD after first-line treatment may be clinically useful to decide whether an adjuvant treatment is requested in order to avoid any possibility of disease recurrence [27].

In the perspective of a painless and noninvasive monitoring of the disease over time, liquid biopsies can be easily used as a feasible tool to monitor MRD also in breast cancer. In particular, MRD represents a higher challenging clinical condition in early-stage tumors (nonmetastatic), while the spread of circulating biomarkers (ctDNA, CTCs) from primary tumor is still not massive. To date, big efforts are still needed to identify which patients, among those who underwent to curative surgery, are completely disease-free from those who still present hidden residual disease that causes relapse. Moreover, a proper evaluation of MRD could spare disease-free patients from receiving useless but still aggressive adjuvant chemotherapy [28]. Therefore, the detection of ctDNA prior and after surgery and/or radiotherapeutic intervention would be fundamental in predicting residual disease [29]. In 2014, Beaver and its group attempted for the first time to highlight the use of liquid biopsy for stratifying patients on the basis of the risk of recurrence in a relatively small cohort of 30 early-stage breast cancer patients. Indeed, by using droplet digital PCR (ddPCR), PIK3CA exon 9 and 20 mutations have been assessed in primary breast tumors and paired pre- and post-surgery plasma samples of ER+/PR+ early-stage breast cancer patients (Fig. 9.4). The presurgery tissue samples have been firstly analyzed by Sanger sequencing for PIK3CA mutations and then confirmed by ddPCR. The digital approach showed five more patients (15/30) positive for

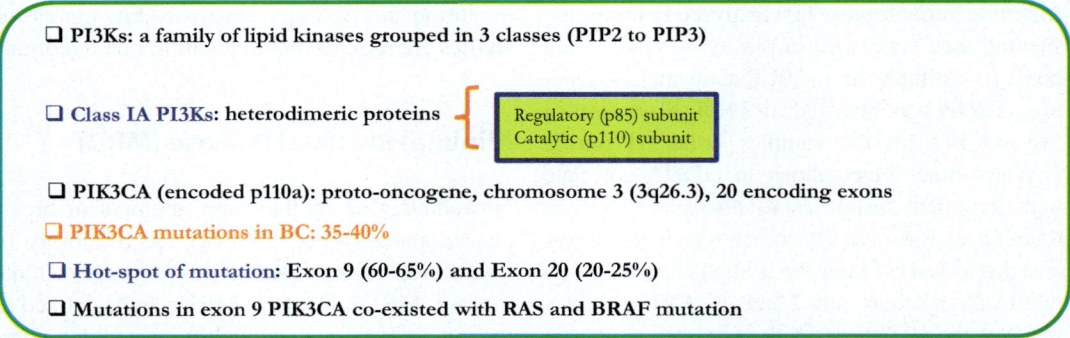

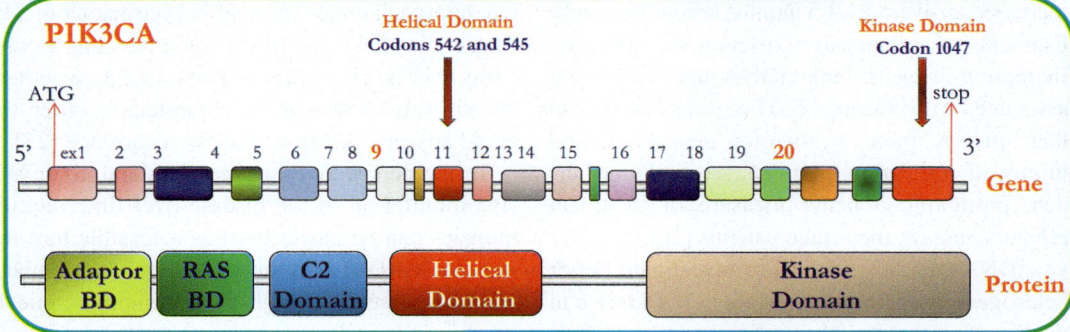

Fig. 9.4 Molecular and biochemical characteristics of PIK3CA domains

PIK3CA mutation with respect to the previous approach. Circulating plasma DNA has been then extracted from pre- and postsurgery blood samples. PIK3CA mutational analysis through ddPCR on presurgery plasma samples showed that of the 15 PIK3CA mutations previously detected in FFPE samples, 14 mutations have been also found in the paired plasma samples with high sensitivity (93.3%) and specificity (100%). Postsurgery plasma samples have been collected, at times ranging from 15 to 72 days after surgery, from 10/15 patients with PIK3CA mutations detected in plasma DNA before surgery. Indeed, five patients had detectable ctDNA demonstrating a still-residual disease despite any clinical or radiological evidence of disease [30]. More recently, Garcia-Murillas et al. have traced PIK3CA mutation in plasma samples to predict relapse in early-stage tumors. In this prospective study, the ddPCR analysis of 55 plasma samples of early breast cancer patients under neoadjuvant chemotherapy was able to anticipate almost

8 months the clinical evidence of metastatic relapse [31]. In 2016, the group of Riva et al. focused on the feasibility of liquid biopsy for the detection of MRD in a cohort of nonmetastatic TBNC patients during neoadjuvant chemotherapy (NCT). Plasma samples were collected at four different time points: before NCT, after one cycle, presurgery, and postsurgery for 36/40 TNBC patients. The analysis of ctDNA has been performed through ddPCR, analyzing TP53 mutations, one of the most common genetic alterations in TNBC. ddPCR analysis showed that before NCT, ctDNA was detected in 27/36 patients, and its levels were significantly correlated with tumor size, tumor stage, as well as mitotic index. After the first NCT cycle, a remarkable decrease of ctDNA levels has been showed for all patients except for one who instead showed increased ctDNA levels. Interestingly, this patient experienced disease progression during chemotherapy. Furthermore, no patients showed detectable ctDNA after surgery [32]. Therefore, liquid

biopsy seems to represent a valuable option in the management and monitoring of breast cancer patients. In particular, in minimal residual disease, the detectability of circulating biomarkers in early-stage disease would open thus the possibility to enroll these patients in specific surveillance programs and consequently get future benefits through longer-term follow-up.

Circulating Tumor Cells (CTCs)

The hematogenous spread of single tumor cells from the primary tumor was first demonstrated in the nineteenth century. In the beginning, the aim was to investigate disseminated tumor cells (DTCs) in the bone marrow. Indeed, in 2005, it was first published a multicenter pooled meta-analysis that assessed the prognostic significance of DTCs in the bone marrow at the time of diagnosis. In particular, the study included 4703 patients diagnosed with stage I, II, and III breast cancer and followed over a 10-year follow-up period. This study highlighted for the first time that patients with bone marrow micrometastasis have larger tumors and tumors with a higher histological grade. Moreover, those patients have lymph node metastasis and hormone-receptor negative tumors. The presence of micrometastasis was a significant prognostic factor with respect to poor overall survival and breast cancer-specific survival (univariate mortality ratios, 2.15 and 2.44, respectively; $p < 0.001$ for both outcomes) and poor disease-free survival and distant-disease-free survival during the 10-year observation period (incidence rate ratios, 2.13 and 2.33, respectively; $p < 0.001$ for both outcomes) (reference).

Nowadays, big efforts are still needed to improve the molecular characterization of a highly heterogeneous tumor. Indeed, studying CTCs would be helpful to improve clinical outcome in particular in triple-negative breast cancer (TNBC). Recently, Angelaki et al. studied CTC phenotype in a cohort including early-stage and metastatic TNBC and hormone-positive breast cancers before and after adjuvant chemotherapy. Expression of ER, PR, CK, HER2, and EGFR on CTCs has been assessed through immunochemistry. In early-stage TNBC, before any adjuvant chemotherapy, the predominant CTC phenotypes were ER+ (24.4%), PR+ (24.4%), CK+/HER2+ (20%), and CK+/EGFR+ (40%). Moreover, in early-stage TNBC, a high risk of relapse is correlated with the CK+/HR- phenotype, and, in particular, the CK+/PR- phenotype is often accompanied by decreased DFI ($p = 0.04$) and OS ($p = 0.032$), demonstrating that these cells may have an aggressive metastatic potential. This study also focused on characterizing CTC subpopulation after adjuvant treatment. Indeed, immunochemistry showed a decreased isolation of HER2-positive CTCs in comparison to ER/PR CTCs. In fact, we can speculate that chemotherapy does not have the same efficacy against all CTC subpopulations. Otherwise, in metastatic cancer, the incidence of CK+/HER2+ CTCs was higher than the early-stage counterpart. Indeed, this finding can predict a more aggressive behavior during disease evolution [33]. The prognostic value of CTC count with respect to the most known unfavorable prognostic factors as progression-free survival (PFS) and overall survivor (OS) has been deeply evaluated in breast cancer. In the study from Bidard et al., CTC count has been evaluated through the CellSearch method before starting a new treatment and after 3–5 and 6–8 weeks after the treatment in a cohort of 2400 patients recruited among 19 different centers. In fact, they demonstrated that a number of five CTCs per 7.5 mL or higher are often associated with decreased PFS and OS if compared with patients with a number of CTCs less than 5 per 7.5 mL. Moreover, increased CTC number both at time 3–5 and 6–8 weeks after the new treatment is significantly correlated with shortened PFS and OS and overall to poorer prognosis [34].

References

1. Ferlay J, Soerjomataram I, Dikshit R, et al. Cancer incidence and mortality worldwide: sources, methods and major patterns in GLOBOCAN 2012. Int J Cancer. 2015;136(5):E359–86.
2. Reis-Filho JS, Pusztai L. Gene expression profiling in breast cancer: classification, prognostication, and prediction. Lancet. 2011;378(9805):1812–23.

3. Network CGA. Comprehensive molecular portraits of human breast tumours. Nature. 2012;490(7418):61–70.

4. Eroles P, Bosch A, Pérez-Fidalgo JA, Lluch A. Molecular biology in breast cancer: intrinsic subtypes and signaling pathways. Cancer Treat Rev. 2012;38(6):698–707.

5. Bedard PL, Hansen AR, Ratain MJ, Siu LL. Tumour heterogeneity in the clinic. Nature. 2013;501(7467): 355–64.

6. Burrell RA, McGranahan N, Bartek J, Swanton C. The causes and consequences of genetic heterogeneity in cancer evolution. Nature. 2013;501(7467): 338–45.

7. Curtit E, Nerich V, Mansi L, et al. Discordances in estrogen receptor status, progesterone receptor status, and HER2 status between primary breast cancer and metastasis. Oncologist. 2013;18(6):667–74.

8. De Mattos-Arruda L, Weigelt B, Cortes J, et al. Capturing intra-tumor genetic heterogeneity by de novo mutation profiling of circulating cell-free tumor DNA: a proof-of-principle. Ann Oncol. 2014;25(9): 1729–35.

9. De Mattos-Arruda L, Caldas C. Cell-free circulating tumour DNA as a liquid biopsy in breast cancer. Mol Oncol. 2016;10(3):464–74.

10. Diehl F, Schmidt K, Choti MA, et al. Circulating mutant DNA to assess tumor dynamics. Nat Med. 2008;14(9):985–90.

11. Loman N, Saal LH. The state of the art in prediction of breast cancer relapse using cell-free circulating tumor DNA liquid biopsies. Ann Transl Med. 2016;4(Suppl 1):S68.

12. Catarino R, Ferreira MM, Rodrigues H, et al. Quantification of free circulating tumor DNA as a diagnostic marker for breast cancer. DNA Cell Biol. 2008;27(8):415–21.

13. Canzoniero JV, Park BH. Use of cell free DNA in breast oncology. Biochim Biophys Acta. 2016; 1865(2):266–74.

14. Chimonidou M, Tzitzira A, Strati A, et al. CST6 promoter methylation in circulating cell-free DNA of breast cancer patients. Clin Biochem. 2013;46(3): 235–40.

15. Dulaimi E, Hillinck J. Ibanez de Caceres I, Al-Saleem T, cairns P. Tumor suppressor gene promoter hypermethylation in serum of breast cancer patients. Clin Cancer Res. 2004;10(18 Pt 1):6189–93.

16. Oshiro C, Kagara N, Naoi Y, et al. PIK3CA mutations in serum DNA are predictive of recurrence in primary breast cancer patients. Breast Cancer Res Treat. 2015;150(2):299–307.

17. Board RE, Wardley AM, Dixon JM, et al. Detection of PIK3CA mutations in circulating free DNA in patients with breast cancer. Breast Cancer Res Treat. 2010;120(2):461–7.

18. Bettegowda C, Sausen M, Leary RJ, et al. Detection of circulating tumor DNA in early- and late-stage human malignancies. Sci Transl Med. 2014;6(224):224ra224.

19. Iqbal S, Vishnubhatla S, Raina V, et al. Circulating cell-free DNA and its integrity as a prognostic marker for breast cancer. Springerplus. 2015;4:265.

20. Bechmann T, Andersen RF, Pallisgaard N, et al. Plasma HER2 amplification in cell-free DNA during neoadjuvant chemotherapy in breast cancer. J Cancer Res Clin Oncol. 2013;139(6):995–1003.

21. Madic J, Kiialainen A, Bidard FC, et al. Circulating tumor DNA and circulating tumor cells in metastatic triple negative breast cancer patients. Int J Cancer. 2015;136(9):2158–65.

22. Forshew T, Murtaza M, Parkinson C, et al. Noninvasive identification and monitoring of cancer mutations by targeted deep sequencing of plasma DNA. Sci Transl Med. 2012;4(136):136ra168.

23. Dawson SJ, Tsui DW, Murtaza M, et al. Analysis of circulating tumor DNA to monitor metastatic breast cancer. N Engl J Med. 2013;368(13):1199–209.

24. Arnedos M, Vicier C, Loi S, et al. Precision medicine for metastatic breast cancer--limitations and solutions. Nat Rev Clin Oncol. 2015;12(12):693–704.

25. Martelotto LG, Ng CK, Piscuoglio S, Weigelt B, Reis-Filho JS. Breast cancer intra-tumor heterogeneity. Breast Cancer Res. 2014;16(3):210.

26. Aparicio S, Caldas C. The implications of clonal genome evolution for cancer medicine. N Engl J Med. 2013;368(9):842–51.

27. Tachtsidis A, McInnes LM, Jacobsen N, Thompson EW, Saunders CM. Minimal residual disease in breast cancer: an overview of circulating and disseminated tumour cells. Clin Exp Metastasis. 2016;33(6):521–50.

28. Siravegna G, Bardelli A. Minimal residual disease in breast cancer: in blood veritas. Clin Cancer Res. 2014a;20(10):2505–7.

29. Siravegna G, Bardelli A. Genotyping cell-free tumor DNA in the blood to detect residual disease and drug resistance. Genome Biol. 2014b;15(8):449.

30. Beaver JA, Jelovac D, Balukrishna S, et al. Detection of cancer DNA in plasma of patients with early-stage breast cancer. Clin Cancer Res. 2014;20(10):2643–50.

31. Garcia-Murillas I, Schiavon G, Weigelt B, Ng C, Hrebien S, Cutts RJ, Cheang M, Osin P, Nerurkar A, Kozarewa I, Garrido JA, Dowsett M, Reis-Filho JS, Smith IE, Turner NC. Mutation tracking in circulating tumor DNA predicts relapse in early breast cancer. Sci Transl Med. 2015 Aug 26;7(302):302ra133.

32. Riva F, Bidard FC, Houy A, et al. Patient-specific circulating tumor DNA detection during neoadjuvant chemotherapy in triple-negative breast cancer. Clin Chem. 2017 Mar;63(3):691–9.

33. Agelaki S, Dragolia M, Markonanolaki H, et al. Phenotypic characterization of circulating tumor cells in triple negative breast cancer patients. Oncotarget. 2017 Jan 17;8(3):5309–22.

34. Bidard FC, Peeters DJ, Fehm T, et al. Clinical validity of circulating tumour cells in patients with metastatic breast cancer: a pooled analysis of individual patient data. Lancet Oncol. 2014;15(4):406–14.

Liquid Biopsy in Gynecological Cancers

10

M. Castiglia, A. Listì, L. Incorvaia, V. Chiantera, and Antonio Russo

Introduction

Gynecological cancers originate in woman's reproductive organs, including ovarian, uterine or endometrial, cervical, vulvar, and vaginal cancers (Fig. 10.1). These tumors represent a leading health problem in women accounting for more than the 20% of new cases and cancer-related deaths worldwide [1]. The American Cancer Society estimated that in 2017, there will be 22,440 new cases of ovarian cancer with 14,080 associated deaths; 12,820 new diagnosis and 4210 related deaths have been estimated for cervical cancer, as well as 61,380 new cases and 10,920 deaths for endometrial cancer. Finally, they expect around 6020 new diagnosis and 1150 deaths for vulvar cancer and 4810 new cases and 1240 deaths for vaginal cancers. Among this wide spectrum of tumors, endometrial cancer has the highest incidence, while ovarian cancer has the highest mortality (Figs. 10.2 and 10.3). However,

the gynecological cancers have a heterogeneous distribution worldwide, especially HPV-related cancers, for which the major incidence and mortality have been recorded in sub-Saharan Africa, Asia, and Central and South America, but also in Hispanic, African, and Indian minorities in the USA, the UK, and Canada [2]. Particularly this distribution highlights a great disparity of safety rate for women who live in low developed countries in which the local organizations and investments in health care do not ensure early diagnosis and access to optimal treatments to prevent and control such disease and ultimately increase patients' survival [3].

Gynecological cancers are characterized by an aggressive biological behavior with a clinical presentation often in advanced stage of disease. Since the diagnosis is usually performed late, the survival rate associated with these tumors is very low also because the treatment regimens are not much effective. Gynecological cancers include different types of disease, which are classified by the International Classification of Diseases (ICD), in which the malignant neoplasms of

M. Castiglia and A. Listì authors contributed equally to this work.

M. Castiglia • A. Listì • L. Incorvaia
Department of Surgical, Oncogical and Oral Sciences, Section of Medical Oncology, University of Palermo, Via del Vespro 127, Palermo 90127, Italy

V. Chiantera
Department of Gynaecology, Charité University, Hindenburgdamm, Berlin, Germany

Department of Gynecology Oncology, University Hospital "Paolo Giaccone", Palermo, Italy

A. Russo (✉)
Department of Surgical, Oncogical and Oral Sciences, Section of Medical Oncology, University of Palermo, Via del Vespro 127, Palermo 90127, Italy

Institute for Cancer Research and Molecular Medicine and Center of Biotechnology, College of Science and Biotechnology, Philadelphia, PA, USA
e-mail: antonio.russo@usa.net

© Springer International Publishing AG 2017
A. Giordano et al. (eds.), *Liquid Biopsy in Cancer Patients*, Current Clinical Pathology,
DOI 10.1007/978-3-319-55661-1_10

female genital organs are coded from C51 to C58 (Table 10.1). To define both the site of origin and histology of the gynecological cancers, it'is used the International Classification of Diseases for Oncology (ICD-O-3), a multi-axel classification obtained from a pathology report. Furthermore, another classification is used as cancer staging system to describe the anatomical extent of tumors, the so-called Tumour Node Metastasis Classification of Malignant Tumours (TNM-6) approved by the International Federation of Gynecology and Obstetrics (FIGO).

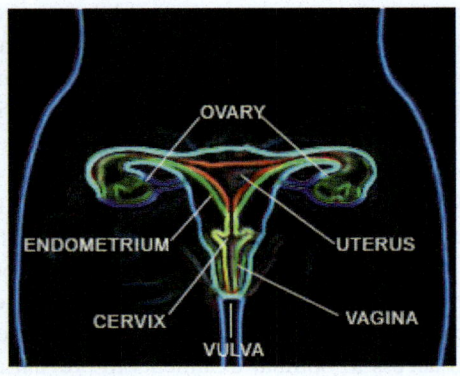

Fig. 10.1 Anatomical districts of female reproductive organs

Vulvar Cancer

The majority of cancers of the vulva are squamous cell carcinomas, including the keratinizing type, which usually develops in older women and is not linked to human papilloma virus (HPV) infections, and the rare basaloid type, which is most commonly detected in young women with HPV infections. The 5-year survival rate is strictly related to the clinical stage of presentation, ranging from 86% to 16% in patients with local and advanced diseases, respectively. Surgery is the gold standard for localized disease, while both radiotherapy and platinum-based chemotherapy can be combined with surgery to treat more advanced-stage cancers [4].

Vaginal Cancer

About 70% of vaginal cancers are squamous cell carcinomas originating from the squamous cells of epithelial lining of the vagina, while only a minority of them are adenocarcinomas. Squamous cell carcinoma usually occurs in older (>70 years or older), and their 5-year survival rate ranges from 84% for localized disease to

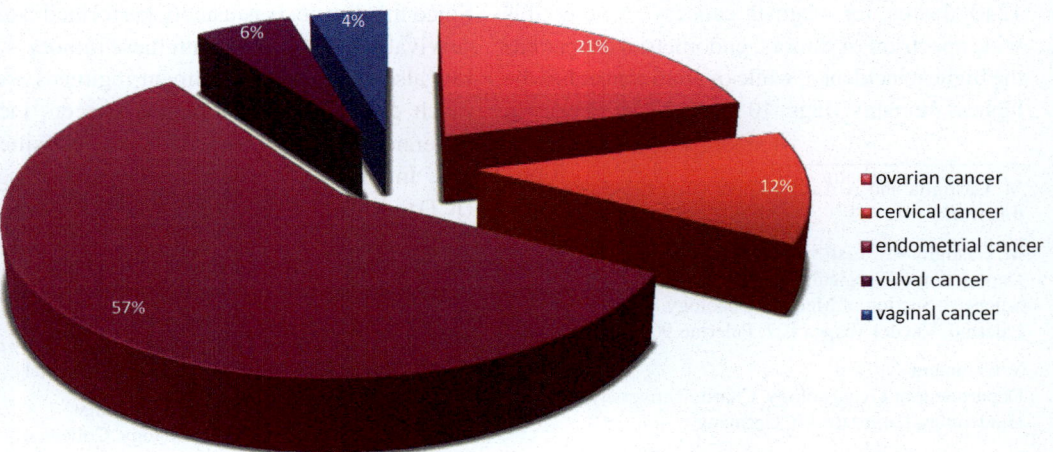

Fig. 10.2 Incidence of gynecological cancers estimated for 2017 (American Cancer Society)

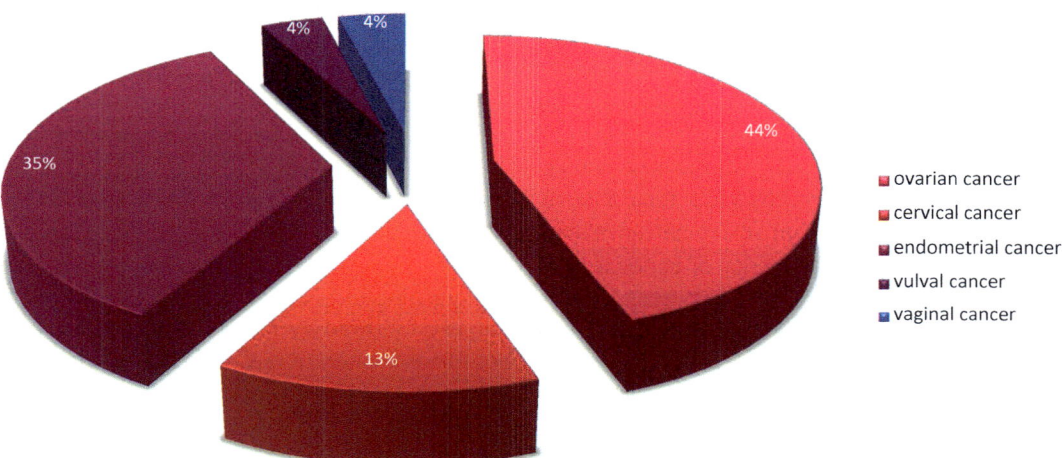

Deaths estimated for 201 7

- ovarian cancer
- cervical cancer
- endometrial cancer
- vulval cancer
- vaginal cancer

Fig. 10.3 Mortality associated with gynecological cancers estimated for 2017 (American Cancer Society)

Table 10.1 International Classification of Diseases (ICD) for gynecological cancers, new cases, and deaths recorded for gynecological cancer in 2016

ICD	Cancer site	New cases estimated 2016	Death estimated 2016
C53	Cervix (uterus)	12,990	4120
C54	Endometrius (uterus)	60,050	10,470
C56	Ovary	22,280	14,240
C51	Vulva	5950	1110
C52/C57	Vagina and other female genital organs	4620	950

57% for advanced-stage III–IV diseases. Radiotherapy represents the most common treatment of vaginal cancer, while surgery is limited to early stage I diseases and for patients who are not eligible to radiation. Particularly combining both external radiotherapy and intracavitary brachytherapy with or without low-dose chemotherapy represents the most effective treatment approach [5].

Cervical Cancer

Cervical cancer originates from the cervix, which connects the vagina with the body of the uterus. The main cause of squamous cell carcinomas is a persistent sexually transmitted infection caused by the human papilloma virus (HPV). HPV infects the basal cells of the cervical epithelium and other epithelial tissues upon microtrauma of tissues and cells. Approximately 100 types of HPV virus have been identified and considered as oncogenic; particularly the 6, 11, 16, and 18 types of HPV are responsible for the occurrence of the majority of cervical, as well as penile, vulvar, vaginal, anal, and oropharyngeal cancers.

Two main strategies, including the regular screening test and the HPV (bivalent or quadrivalent) vaccines, have been adopted by the national health systems in developed countries, in order to identify the high-risk population and to prevent cancer development. The two screening tests adopted to favor early diagnosis of cervical cancer are the PAP test, starting at 21 years old, which aims to identify precancerous lesions on the cervix which may be suitable to radical treatment, and the HPV-DNA test, starting at 30 or older, which is used to identify the presence of HPV infection that predisposes to cancer development. To date a key role on the prevention is played by the vaccine [6]. Thanks to the advent of cervical screening test, the cervical cancer death rate has gone down by more than 50% in the last years, with about 4210 cancer-related expected in 2017. The majority of cervical cancers occur in young women between 20 and 50 years old, but about 20% of cases are currently detected in women older than 65. Surgery is a curative treatment for early diseases. There are several types of surgery, including cryosurgery, laser surgery, and conization, which are currently used to treat squamous cell carcinoma in situ, while radical hysterectomy is the gold standard for invasive localized cancers. Cisplatin-based chemotherapy with or without radiotherapy represents the main treatment option for patients in advanced clinical stages [7].

Liquid Biopsy in Cervical Cancer

Since HPV is the main cause of cervical cancer, it has been recently investigated whether HPV-DNA can be detected in blood for a better patient clinical monitoring. Nevertheless, the data concerning human circulating HPV-DNA have provided inconsistent results mainly due to technical reasons. Indeed the detection techniques used until now were not sensitive enough for the identification of small-sized tumors. With the advent of more sensitive methods, such as droplet digital PCR (ddPCR), it is becoming easier to work with material that requires an adequate sensitivity. In a recent paper, 70 serum specimens were retrospectively analyzed in patients with HPV-16 or HPV-18 carcinomas. They investigated whether ddPCR was able to detect HPV-DNA in serum, reporting that in 61 out of 70 serum samples, HPV-DNA was detectable, and therefore this innovative technique is a promising method for cervical cancer patient monitoring [8].

Endometrial Cancer

The two types of cancer that may affect uterus are endometrial carcinoma and uterine sarcoma. The majority of endometrial carcinomas are adenocarcinoma defined also as endometrioid cancers and are usually detected in women older than 60 years. The endometrium is an inner lining of the uterus, and it is hormonally sensitive; thus, both estrogens and progesterone are needed to maintain its cyclical operations. To date there are no screening tests approved for early diagnosis. Surgery followed by radiotherapy with or without chemotherapy represents the optimal treatment for patients with localized disease. Platinum-based chemotherapy is the standard treatment for advanced stages [9].

Ovarian Cancer

Ovarian cancer is the second most common gynecological malignancy often diagnosed at advanced stages (75–80% of cases) with overall 5-year survival rate around 40% despite significant improvements in surgical and systemic management of patients. Epithelial ovarian cancers (EOCs) are the most common subtype, classified according to the grade of malignancy as high-/low-grade or borderline tumors. Unfortunately, 70% of EOC are diagnosed at advanced stage and are characterized by a very poor prognosis. The reasons of delayed diagnosis are partly due to lack of sensitive signs and symptoms and effective screening methods [10]. Ovarian carcinomas represent about 85–90% of ovarian tumors and are further classified according to histological criteria as serous (the most frequent), clear cell, endometrioid, and mucinous carcinomas. The treatment of EOC consists in both cytoreductive surgery (whenever possible) and platinum-based chemotherapy [11, 12]. Platinum-based chemotherapy may be used as adjuvant/neoadjuvant treatment for early stages or as first-line therapy for metastatic disease, with 5-year survival rates ranging from 90% (stage I) to 20% (stage IV). Anti-angiogenic agents, such as bevacizumab, may be combined with chemotherapy both in first-line and at recurrence to further improve patients' outcomes. The majority of ovarian carcinomas are sporadic. An inherited susceptibility to EOC is present in at least 15% of patients, the vast majority of which are caused by germline mutations in BRCA1 or BRCA2 genes that define the hereditary breast and ovarian cancer syndrome (HBOC) [13]. Heterozygous carriers of germline BRCA1 or BRCA2 mutations have an increased lifetime risk of developing ovarian cancer, respectively, of 40–60% and 11–30%. Other genes can be involved in HBOC susceptibility including some genes encoding for proteins involved in homologous recombination (HR) DNA repair pathway, such as RAD50, RAD51C, RAD51D, PALB2, CHEK2, MRE11A, BARD1, BRIP 1, NBS1, and ATM [14].

Ovarian cancer in patients with a BRCA1 or BRCA2 germline mutation is associated with several clinical characteristics including an increased likelihood of platinum sensitivity and improved survival compared with those with non-BRCA-related ovarian cancer. Furthermore, poly(ADP-ribose) polymerase (PARP) inhibitors have shown exceptional clinical activity in this subgroup of patients [15, 16]. PARP inhibitors exploit the concept of "synthetic lethality," which describes the situation when a mutation in either of two genes individually has no effect, but in combination leads to cell death. The clinical relevance is that the significant activity of PARP inhibitors may not be limited to germline BRCA-mutated ovarian cancer, but indeed extends to a larger group of sporadic ovarian cancer patients with homologous recombination deficiency (HRD) [17]. To date, BRCA1 and BRCA2 mutations are the most significant molecular aberrations, which have shown both prognostic and predictive value in ovarian cancer patients.

To date, the cancer antigen-125, (CA-125) is the most common biomarker used to monitor the response to therapy and identify the disease relapse/progression in ovarian cancer patients. However, because of its low sensitivity (50–62% for early-stage epithelial ovarian cancer) and specificity (94–98.5%), CA-125 is not usable as screening tool in asymptomatic women.

Moreover, CA-125 has a limited application in guiding treatment choice and does not provide any predictive information [18]. Therefore, new markers for early detection, improved knowledge of the molecular biology, better innovative treatment options, and predictive biomarkers are urgently requested in EOC. As for other tumor types, also for EOC liquid biopsy may become a valid and easy method for a better patient management from diagnosis to treatment.

Circulating Tumor Cells (CTC) in EOC

Prognostic and Predictive Value

Several studies have demonstrated that tumor cell dissemination may occur in gynecological cancer and may affect clinical outcome. In particular disseminated tumor cells detected in bone marrow have been shown to correlate with shorter disease-free survival in 25% of EOC patients [19]. Nevertheless, bone marrow sampling is not easy and not always feasible. Otherwise, the identification of CTCs in peripheral blood is always feasible, and it is repeatable at different time points during treatment.

CTC assessment remains difficult because they are outnumbered by white blood cells (WBC) by at least a factor of 10^6 [20, 21]. The mostly used approach for CTC detection is, nowadays, the positive immunomagnetic enrichment based on frequently expressed surface markers. Indeed the CellSearch™ system, the first FDA-approved method for CTC isolation, is based on immunomagnetic enrichment using anti-EpCAM together with a depletion of white blood cells through anti-CD45 antibody. These methods are often coupled with reverse transcription polymerase chain reaction (RT-PCR) or immunocytochemistry (ICC) for visualization and quantification of CTCs.

In a recent meta-analysis, it has been evaluated the association between CTC and DTCs with different clinical pathological features in ovarian cancer [22]. The meta-analysis included 16 studies for a total of 1623 patients but with different detection methods (RT-PCR,

CellSearch, cell invasion assay, IHC); the study revealed that CTC/DTC are not significantly associated with tumor histology (OR = 0.71 [0.49, 1.05]), lymph node metastasis (OR 1.14 [0.67, 1.93]), and optimal or suboptimal surgery (OR 1.45 [0.90, 2.34]). On the contrary an increased number of CTC/DTC is associated with advanced tumor stage (III–IV stages; OR = 1.90 [1.02, 3.56]) and both OS (HR 1.94 [1.56–2.40]) and PFS/DFS (HR 1.99 [1.59–2.50]). In two of the 16 studies included in the meta-analysis, it was questioned the relationship between CTCs and treatment response suggesting that a reduction of CTCs after treatment strongly correlates with better response (pooled OR = 0.55; 95% CI: 0.34–0.90) [22].

Another meta-analysis, based on 11 publications for a total of 1129 patients, evaluated the prognostic value of CTC in ovarian cancer patients, but they also make a subgroup analysis according to the isolation techniques used ("RT-PCR," "CellSearch," and "other ICC" subgroup). They showed that both OS and PFS/DFS are significantly associated with CTC status (HR, 1.61; 95% CI, 1.22–2.13; HR, 1.44; 95% CI, 1.18–1.75, respectively). Moreover, the subgroup analysis revealed that the value of CTC status in OS was significant in the "RT-PCR" subgroup (HR, 2.02; 95% CI, 1.34–3.03), whereas it was not significant in "CellSearch" subgroup (HR, 1.15; 95% CI 0.45–2.92) and "other ICC" subgroup (HR, 1.09; 95% CI 0.62–1.90) [23].

These meta-analyses were conducted mainly in advanced ovarian cancer population, but what it needed is to improve the detection method also for early-stage disease. Indeed it has been recently developed a CAM-initiated CTC enrichment/identification method for invasive CTC (iCTCs) also in early EOC stages. The reported sensitivity and specificity was 41.2% and 95.1%, respectively, for stage I and II malignancy. When all stages of EOC were considered, sensitivity increased to 83%, with 97.3% positive predictive value (PPV). Moreover, it is shown that elevated iCTCs better correlate to OS, PFS, and other clinical factors (tumor stage, debulking, and platinum sensitivity) than CA-125 serum marker [24].

CTCs can also be used for treatment monitoring of EOC patients; indeed the study proposed by Pearl et al. aimed at the evaluation of iCTC in monitoring EOC patient response to treatment compared with CA-125 serum marker [25]. In this study iCTCs were detected in each of the 31 patients monitored. Furthermore, an increase in iCTC was reported to be more sensitive than CA-125 in predicting PD or relapse [25].

CTC may also be used in the identification of treatment-resistant patients at diagnosis. In particular in a recent study, ERCC1-positive CTCs have been reported to predict platinum resistance in EOC patients. CTCs were first immunomagnetically enriched (using EpCAM and MUC1 antigens) and then characterized by RT-PCR to detect the transcripts of EPCAM, MUC1, CA-125, and ERCC1. At primary diagnosis, the presence of CTC was observed in 14% of patients and constituted an independent predictor of OS. ERCC1-positive CTCs were observed in 8% of patients and constituted an independent predictor, not only for OS but also for PFS. Interestingly the presence of ERCC1-positive CTC at primary diagnosis was shown to be likewise an independent predictor of platinum resistance [26].

Circulating Tumor DNA (ctDNA) in EOC

Circulating tumor DNA represents a powerful biomarker for detecting occult disease in EOC; indeed no currently used biomarkers or imaging techniques can predict outcome following initial treatment. Therefore, several research groups are investigating the use of personalized ctDNA markers as both a surveillance and a prognostic biomarker in gynecological cancers and compared this to current FDA-approved surveillance tools. It is fundamental to develop more sensitive and accurate biomarkers for both an earlier diagnosis and for a more effective surveillance in the posttreatment setting. We already know that EOC is frequently diagnosed in advanced stages and patients are managed by surgical resection followed by a combination of platinum- and taxane-based chemotherapy. Moreover, using the current detection technologies, around 80% of these patients will appear to have a complete clinical response to therapy even if more than half will relapse within 18 months. Both CA-125 and imaging modalities (e.g., computed tomography) lack sensitivity and often remain inconclusive or delayed in demonstrating PD [27–29]. ctDNA as well as CTC may represent a valid tool for diagnosis and monitoring. The first studies exploring cell-free DNA in gynecological malignances were first published more than 10 years ago [30, 31]. In these early papers, the aim was only to quantify cell-free DNA (cfDNA) and its absolute concentration with disease stage [31]. By then new sequencing technologies and analytical techniques have definitely improved the ability to detect ctDNA and to monitor disease molecular changes over time. In 2014 a very interesting case report demonstrated the ability to serially track disease over time [32]. In the study was reported the case of a single patient with a tumor-specific fusion event in which ctDNA analysis was more sensitive than CA-125. The patient was monitored for 4 years during which she underwent to primary debulking surgery and chemotherapy, tumor recurrences, and multiple chemotherapeutic regimens. During this follow-up period, CA-125 levels were elevated only three times in 28 measurements, whereas the tumor-specific fusion event was readily detectable in ctDNA by quantitative real-time reverse transcription polymerase chain reaction (PCR) in the same blood samples and in the tumor recurrence [32]. Then the same group performed a larger study in a cohort of 44 patients including ovarian and other gynecological malignancies. Tumor mutation profiles were first obtained through whole exome sequencing (WES) and directed gene sequencing panel and afterward used to generate patient-derived panels of ctDNA biomarkers to be tested using droplet digital PCR (ddPCR). The results demonstrated that serial measurement of ctDNA is as sensitive and specific as CA-125, with the advantage to enable disease relapse detection months earlier

than CT scanning. Moreover, the measurement of ctDNA levels at the time of completion of initial therapy, debulking surgery, and combination platinum/taxane doublet chemotherapy provides prognostic information. Indeed, undetectable levels of ctDNA were associated with both improved PFS and OS [33].

Aside from analyzing point mutation, ctDNA offers the possibility to identify also chromosomal rearrangements. These rearrangements have to be first detected in tumor tissue and subsequently investigated in plasma samples using real-time PCR techniques. This approach was recently used by Harris et al. in a series of ten EOC patients with stage IIIC-IV disease [34]. Primary tumor samples were first analyzed through next-generation sequencing (NGS) in order to identify genomic rearrangements; once the specific alterations were recorded, individualized monitoring panels were developed and used for ctDNA analysis. Using this approach, it was possible to monitor cancer patients for relapse and therapeutic efficacy using cfDNA [34].

Exosome and Circulating miRNA in EOC

It has been shown that exosomes can be detected in ovarian cancer patients' plasma, serum, and ascites [35, 36] and multiple components of cancer exosomes have the potential to be used as biomarkers and therapeutic targets for the disease [37]. In particular exosomes contain miRNA that have been shown to be functional; moreover, exosomal miRNAs have a characteristic signature. Indeed exosomal miRNA profile is similar to miRNA profile of tumor cells, and it is unique compared to exosomes isolated from patients with benign ovarian tumors [38, 39].

Exosomes can be used as diagnostic/screening tool but also as prognostic and predictive biomarker for response to treatment in EOC patients. In 2016 it has been investigated the diagnostic and prognostic relevance of exosomal miR-373, miR-200a, miR-200b, and miR-200c and circulating exosomes in a cohort of 163 EOC patients [40]. Compared to healthy women, levels of miR-373, miR-200a, miR-200b, and miR-200c and circulating exosomes were significantly increased in EOC patients; moreover, the levels of miR-200a, miR-200b, and miR-200c were able to distinguish between malignant and benign ovarian tumors. Looking at stages, it was shown that miR-373 and miR-200a were increased in all tumor stages, while miR-200c and miR-200b were higher in stages III–IV and then stages I–II. These miRNAs were also validated in a subgroup of 112 high-grade ovarian cancers.

Resistance is the main cause for treatment failure and it is important to identify markers for patient's stratification. It has been reported that exosomes are able to pack cisplatin and to export the drug out from cancer cells leading to treatment inefficacy [41]. In addition, exosomes released from platinum-resistant ovarian cancer cells are able to transfer resistance to platinum-sensitive cells; this effect seems to be mediated by miR-21-3p contained and vehicled by exosomes [42]. Exosomal miR-433 contributes to paclitaxel resistance in A2780 ovarian cancer cells by inhibiting apoptosis and inducing cellular senescence [43]. Another resistance mechanism that seems mediated by exosomes is the seizure/sequestration of immunotherapeutic agents. In particular it has been recently reported that exosomes secreted from HER2-overexpressing cancer cells expressed HER2 on their surface; they can therefore bind to anti-HER2 monoclonal antibody (trastuzumab) interfering with the drug activity [44]. It is therefore plausible that an analysis of the concentration, content, and activity of exosomes could be used as a predictive marker for response to treatment.

Despite the promising expectations for exosome application in the management of EOC patients, there are still several challenges that need to be met before the definitive introduction in clinical practice. It is primarily requested a standardization of methods used for exosome isolation from peripheral blood and for the separation from normal physiologic circulating exosomes. Moreover, it is still needed a clinical validation of exosome analysis that would be achieved through big clinical trial developments.

References

1. Ferlay J, Steliarova-Foucher E, Lortet-Tieulent J, et al. Cancer incidence and mortality patterns in Europe: estimates for 40 countries in 2012. Eur J Cancer. 2013;49(6):1374–403.
2. Zhou Y, Irwin ML, Ferrucci LM, et al. Health-related quality of life in ovarian cancer survivors: results from the American Cancer Society's study of cancer survivors - I. Gynecol Oncol. 2016;141(3):543–9.
3. Ferlay J, Soerjomataram I, Dikshit R, et al. Cancer incidence and mortality worldwide: sources, methods and major patterns in GLOBOCAN 2012. Int J Cancer. 2015;136(5):E359–86.
4. Gentileschi S, Servillo M, Garganese G, et al. Surgical therapy of vulvar cancer: how to choose the correct reconstruction? J Gynecol Oncol. 2016;27(6):e60.
5. Prameela CG, Ravind R, Gurram BC, Sheejamol VS, Dinesh M. Prognostic factors in primary vaginal cancer: a single institute experience and review of literature. J Obstet Gynaecol India. 2016;66(5):363–71.
6. Sangar VC, Ghongane B, Mathur G. Development of human papillomavirus (HPV) vaccines: a review of literature and clinical update. Rev Recent Clin Trials. 2016;11(4):284–9.
7. Ginsburg O, Bray F, Coleman MP, et al. The global burden of women's cancers: a grand challenge in global health. Lancet. 2017;389(10071):847–60.
8. Jeannot E, Becette V, Campitelli M, et al. Circulating human papillomavirus DNA detected using droplet digital PCR in the serum of patients diagnosed with early stage human papillomavirus-associated invasive carcinoma. J Pathol Clin Res. 2016;2(4):201–9.
9. Brasseur K, Gévry N, Asselin E. Chemoresistance and targeted therapies in ovarian and endometrial cancers. Oncotarget. 2016;8:4008–42.
10. Jacobs IJ, Menon U. Progress and challenges in screening for early detection of ovarian cancer. Mol Cell Proteomics. 2004;3(4):355–66.
11. Ozols RF, Bundy BN, Greer BE, et al. Phase III trial of carboplatin and paclitaxel compared with cisplatin and paclitaxel in patients with optimally resected stage III ovarian cancer: a gynecologic oncology group study. J Clin Oncol. 2003;21(17):3194–200.
12. Yap TA, Carden CP, Kaye SB. Beyond chemotherapy: targeted therapies in ovarian cancer. Nat Rev Cancer. 2009;9(3):167–81.
13. Candido-dos-Reis FJ, Song H, Goode EL, et al. Germline mutation in BRCA1 or BRCA2 and ten-year survival for women diagnosed with epithelial ovarian cancer. Clin Cancer Res. 2015;21(3):652–7.
14. Incorvaia L, Passiglia F, Rizzo S, et al. "Back to a false normality": new intriguing mechanisms of resistance to PARP inhibitors. Oncotarget. 2016; doi:10.18632/oncotarget.14409.
15. Ledermann JA, Harter P, Gourley C, et al. Overall survival in patients with platinum-sensitive recurrent serous ovarian cancer receiving olaparib maintenance monotherapy: an updated analysis from a randomised, placebo-controlled, double-blind, phase 2 trial. Lancet Oncol. 2016a;17(11):1579–89.

16. Ledermann J, Harter P, Gourley C, et al. Olaparib maintenance therapy in patients with platinum-sensitive relapsed serous ovarian cancer: a preplanned retrospective analysis of outcomes by BRCA status in a randomised phase 2 trial. Lancet Oncol. 2014; 15(8):852–61.

17. Ledermann JA, Drew Y, Kristeleit RS. Homologous recombination deficiency and ovarian cancer. Eur J Cancer. 2016b;60:49–58.

18. Sölétormos G, Duffy MJ, Othman Abu Hassan S, et al. Clinical use of cancer biomarkers in epithelial ovarian cancer: updated guidelines from the European group on tumor markers. Int J Gynecol Cancer. 2016;26(1):43–51.

19. Banys M, Solomayer EF, Becker S, et al. Disseminated tumor cells in bone marrow may affect prognosis of patients with gynecologic malignancies. Int J Gynecol Cancer. 2009;19(5):948–52.

20. Banys-Paluchowski M, Krawczyk N, Meier-Stiegen F, Fehm T. Circulating tumor cells in breast cancer-current status and perspectives. Crit Rev Oncol Hematol. 2016;97:22–9.

21. Mostert B, Sleijfer S, Foekens JA, Gratama JW. Circulating tumor cells (CTCs): detection methods and their clinical relevance in breast cancer. Cancer Treat Rev. 2009;35(5):463–74.

22. Cui L, Kwong J, Wang CC. Prognostic value of circulating tumor cells and disseminated tumor cells in patients with ovarian cancer: a systematic review and meta-analysis. J Ovarian Res. 2015;8:38.

23. Zhou Y, Bian B, Yuan X, Xie G, Ma Y, Shen L. Prognostic value of circulating tumor cells in ovarian cancer: a meta-analysis. PLoS One. 2015;10(6): e0130873.

24. Pearl ML, Zhao Q, Yang J, et al. Prognostic analysis of invasive circulating tumor cells (iCTCs) in epithelial ovarian cancer. Gynecol Oncol. 2014;134(3):581–90.

25. Pearl ML, Dong H, Tulley S, et al. Treatment monitoring of patients with epithelial ovarian cancer using invasive circulating tumor cells (iCTCs). Gynecol Oncol. 2015;137(2):229–38.

26. Kuhlmann JD, Wimberger P, Bankfalvi A, et al. ERCC1-positive circulating tumor cells in the blood of ovarian cancer patients as a predictive biomarker for platinum resistance. Clin Chem. 2014;60(10): 1282–9.

27. Buys SS, Partridge E, Black A, et al. Effect of screening on ovarian cancer mortality: the prostate, lung, colorectal and ovarian (PLCO) cancer screening randomized controlled trial. JAMA. 2011;305(22): 2295–303.

28. Meyer T, Rustin GJ. Role of tumour markers in monitoring epithelial ovarian cancer. Br J Cancer. 2000;82(9):1535–8.

29. Testa AC, Di Legge A, Virgilio B, et al. Which imaging technique should we use in the follow up of gynaecological cancer? Best Pract Res Clin Obstet Gynaecol. 2014;28(5):769–91.

30. Chang HW, Lee SM, Goodman SN, et al. Assessment of plasma DNA levels, allelic imbalance, and CA 125 as diagnostic tests for cancer. J Natl Cancer Inst. 2002;94(22):1697–703.

31. Kamat AA, Sood AK, Dang D, Gershenson DM, Simpson JL, Bischoff FZ. Quantification of total plasma cell-free DNA in ovarian cancer using real-time PCR. Ann N Y Acad Sci. 2006;1075:230–4.

32. Martignetti JA, Camacho-Vanegas O, Priedigkeit N, et al. Personalized ovarian cancer disease surveillance and detection of candidate therapeutic drug target in circulating tumor DNA. Neoplasia. 2014;16(1):97–103.

33. Pereira E, Camacho-Vanegas O, Anand S, et al. Personalized circulating tumor DNA biomarkers dynamically predict treatment response and survival in gynecologic cancers. PLoS One. 2015;10(12):e0145754.

34. Harris FR, Kovtun IV, Smadbeck J, et al. Quantification of somatic chromosomal rearrangements in circulating cell-free DNA from ovarian cancers. Sci Rep. 2016;6:29831.

35. Runz S, Keller S, Rupp C, et al. Malignant ascites-derived exosomes of ovarian carcinoma patients contain CD24 and EpCAM. Gynecol Oncol. 2007;107(3):563–71.

36. Shender VO, Pavlyukov MS, Ziganshin RH, et al. Proteome-metabolome profiling of ovarian cancer ascites reveals novel components involved in intercellular communication. Mol Cell Proteomics. 2014;13(12):3558–71.

37. Li M, Rai AJ, DeCastro GJ, et al. An optimized procedure for exosome isolation and analysis using serum samples: application to cancer biomarker discovery. Methods. 2015;87:26–30.

38. Taylor DD, Gercel-Taylor C. MicroRNA signatures of tumor-derived exosomes as diagnostic biomarkers of ovarian cancer. Gynecol Oncol. 2008;110(1):13–21.

39. Tang MK, Wong AS. Exosomes: emerging biomarkers and targets for ovarian cancer. Cancer Lett. 2015;367(1):26–33.

40. Meng X, Müller V, Milde-Langosch K, Trillsch F, Pantel K, Schwarzenbach H. Diagnostic and prognostic relevance of circulating exosomal miR-373, miR-200a, miR-200b and miR-200c in patients with epithelial ovarian cancer. Oncotarget. 2016;7(13): 16923–35.

41. Safaei R, Larson BJ, Cheng TC, et al. Abnormal lysosomal trafficking and enhanced exosomal export of cisplatin in drug-resistant human ovarian carcinoma cells. Mol Cancer Ther. 2005;4(10):1595–604.

42. Pink RC, Samuel P, Massa D, Caley DP, Brooks SA, Carter DR. The passenger strand, miR-21-3p, plays a role in mediating cisplatin resistance in ovarian cancer cells. Gynecol Oncol. 2015;137(1):143–51.

43. Weiner-Gorzel K, Dempsey E, Milewska M, et al. Overexpression of the microRNA miR-433 promotes resistance to paclitaxel through the induction of cellular senescence in ovarian cancer cells. Cancer Med. 2015;4(5):745–58.

44. Ciravolo V, Huber V, Ghedini GC, et al. Potential role of HER2-overexpressing exosomes in countering trastuzumab-based therapy. J Cell Physiol. 2012; 227(2):658–67.

Liquid Biopsy in Prostate Cancer

11

A. Galvano, K. Papadimitriou, B. Di Stefano, M. Castiglia, and Christian Rolfo

Introduction

Until few years ago, the treatment of prostate cancer (PCa) in advanced stage was based exclusively on the use of chemotherapy, showing very modest outcomes. The understanding of the molecular mechanisms that regulate the pathogenesis and progression of PCa (from the hormone sensitivity to the castration resistance phase) has paved the way to new-generation hormone drugs (abiraterone and enzalutamide) and new chemotherapeutic agents (cabazitaxel) that have become part of our daily clinical practice because of their ability to improve significantly the most important oncological clinical outcomes (PFS and OS). The use of these targeted therapies today is based on the ability to separate patients according to their disease prognosis and on the capacity to predict the response to drugs. In view of the huge tumor heterogeneity and the continuing evolution of neoplastic clones, continuous monitoring of the disease has now become an absolute need in oncology. For these and other reasons, liquid biopsy represents a useful noninvasive method for the study of all solid tumors, including PCa.

Circulating Tumor Cells (CTCs)

Circulating tumor cells (CTCs) are known for a long time, since their first description dates back to the mid-1800s, where they were described as particles very similar to cancer cells [1]. One of the most used technologies for their isolation is represented by FDA-approved CellSearch® CTC assay. Many recent studies have suggested that the CTCs can be used in clinical purposes because of their ability to guide therapeutic decisions in patients with solid tumors, including prostate cancer (PCa). Although results are not yet strong enough to lead to such a change in the daily management, the possible applications field of CTCs in metastatic castration-resistant prostate cancer (mCRPC) include the treatment choice (second generation hormonal agents versus chemotherapy), the detection of early treatment resistance and also defining prognosis. From this point of view, one of the first parameters to be studied was the CTC-derived PSA using RT-PCR technique, aiming to determine drug resistance and to predict outcomes [2, 3]. In a study by Allard WJ et al., the CTCs were isolated from blood (7.5 mL of blood) of healthy patients, suffering from non-oncological diseases and cancer patients with

A. Galvano • B. Di Stefano • M. Castiglia
Department of Surgical, Oncological and Oral Sciences, Section of Medical Oncology, University of Palermo, Via del Vespro 129, 90127 Palermo, Italy

K. Papadimitriou • C. Rolfo, MD, PhD (✉)
Department of Oncology, Antwerp University Hospital, Wilrijkstraat 10, 2650 Edegem, Belgium
e-mail: christian.rolfo@uza.be

© Springer International Publishing AG 2017
A. Giordano et al. (eds.), *Liquid Biopsy in Cancer Patients*, Current Clinical Pathology,
DOI 10.1007/978-3-319-55661-1_11

advanced disease, using CellSearch platform, proving to be greater in the latter cohort (mean, 60 ± 693 CTCs for 7.5 mL) compared to the other two categories (mean, 0.1 ± 0.2 and 0.1 ± 0.3 CTCs to 7.5 mL, respectively), also demonstrating that the sensitivity of the method was high, more than 90% [4]. Another prospective study performed successively on mCRPC allowed to identify a PCa CTC median value of 16 (CTCs positive for biomarkers such as prostate-specific amplification of AR), confirming a possible prognostic role for CTCs [5]. De Bono et al. have also suggested CTC number can influence the outcome of patients suffering from mCRPC finding that CTC count ≥ 5 per 7.5 mL of blood showed worse median overall survival (mOS; 21.7 mo vs. 11.5 mo – p value <0.0001). If compared with PSA decline after a course of standard chemotherapy (3–4 months), CTCs have been shown to have a greater ability to predict prognosis, so as to apply as a reliable independent prognostic biomarker in this context (AUC 0.82) [6]. This hypothesis has been validated in a large prospective randomized phase III trial (SWOG S0421) in which patients who had a CTC count ≥ 5 per 7.5 mL of blood were at high risk of having greater values of PSA, visceral metastases, bone metastases, alkaline phosphatase, and lower hemoglobin. In addition, these patients had a lower response rate to chemotherapy (44% vs. 63%), demonstrating that CTC enumeration is an independent prognostic factor, in addition to PSA values and the radiological assessment [7]. The validation of the number of CTCs as an independent prognostic factor has allowed the construction of multiple biomarker panels, in order to increase the efficiency of the test. The LDH-CTC panel is indeed considered one of the most studied in this context, particularly as regards the evaluation of the effectiveness of the chemotherapy treatment (CT), since patients with high levels of CTCs and LDH post CT would have worse prognosis compared to those with biomarker decrease [8]. The CTC/LDH panel was also assessed in a secondary analysis of the COU-AA-301 prospective randomized phase III study in which abiraterone, an inhibitor of CYP 17 plus prednisone, was compared to placebo plus prednisone in mCRPC patients, showing that the CTC (≥ 5) and LDH (<250 U/L) combination was able to select a group of patients with extremely lower 2-year survival rate (2% vs. 46%) [9]. Although the results described above are to be considered very promising, there are no sufficient recommendations to define a course of treatment based on information from the panel, and above all there are no suggestions on how to treat the worse prognosis category of patients. Unfortunately, the large-scale use of CellSearch assay has some important limitations, among which the inability to identify cells not expressing EpCAM (dedifferentiated or stemlike). Furthermore, since their number is directly proportional to the load of neoplastic disease, there is a higher probability that their presence reaches a sufficiently high number when the mCRPC is resistant to hormonal treatments or CT. As mentioned previously, the predictive significance of CTCs is one of the most investigated for patient's clinical management [2, 10–12]. The role of CTCs in this context has been studied in combination to the androgen receptor (AR). The aim is to obtain a test capable to identify the AR receptor splice variants (AR-V7) in order to get a noninvasive negative predictive biomarker of response to the new-generation hormone treatments. Antonarakis ES et al. evaluated two cohorts of patients mCRPC (n1 = 31, n2 = 31, respectively), treated with abiraterone and enzalutamide pointing out that those who carried the AR-V7 in CTCs identified by qRT-PCR technique had a significant reduction in median progression-free survival (mPFS), in median overall survival (mOS), and in PSA response showing a possible predictive role of CTCs in detecting abiraterone and enzalutamide resistance [13] (Fig. 11.1). The same author has recently published the updated results of this study which included a total of 202 patients and showed not only that patients who were AR-V7+ had worst mPFS and mOS, but that patients identified as CTC+/AR-V7+ have a worse prognosis, suggesting a possible prognostic role of CTCs in detection [14]. These secondary analyses, although from large clinical trials, are not strong enough to change the current clinical practice.

Fig. 11.1 Negative predictive role of androgen receptor splicing variant 7 (AR-V7) in metastatic castration-resistant prostate cancer (mCRPC). (**a**) The AR expression does not affect the response to chemotherapy and hormone therapy. (**b**) The expression of AR-V7 would affect the response to hormone therapy without interfering with chemotherapy

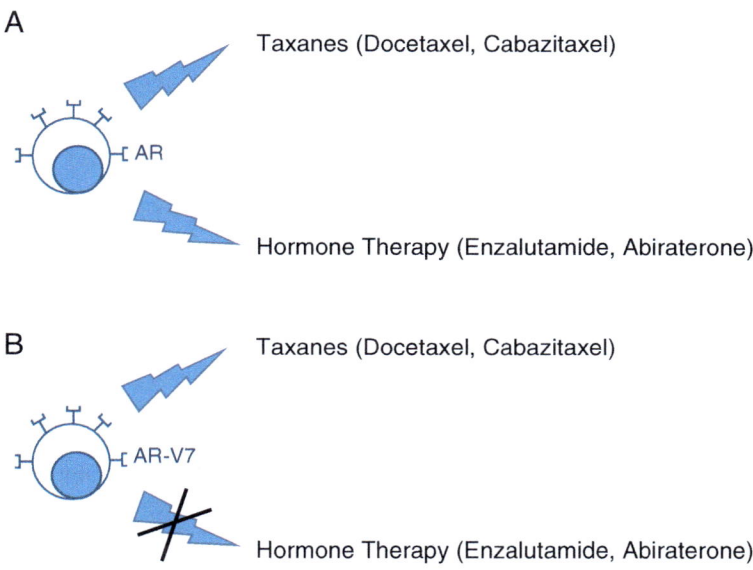

A

Taxanes (Docetaxel, Cabazitaxel)

AR

Hormone Therapy (Enzalutamide, Abiraterone)

B

Taxanes (Docetaxel, Cabazitaxel)

AR-V7

Hormone Therapy (Enzalutamide, Abiraterone)

For these reasons, a number of ongoing clinical trials are evaluating the impact of these results by trying to select a cohort of patient candidates for other options (cabazitaxel – NCT02379390). Equally suggestive is the hypothesis that treatment resistance may be due to receptor switch (AR-V7 negative to positive; AR-V7 positive to negative), as the continuous monitoring of CTCs may represent a useful tool in the next future for the clinical management of mCRPC [15]. Cabazitaxel and CTCs were studied also in further investigations by Onstenk W. et al. in which patients with mCRPC were subjected to cabazitaxel to evaluate the association between CTC AR-V7 status and the objective response rate. The results of this study suggested that the response to chemotherapy was substantially independent of the state of AR-V7, proposing cabazitaxel as a valid therapeutic option in this disease setting, although the data come from a small sample size [16]. Finally, the role of AR-V7 has been investigated in mCRPC patients who were enrolled for CT (docetaxel or cabazitaxel) or new-generation hormone therapy (abiraterone or enzalutamide) substantially confirming what has already been described in previous works. In particular, authors do not describe significant differences in PSA response rate in the AR-V7-positive or -negative patients who underwent both CTs (41% vs. 65%, $p = 0.19$, respectively), while among the AR-V7-positive CTs cause a significant reduction in PSA response compared with HT (41% vs. 0%, $p < 0.001$) [17]. Scher HI et al. have indeed recently demonstrated on a large series of 161 cases treated at the Memorial Sloan Kettering Cancer Center that the subgroup of patients who were CTC+/AR-V7+ before hormone therapy had lower PSA response rate, a lower radiological PFS, and OS less than other AR-V7-negative patients, while for those who underwent chemotherapy with taxanes, the difference was significant in terms of OS but not considering the other endpoints [18]. Although the results of the studies described above should be confirmed in a large series, these results also suggest that the use of CTCs may become in the next future a large clinical resource for evaluating the prognosis and the effectiveness of treatments with the ability to assess the state of AR (especially AR-V7) which could serve as a negative predictor of response to HT. The CTCs seem also useful in the evaluation of other molecules that may play a key role in the management of prostate cancer. These include the TMPRSS2-ERG rearrangements, which would seem to predict the response to HT (abiraterone) and were reported in more than 50% of the cases of hormone-sensitive cancer (ranging 20–60%), although in some experiments the results are discordant probably because of the different techniques used for the characterization of the CTCs (qRT-PCR. vs. FISH). Other studies have investigated the role of Ki-67, a biomarker of cell proliferation. Several authors have associated the expression of Ki-67 in CTCs with PCa in progression and with the nuclear localization of AR, suggesting that it may be a marker of resistance to treatments [19, 20]. Other experiences have instead suggested a possible role of telomerase, an enzyme whose main role is to protect cells from apoptosis, as a prognostic marker in prostate cancer. Goldkom A. et al. in a retrospective analysis underlined that the group with CTC count ≥5 and high levels of telomerase had a worse mOS (HR: 1.14) [21]. Loss of PTEN [22], insulin-like growth factor 1 receptor (IGF1R) expression [23], the enhancer of zest homolog 2 (EZH2) expression [24] and EGFR alterations [5] are subject to further investigations to study their potentiality in mCRPC as possible biomarkers.

Circulating Tumor DNA (ctDNA)

Another component of the liquid biopsy is the circulating tumor DNA (ctDNA) that consists of fragments of 140–180 base pair long DNA, found in low amounts (0–50 ng/ml) in the blood of healthy subjects and in larger quantities (50–5000 ng/ml) in neoplastic situations or other benign conditions (exercise, inflammation) [25, 26]. The ctDNA also represents a small proportion (0.1 –10%) of circulating free DNA (cfDNA) in the blood and derives mainly from lysed cells or apoptosis. This small percentage is difficult to analyze for the technical difficulties that characterize the identification of these particles. Nowadays, extremely sensitive methods are available and able at least partially to solve the above limitations. These new tools are the PCR (BEAming and Droplet Digital) and more recently the next-generation sequencing (NGS) techniques with massive parallel sequencing [27–32]. Numerous small trials provided preliminary results about the cfDNA ability to be a marker of prostate cancer like PSA. Although

with limitations due to the heterogeneity between the different trials, a recent meta-analysis has tried to evaluate the diagnostic value of cfDNA in PCa. Although the qualitative analysis of cfDNA has shown promising results with a sensitivity of 0.34 (95% CI, 0.22–0.48), a specificity of 0.99 (95% CI, 0.97–1.00), and AUC (area under curve) 0.91 (95% CI, 0.88–0.93), the authors concluded that the cfDNA should still be used in combination with the traditional PSA, for the screening of the PCa [33]. As for the CTCs, also the amount of cfDNA would seem to be correlated with tumor burden and with prognosis. H Schwarzenbach et al. evaluated the amount of cfDNA using fluorescence-labeled PCR in 81 patients suffering from PCa, showing that the cfDNA values increase in accordance with the deterioration of the tumor stage (median 186 ng/mL vs. 562 ng/ml; $p = 0.03$), although the values were still significantly different compared to those reported in the cohort of healthy patients (21 ng/ml) [34]. Several studies have shown that the metastatic cancer has a higher frequency of mutations and genomic instability if compared to tumors of localized stage. These alterations also characterized the castration resistance phase correlated to the selection of clones caused by tumor microenvironment (selective pressure). Among these, one of the most known is the AR mutation, which constitutes a target for the new-generation hormonal therapies (enzalutamide and abiraterone). Although several experiences had concluded that the AR alterations could be drivers for disease management in advanced-stage PCa [35], researchers using whole-genome sequencing techniques have suggested a more probable role of AR alterations as resistance factor to the abovementioned hormonal therapies. For this reason, accurate identification methods, also noninvasive and low-cost, can be considered today as a priority in the field of precision medicine [36–39]. Interestingly, a recent study also evaluated the possible predictive role of cfDNA in a cohort of 59 mCRPC patients who underwent a taxane-containing regimen in which patients with cfDNA values greater than 55 ng/ml were associated with lower PSA response rate ($p = 0.005$), showing to be a possible independent prognostic factor for OS ($p = 0.032$) [40]. Like CTCs, ctDNA can be a useful tool to identify genomic aberrations and the AR mutations in mCRPC patients undergoing HT. In particular, Romanel A. et al. have sequenced 274 blood samples from 97 patients suffering from mCRPC treated with abiraterone, highlighting the appearance of a mutation of AR (L702H or T878A). The group in which the AR mutation was present in ctDNA before starting treatment (45%) had a chance to have a PSA response rate < 50%, 4.9 times lower with worse OS (HR 7.33; 95% CI 3.51–15.34) and PFS (HR 3.73; 95% CI 2.17–6.41), and these results were also confirmed using multivariate analysis [39]. Abiraterone [41] and enzalutamide [42] were also investigated in two clinical trials in which aberrations of CYP17-A1 and AR were analyzed, showing that an increase of mutations in these genes' ctDNA, after drug exposure, was responsible for poor clinical outcomes in terms of mPFS (abi 2.8 mo vs. 9.2 mo; enza 2.3 mo vs. 7.0 mo) and mOS (abi 5.0 mo vs. 21.9 mo) compared with patients with no gain in mutation. The importance of monitoring somatic genetic mutations has been recently further confirmed by the results by Frênel JS et al. They recorded that genetic alterations in the course of phase I trials (including prostate cancer) which were mainly directed against the PI3K-AKT-mTOR suggested mutations correlate to drug response, thus enhancing the usefulness of cftDNA even during the design of every new pivotal clinical trial [43]. In a similar study, Wyatt AW et al. evaluated the copy number variation and mutation rate of AR and other genes (MYC, RB1, and MET) before and after treatment with enzalutamide showing how they (mutations ≥ 2, amplifications, RB loss) were associated with worse mPFS.

Exosomes and MicroRNAs (miRNAs)

Exosomes are a family of vesicles derived from cells (30–100 nm) that can be detected in body fluids. Numerous studies have evaluated the role of exosomes in PCa, focusing on relations with the progression of the disease, biomarkers, and [44] immune system [45–50]. One of the most

significant challenges in the PCa management is the early localized PCa detection to avoid overtreatment. Exosomes could potentially guarantee not only a reduction of unnecessary interventions but also an indolent monitoring and effective in patients who are candidates for active surveillance protocols, stratifying patients who are high or low risk for progressing. There are currently various biomarkers used in early diagnosis of PCa. These include the PSA and more recently the prostate cancer antigen 3 (PCA3), a noncoding upregulated RNA specific for PCa. The protein kinase C α (PKCA) is still under systematic validation. Although these and other potential biomarkers in the blood, urine, and seminal fluid (DNA or RNA fragments) have been studied by means of innovative techniques (next-generation sequencing), most of them still do not guarantee sufficient specificity and sensitivity levels. For these reasons, the information contained into exosomes are interesting and deserve further investigations, since in preliminary studies on PCa cell lines and tissue were found cancer-derived exosomes [51–54].

In plasma-derived exosomes, for example, were found specific PCa-related proteins as PTEN and survivin that were not reported in high levels in patients with benign prostatic hyperplasia (PBH) or in healthy subjects. In particular, Hosseini-Beheshti E. et al. using mass spectrometry aimed to evaluate the exosome content in AR-negative and A-positive cells of six PCa cell lines to identify potential biomarker proteins for PCa in different stages (as FOLH1, ANXA1, FASN, CLSTN1, FLNC, and GDF15). Similarly, another research team was able to detect the presence of another possible biomarker (XPO140) from multiple cell lines of PCa [52, 55]. Even fragments of noncoding microRNAs (miRNAs) have been found inside the exosomes, 20–25 nucleotides long, which negatively regulate target genes. In another experience, Bryant RJ et al. have found on plasma, serum, and urine sample of patients with advanced PCa 12 different miRNAs upregulated significantly if compared to early-stage PCa. In particular, miR-141 could help to distinguish PCa patients from healthy subjects [56]. Despite the promising role of miR-NAs as biomarkers with diagnostic value, many of them do not reach a sufficient value in a urine sample to be detected and therefore require further analysis to provide robust information to be transferred in current clinical practice [57]. Numerous experiences have evaluated the expression of exosomes even on prostate-derived fluids and urine tests, finding different levels of N-glycoproteins correlated with the various stages of PCa [58–60]. Additionally, subsequent studies have identified within urinary exosomes from patients with PCa increased levels of alpha-1, beta-1 integrin, and delta-catenin compared to levels in healthy patients or those with non-oncological diseases [61–63]. Some gene transcripts permanently linked to PCa are reported within the urinary exosomes (PCA3 and TMPRSS2), and their study could serve as a source in a short time, yet little explored, of novel biomarkers since the urinary sample should serve as an ideal tool because it is less complex to be analyzed with modern instruments [53, 57]. Furthermore, beyond their influence on the prognosis, preliminary research has suggested how exosomes may contribute to the CT resistance, as demonstrated in a study in which they were isolated from plasma of patients affected by taxane-resistant PCa, probably due to an exosomal MDR-1/P-gp transfer [64]. In addition, exosomes could be decisive in the modulation of enzalutamide or abiraterone on PCa. Del Re M. et al. have used a new-generation method able to facilitate analysis of the RNA fragment coding for the AR-V7 (digital droplet polymerase chain reaction – ddPCR) of the plasma-derived exosomes, since the presence of AR-V7 was related to the resistance to these molecules and significantly lower mPFS and mOS outcomes suggesting AR-V7 as possible predictive biomarker of resistance to HT [65].

In addition, some authors reported preliminary evidence on the role of exosomes in lymphocyte-mediated immune evasion mechanisms, through the inhibition of NKG2D receptor expressed on CD8+ T lymphocytes and natural killer cells [45]. Although exosomes provided clear preliminary results on their clinical possible utility, there are significant limitations that still are maintained, mainly of technical nature. There will be a call for great commitment by the research in this context

hoping that new resources would allow in the near future to be able to speed up and standardize the isolation of exosomes and also try to maintain the specificity of avoiding contamination from material not useful for research.

References

1. Ashworth TR. A case of cancer in which cells similar to those in the tumors were seen in the blood after death. Aus Med J. 1869;14:146–9.
2. Armstrong AJ, et al. Circulating tumor cells from patients with advanced prostate and breast cancer display both epithelial and mesenchymal markers. Mol Cancer Res. 2011;9:997–1007.
3. Bitting RL, et al. Development of a method to isolate circulating tumor cells using mesenchymal-based capture. Methods. 2013;64:129–36.
4. Allard WJ, et al. Tumor cells circulate in the peripheral blood of all major carcinomas but not in healthy subjects or patients with nonmalignant diseases. Clin Cancer Res. 2004;10:6897–904.
5. Shaffer DR, et al. Circulating tumor cell analysis in patients with progressive castration-resistant prostate cancer. Clin Cancer Res. 2007;13:2023–9.
6. de Bono JS, et al. Circulating tumor cells predict survival benefit from treatment in metastatic castration-resistant prostate cancer. Clin Cancer Res. 2008;14:6302–9.
7. Goldkorn A, et al. Circulating tumor cell counts are prognostic of overall survival in SWOG S0421: a phase III trial of docetaxel with or without atrasentan for metastatic castration-resistant prostate cancer. J Clin Oncol. 2014;32:1136–42.
8. Scher HI, et al. Circulating tumour cells as prognostic markers in progressive, castration-resistant prostate cancer: a reanalysis of IMMC38 trial data. Lancet Oncol. 2009;10:233–9.
9. Scher HI, et al. Circulating tumor cell biomarker panel as an individual-level surrogate for survival in metastatic castration-resistant prostate cancer. J Clin Oncol. 2015;33:1348–55.
10. Sieuwerts AM, et al. Anti-epithelial cell adhesion molecule antibodies and the detection of circulating normal-like breast tumor cells. J Natl Cancer Inst. 2009;101:61–6.
11. Yu M, et al. Circulating breast tumor cells exhibit dynamic changes in epithelial and mesenchymal composition. Science. 2013;339:580–4.
12. Pecot CV, et al. A novel platform for detection of CK+ and CK- CTCs. Cancer Discov. 2011;1:580–6.
13. Antonarakis ES, et al. AR-V7 and resistance to enzalutamide and abiraterone in prostate cancer. N Engl J Med. 2014;371:1028–38.
14. Antonarakis ES, et al. AR-V7 and efficacy of abiraterone (Abi) and enzalutamide (Enza) in castration-resistant prostate cancer (CRPC): expanded analysis

of the Johns Hopkins cohort. J Clin Oncol. 2016;34(suppl; abstr 5012).

15. Nakazawa M, et al. Serial blood-based analysis of AR-V7 in men with advanced prostate cancer. Ann Oncol. 2015;26:1859–65.

16. Onstenk W, et al. Efficacy of cabazitaxel in castration-resistant prostate cancer is independent of the presence of AR-V7 in circulating tumor cells. Eur Urol. 2015;68:939–45.

17. Antonarakis ES, et al. Androgen receptor splice variant 7 and efficacy of taxane chemotherapy in patients with metastatic castration-resistant prostate cancer. JAMA Oncol. 2015;1:582–91.

18. Scher HI, et al. Association of AR-V7 on circulating tumor cells as a treatment-specific biomarker with outcomes and survival in castration-resistant prostate cancer. JAMA Oncol. 2016;2:1441–9.

19. Stott SL, et al. Isolation and characterization of circulating tumor cells from patients with localized and metastatic prostate cancer. Sci Transl Med. 2010;2:25ra23.

20. Reyes EE, et al. Quantitative characterization of androgen receptor protein expression and cellular localization in circulating tumor cells from patients with metastatic castration-resistant prostate cancer. J Transl Med. 2014;12:313.

21. Goldkorn A, et al. Circulating tumor cell telomerase activity as a prognostic marker for overall survival in SWOG 0421: a phase III metastatic castration resistant prostate cancer trial. Int J Cancer. 2015;136:1856–62.

22. Punnoose EA, et al. PTEN loss in circulating tumour cells correlates with PTEN loss in fresh tumour tissue from castration-resistant prostate cancer patients. Br J Cancer. 2015;113:1225–33.

23. de Bono JS, et al. Potential applications for circulating tumor cells expressing the insulin-like growth factor-I receptor. Clin Cancer Res. 2007;13:3611–6.

24. Cho KS, Oh HY, Lee EJ, Hong SJ. Identification of enhancer of zeste homolog 2 expression in peripheral circulating tumor cells in metastatic prostate cancer patients: a preliminary study. Yonsei Med J. 2007;48:1009–14.

25. Perkins G, et al. Multi-purpose utility of circulating plasma DNA testing in patients with advanced cancers. PLoS One. 2012;7:e47020.

26. Leon SA, Shapiro B, Sklaroff DM, Yaros MJ. Free DNA in the serum of cancer patients and the effect of therapy. Cancer Res. 1977;37:646–50.

27. Dressman D, Yan H, Traverso G, Kinzler KW, Vogelstein B. Transforming single DNA molecules into fluorescent magnetic particles for detection and enumeration of genetic variations. Proc Natl Acad Sci U S A. 2003;100:8817–22.

28. Pekin D, et al. Quantitative and sensitive detection of rare mutations using droplet-based microfluidics. Lab Chip. 2011;11:2156–66.

29. Heitzer E, Ulz P, Geigl JB. Circulating tumor DNA as a liquid biopsy for cancer. Clin Chem. 2015;61:112–23.

30. Vogelstein B, Kinzler KW. Digital PCR. Proc Natl Acad Sci U S A. 1999;96:9236–41.

31. Forshew T, et al. Noninvasive identification and monitoring of cancer mutations by targeted deep sequencing of plasma DNA. Sci Transl Med. 2012;4:136ra168.

32. Newman AM, et al. An ultrasensitive method for quantitating circulating tumor DNA with broad patient coverage. Nat Med. 2014;20:548–54.

33. Yin C, et al. Quantitative and qualitative analysis of circulating cell-free DNA can be used as an adjuvant tool for prostate cancer screening: a meta-analysis. Dis Markers. 2016;2016:3825819.

34. Schwarzenbach H, et al. Cell-free tumor DNA in blood plasma as a marker for circulating tumor cells in prostate cancer. Clin Cancer Res. 2009;15:1032–8.

35. Network CGAR. The molecular taxonomy of primary prostate cancer. Cell. 2015;163:1011–25.

36. Carreira S, et al. Tumor clone dynamics in lethal prostate cancer. Sci Transl Med. 2014;6:254ra125.

37. Gundem G, et al. The evolutionary history of lethal metastatic prostate cancer. Nature. 2015;520:353–7.

38. Hong MK, et al. Tracking the origins and drivers of subclonal metastatic expansion in prostate cancer. Nat Commun. 2015;6:6605.

39. Romanel A, et al. Plasma AR and abiraterone-resistant prostate cancer. Sci Transl Med. 2015;7:312re310.

40. Kwee S, Song MA, Cheng I, Loo L, Tiirikainen M. Measurement of circulating cell-free DNA in relation to 18F-fluorocholine PET/CT imaging in chemotherapy-treated advanced prostate cancer. Clin Transl Sci. 2012;5:65–70.

41. Salvi S, et al. Circulating cell-free AR and CYP17A1 copy number variations may associate with outcome of metastatic castration-resistant prostate cancer patients treated with abiraterone. Br J Cancer. 2015;112:1717–24.

42. Azad AA, et al. Androgen receptor gene aberrations in circulating cell-free DNA: biomarkers of therapeutic resistance in castration-resistant prostate cancer. Clin Cancer Res. 2015;21:2315–24.

43. Frenel JS, et al. Serial next-generation sequencing of circulating cell-free DNA evaluating tumor clone response to molecularly targeted drug administration. Clin Cancer Res. 2015;21:4586–96.

44. Abusamra AJ, et al. Tumor exosomes expressing fas ligand mediate CD8+ T-cell apoptosis. Blood Cells Mol Dis. 2005;35:169–73.

45. Lundholm M, et al. Prostate tumor-derived exosomes down-regulate NKG2D expression on natural killer cells and CD8+ T cells: mechanism of immune evasion. PLoS One. 2014;9:e108925.

46. Bryant RJ, et al. Changes in circulating microRNA levels associated with prostate cancer. Br J Cancer. 2012;106:768–74.

47. Lázaro-Ibáñez E, et al. Different gDNA content in the subpopulations of prostate cancer extracellular vesicles: apoptotic bodies, microvesicles, and exosomes. Prostate. 2014;74:1379–90.

48. Hessvik NP, Phuyal S, Brech A, Sandvig K, Llorente A. Profiling of microRNAs in exosomes released from PC-3 prostate cancer cells. Biochim Biophys Acta. 2012;1819:1154–63.

49. Di Vizio D, et al. Large oncosomes in human prostate cancer tissues and in the circulation of mice with metastatic disease. Am J Pathol. 2012;181:1573–84.

50. Khan S, et al. Plasma-derived exosomal survivin, a plausible biomarker for early detection of prostate cancer. PLoS One. 2012;7:e46737.

51. Ronquist G. Prostasomes are mediators of intercellular communication: from basic research to clinical implications. J Intern Med. 2012;271:400–13.

52. Hosseini-Beheshti E, Pham S, Adomat H, Li N, Tomlinson Guns ES. Exosomes as biomarker enriched microvesicles: characterization of exosomal proteins derived from a panel of prostate cell lines with distinct AR phenotypes. Mol Cell Proteomics. 2012;11:863–85.

53. Nilsson J, et al. Prostate cancer-derived urine exosomes: a novel approach to biomarkers for prostate cancer. Br J Cancer. 2009;100:1603–7.

54. Tavoosidana G, et al. Multiple recognition assay reveals prostasomes as promising plasma biomarkers for prostate cancer. Proc Natl Acad Sci U S A. 2011;108:8809–14.

55. Duijvesz D, et al. Proteomic profiling of exosomes leads to the identification of novel biomarkers for prostate cancer. PLoS One. 2013;8:e82589.

56. Huang X, Liang M, Dittmar R, Wang L. Extracellular microRNAs in urologic malignancies: chances and challenges. Int J Mol Sci. 2013;14:14785–99.

57. Dijkstra S, et al. Prostate cancer biomarker profiles in urinary sediments and exosomes. J Urol. 2014;191:1132–8.

58. Drake RR, Kislinger T. The proteomics of prostate cancer exosomes. Expert Rev Proteomics. 2014;11:167–77.

59. Principe S, et al. In-depth proteomic analyses of exosomes isolated from expressed prostatic secretions in urine. Proteomics. 2013;13:1667–71.

60. Nyalwidhe JO, et al. Increased bisecting N-acetylglucosamine and decreased branched chain glycans of N-linked glycoproteins in expressed prostatic secretions associated with prostate cancer progression. Proteomics Clin Appl. 2013;7:677–89.

61. Bijnsdorp IV, et al. Exosomal ITGA3 interferes with non-cancerous prostate cell functions and is increased in urine exosomes of metastatic prostate cancer patients. J Extracell Vesicles. 2013;2:1–10.

62. Lu Q, et al. Identification of extracellular delta-catenin accumulation for prostate cancer detection. Prostate. 2009;69:411–8.

63. Fedele C, Singh A, Zerlanko BJ, Iozzo RV, Languino LR. The αvβ6 integrin is transferred intercellularly via exosomes. J Biol Chem. 2015;290:4545–51.

64. Corcoran C, et al. Docetaxel-resistance in prostate cancer: evaluating associated phenotypic changes and potential for resistance transfer via exosomes. PLoS One. 2012;7:e50999.

65. Del Re M, et al. The detection of androgen receptor splice variant 7 in plasma-derived exosomal RNA strongly predicts resistance to hormonal therapy in metastatic prostate cancer patients. Eur Urol. 2017;71(4):680–7.

Liquid Biopsy in Non-Small Cell Lung Cancer (NSCLC)

12

Christian Rolfo, Marta Castiglia, Alessandro Perez,
Pablo Reclusa, Patrick Pauwels, Laure Sober,
Francesco Passiglia, and Antonio Russo

Current Status of Lung Cancer

Lung cancer is the leading cause of cancer deaths worldwide [1], being 85% of those non-small cell lung cancer (NSCLC). The last data published by Cancer Research UK reported the 1-year overall survival rate of 32% for lung cancer patients, while the 5-year survival rate is around 10%. Besides the development of new effective therapies, lung cancer is still today a disease difficult to control.

The advent of targeted agents represents the most important innovation in the treatment of lung cancer over the last years. The discovery of epidermal growth factor receptor (EGFR)-activating mutations in 2004 as oncogene driver in a subgroup of patients with NSCLC led to the development of a new family of biological agents, called EGFR-TKIs, which were able to selectively bind and inhibit the EGFR molecular pathway. About eight phase III randomized clinical trials compared EGFR-TKI gefitinib, erlotinib, or afatinib vs platinum-based chemotherapy as first-line treatment for EGFR-mutated NSCLC patients, all showing a significant survival benefit in favor of EGFR-TKIs. These drugs have revolutionized the clinical management of about 40% Asian and 12% Caucasian NSCLC patients harboring EGFR mutations, whose survival outcomes nearly doubled compared to standard chemotherapy. Later the discovery of the EML4-ALK fusion gene in about 3–8% of patients with NSCLC and the subsequent clinical development of crizotinib represented an amazing success story leading to the recent approval of this compound as new standard first-line treatment in this

C. Rolfo
Phase I-Early Clinical Trials Unit, Oncology Department, Antwerp University Hospital, Wilrijkstraat 10, 2650 Edegem, Belgium

Center for Oncological Research (CORE), Antwerp University, Antwerp, Belgium

M. Castiglia • A. Perez • F. Passiglia • A. Russo (⊠)
Department of Surgical, Oncological and Oral Sciences, Section of Medical Oncology, University of Palermo, Via del Vespro 129, 90127, Palermo, Italy
e-mail: antonio.russo@usa.net

P. Reclusa
Phase I-Early Clinical Trials Unit, Oncology Department, Antwerp University Hospital, Wilrijkstraat 10, 2650 Edegem, Belgium

Center for Oncological Research (CORE), Antwerp University, Antwerp, Belgium

Center for Oncological Research, Faculty of Medicine and Health Sciences, University of Antwerp, Wilrijk, Belgium

Department of Pathology, Antwerp University Hospital, Edegem, Belgium

P. Pauwels • L. Sober
Center for Oncological Research, Faculty of Medicine and Health Sciences, University of Antwerp, Wilrijk, Belgium

Department of Pathology, Antwerp University Hospital, Edegem, Belgium

© Springer International Publishing AG 2017
A. Giordano et al. (eds.), *Liquid Biopsy in Cancer Patients*, Current Clinical Pathology,
DOI 10.1007/978-3-319-55661-1_12

subgroup of patients [2]. Nevertheless in both cases, despite an initial impressive benefit, patients inevitably experience tumor progression, because the tumor can generate resistance to these treatments through genetic modifications like mutations or amplifications. To avoid this problem, pharmaceutical industries are developing new drugs that are able to overcome resistance mechanisms. New generations of EGFR and ALK inhibitors have been recently investigated in randomized clinical studies, showing a great efficacy and tolerability in patients who failed prior TKIs. Particularly osimertinib is the third-generation EGFR-TKI in most advanced stage of clinical development which is active against both EGFR-sensitizing and EGFR-resistant T790M mutation. The phase III AURA 3 study has recently shown a significant survival benefit in favor of osimertinib over platinum chemotherapy in NSCLC patients who progressed to prior EGFR-TKI and were T790M positive [3]. Similarly the new-generation ALK inhibitors alectinib and ceritinib also demonstrated a significant superiority over platinum chemotherapy in ALK-rearranged patients who failed prior therapy with crizotinib [4]. However, there are already some data showing that resistance mechanisms can occur also for these new-generation drugs [5, 6]. In this scenario biomarker investigations have become one of the most interesting and studied fields of translational lung cancer research with the aim to estimate patients' prognosis, to monitor treatment response and to eventually predict both treatment efficacy and tumor recurrence [7, 8].

The genetic analysis of both EGFR mutations and EML4-ALK translocation is a crucial step at the time of diagnosis, in order to plan the optimal treatment strategy for each patient. Furthermore, the analysis of EGFR mutations has acquired a growing importance also in the follow-up of TKI-treated patients. In fact, almost in nearly 60% of TKI-treated patients, the treatment efficacy fails due to resistance mechanisms. The most common cause of TKI failure depends on the onset of secondary mutations; the exon 20 T790M is the most characterized resistance mutation in EGFR [9].

Therefore EGFR mutational status should be monitored during treatment and mostly at relapse to choose the proper subsequent therapy. To date, the gold standard for the molecular analysis of a patient affected by NSCLC is the tissue biopsy.

Even if there is a big consensus about the use of tissue biopsy as a primary source of genetic information, we still have to face the situation when "the tissue becomes the issue". This may happen when a strict "molecular follow-up" is mandatory to evaluate patient's disease evolution. To solve this problem, liquid biopsy has raised as the "new ambrosia of researchers" as it could help clinicians to identify both prognostic and predictive biomarkers in a more accessible way [10].

The Importance of Liquid Biopsy in NSCLC

One of the new hallmarks of cancer is the "genome instability and mutation" [11]. In lung cancer, it becomes a very relevant issue because of the high heterogeneity of this tumor. Lung cancer is characterized by different driver molecular alterations, with EGFR mutations, ALK-EML4 translocations, and RAS mutation being the most common among others [12, 13]. The new targeted therapies against these driver mutations have nearly doubled patients' survival [14, 15]. However, due to the genomic instability of cancer and its peculiar ability to adapt to the tumor microenvironment, cancer cells usually develop resistance mechanisms such as the EGFR-T790M mutation or the L1196M mutation during first-generation EGFR-TKIs and crizotinib treatment, respectively [16, 17]. Recent evidences showed that the tumor molecular alterations may not be homogeneously distributed within the same lesion and, what is most relevant, the metastasis can present a completely different molecular profile as compared to the primary tumor [18, 19].

Therefore, the molecular analysis of the tumor and/or of the metastatic lesions is becoming more and more requested at the time of PD. Unfortunately, tissue biopsy is a procedure often limited by several features, including its invasiveness, the not easy access to different tumor sites, the high intra-tumor heterogeneity, and not ultimately the low patients' compliance [20]. Thus, in the last decade, many new noninvasive approaches have been studied to overcome the aforementioned issues. Among these, liquid biopsy represents a valuable alternative for the detection of EGFR mutational status once it cannot be performed on tissue samples according to international guidelines. Furthermore a liquid biopsy can be easily repeated at different time points allowing to follow the tumor molecular status during the treatment course [21]. This could help clinicians to predict disease progression over time, to identify new acquired molecular alterations, and to observe how all these characteristics correspond to patient's status.

Liquid Biopsy in Non-small Cell Lung Cancer

As we are describing in this book, there are many definitions of "liquid biopsy". The definition is complex since different body fluids as urine, ascites, saliva, cerebrospinal liquid or plasma can be considered as valuable sources of tumor components.

In this chapter, we are going to focus our attention on the main published studies investigating circulating tumor cells (CTCs), circulating tumor DNA (ctDNA), and exosomes and other extracellular vesicles (EVs) in lung cancer. The last paragraph will be destined to describe the uncommon components of the liquid biopsy such as platelets.

Circulating Tumor Cells (CTCs)

The circulating tumor cells are shed from both primary and metastatic tumor; thus they are representative of the tumor from which they detached. It is known that lung cancer releases a limited number of CTCs, and therefore they were not so far considered a good field of study. Nevertheless, limitations of CTCs detection in

lung cancer were mainly due to the limited available isolation methods. Thanks to the increase of knowledge about CTCs' biological and physical characteristics, detection and isolation methods have been consequently improved. Nowadays, CTCs may become a promising field of study also in lung cancer [22].

CTCs can be used for two different aims: to evaluate the risk of metastasis and as a source of nucleic acid for molecular characterization. Indeed, CTCs are shed to the bloodstream and can play an important role in the metastatic process. Moreover, since CTCs spread directly from the tumor, they might harbor the same mutational landscape that can be investigated through molecular analysis.

The studies on CTCs in lung cancer have shown heterogeneous results, mainly due to the different techniques and criteria used for the experiments. Tanaka et al. demonstrated that the number of CTCs is higher in patients with lung cancer than in those with benign disease, and the number of CTCs is significantly increased in patients with distant metastasis than in the primary ones. In the same study the authors demonstrated a significant correlation between the number of CTCs in the bloodstream and the stage of the disease [23], but other studies have not showed the same results [24, 25]. The number of CTCs can be also a good marker of tumor growth and prognosis. Krebs et al. demonstrated that patients with five or more CTCs in 7.5 mL of total blood, after one cycle of chemotherapy, have a worse prognosis as compared to those with a lower number [26].

The molecular characterization of CTCs is technically challenging mainly because of the limited performance of isolation and detection methods. Moreover, the amount of extracted nucleic acids is always very poor, limiting the downstream applications. Indeed, new highly sensitive techniques, such as next-generation sequencing (NGS), are now available and offer the possibility to analyze the molecular alteration of CTCs in a relatively simple way.

The detection of EGFR-activating mutations in CTCs has revealed contradictory results. Maheswaran et al. first published in 2008 an article describing the identification of EGFR mutations in CTCs, providing exciting results. They analyzed EGFR mutations in both CTCs and ctDNA using a SARMS assay in patients already tested positive in tissue samples. Mutations in CTCs were detected in 19 out of 20 patients with 95% sensitivity; they also detected T790M mutation in 2 out of 6 responding patients and in 9 out of 14 progressive patients. Moreover, in four patients they reported that levels of activating and resistance mutation (exon 19 deletion and exon 20 T790M, respectively) floated according to disease status [27]. However, a study carried by Punnoose et al. showed disparate results. In this paper the authors analyzed the EGFR expression through FISH showing very heterogeneous results. Indeed, they revealed CTCs with very strong signal (3+), others with very low (0), and other with intra-heterogenic results ranging from 3+ to 0, and this expression was not correlated with the EGFR status on tissue. Moreover, when the DNA from CTCs was analyzed to detect EGFR mutations, only one out of eight EGFR-mutated patients was detected [28].

Besides EGFR mutations, it has been proposed that ALK-EML4 translocations are detectable in CTCs using immunohistochemistry and FISH. The results reported in literature showed a high correlation between ALK-EML4 detection in tissue and in CTCs even if the cutoff value was different among the studies due the various techniques used for CTCs isolation [29–31]. Moreover, a study performed by He et al. investigated a new technique for CTC isolation comparing the results with the FDA-approved methods, the CellSearch system. They demonstrated a correlation between the ratio ALK-EML4 rearrangement signal/CTCs and TNM stage, and similarly to other studies, the count of CTCs was related to the disease status [32]. Therefore, CTCs can be useful for disease follow-up as they offer the opportunity to evaluate both EGFR and ALK-EML4 alterations, as a surrogate biomarker for treatment response and to promptly identify resistance mutations responsible for treatment failure.

The CTC study has risen with the implementation of new isolation techniques that allow more reliability and the improvement of the molecular analysis techniques such as one-cell genotyping. However, a standardization of the techniques is needed and a big consensus on how the samples must be analyzed is fully required to make the CTC analysis truth.

Circulating Tumor DNA (ctDNA)

The investigation of ctDNA can hypothetically reveal a wider genomic landscape of a tumor [33]. For this purpose, new sensitive technical approaches are available to analyze EGFR mutational status from plasma-derived ctDNA. In particular, digital PCR (dPCR) and next-generation sequencing (NGS) platforms represent to date the most studied approaches for application in clinical practice. Through the dPCR approach, the DNA sample is partitioned into thousands of single PCR reactions. As in the qPCR approach, analysis software allows to identify a positive or a negative signal indicating the presence or absence of a target sequence. Therefore, a mutated ctDNA can be detected in a wide background of wild-type sequences [34]. The introduction of NGS technologies in clinical practice is the most important revolution that we have experienced since the discovery of polymerase chain reaction (PCR) and Sanger sequencing. Until now we have been working analyzing *one gene at a time* and *one patient at a time*, with NGS techniques this assertion has been revolutionized and we can analyze *multiple genes and multiple patients at a time* with a consistent reduction in time and costs [35]. NGS is a high-throughput technique, based on massive parallel sequencing of thousands of DNA molecules [36]. There are several NGS platforms that differ mainly in the detection chemistry, but they all share some important steps: library preparation, library amplification, sequencing, and data analysis. At the end of the analysis they all provide a plethora of information about the mutational landscape of the analyzed samples that can be used in clinical practice. Another great advantage of NGS compared to Sanger sequencing is the higher sensitivity, which is important when we have to look for somatic and rare mutations. This is the case of liquid biopsy and specifically of circulating tumor DNA (ctDNA) analysis. The information arising from ctDNA analysis will broad from early diagnosis to prognosis as well as response to drug administration and real-time monitoring of the disease.

Diagnostic Role of ctDNA

To date, several studies and meta-analysis deeply highlighted the diagnostic value of plasma-based EGFR testing in NSCLC patients, showing an interesting accuracy of ctDNA in terms of sensitivity and specificity if compared with the gold standard tissue genotyping [37–40]. Therefore, the isolation of ctDNA from plasma or serum would be helpful for EGFR testing in all those patients whose tissue is not available at diagnosis or tissue analysis results are inconclusive. Sacher et al. have recently evaluated the reliability of plasma analysis. This study demonstrated a high specificity (100%) and sensitivity (74–82%) in 80 patients with advanced NSCLC harboring activating EGFR del19/L858R mutations [41] using droplet digital PCR (ddPCR). The same promising results at diagnosis have been also showed within the multicenter ASSESS study in which a similar concordance rate of 89% (sensitivity 46%, specificity 97%) has been found in a cohort of 1162 patients with advanced NSCLC [42]. Furthermore, despite real-time PCR and ddPCR techniques are definitely the most used for ctDNA analysis, NGS is emerging as an important tool that can complement or substitute tissue NGS analysis. Indeed, there are several commercially available NGS panels specifically designed for ctDNA testing in lung cancer. Recently Villaflor et al. assessed the utility of two ctDNA panels in a clinical series of 68 NSCLC patients; the 54-gene panel includes only mutations, whereas the 68-gene panel includes also *ALK, RET*, or *ROS1* fusions [43]. In this paper, it was also investigated the concordance between paired tissue and blood samples whenever possible. The results reported that 80% of patients have detectable ctDNA, with 83% presenting at

least one non-synonymous ctDNA alteration. As expected the most frequent mutations were reported in TP53, KRAS, and EGFR genes [43]. Another recent paper published on December 2016 supports these evidences. NGS was used to characterize 112 plasma samples from 102 patients with advanced NSCLC, detecting 275 alterations in 45 genes in 84% of patients (86 of 102). As well as reported in the paper from Villaflor [43], NGS was able to detect mutations in additional genes for which experimental therapies, including clinical trials, were available. The concordance between tissue and plasma was 79%, and interestingly the concordance increases when a shorter time interval between tissue and blood collection was reported [44]. Moreover, ctDNA sequencing enabled the detection of resistance mutation in eight patients who experienced progressive disease during targeted therapy and for whom tissue analysis was not possible. Finally, Chen et al. prospectively evaluated the detection of ctDNA mutations in early-stage NSCLC patients (IA, IB, and IIA) by targeted sequencing in plasma and paired tissue samples. They found a considerable ctDNA concentration in 52 out of 58 patients, suggesting that ctDNA might be related to tumor cancer spread. Furthermore, plasma ctDNA mutations were identified in 35 out of 58 patient samples, with 50% concordance between plasma and tissue [45]. These results suggest that ctDNA analysis may also be applied in early-stage disease.

Prognostic Role of ctDNA

The prognostic role of ctDNA has been deeply investigated. In 2014 the group of Wang et al. tested the ability of dPCR to identify T790M in plasma ctDNA compared to a non-digital approach (ARMS). They showed a statistical correlation between survival and allele fraction of circulating T790M before and after EGFR-TKI administration. Patients with increasing levels of circulating T790M during EGFR-TKI treatment showed better progression-free survival (PFS) and overall survival (OS) if compared with patients who do not display any significant

T790M variation [46]. Furthermore, in 2016 the same research group confirmed that patients with circulating T790M had a better clinical outcome compared to plasma T790M-negative patients [47]. Recently, Thompson et al. correlated survival with ctDNA levels and number of variants using NGS in plasma specimens of metastatic NSCLC patients. The high levels of ctDNA (>3 ng/mL), irrespective of mutational profile, were associated with decreased survival. Conversely, patients with ctDNA levels lower than 3 ng/mL showed a better median survival (24 months vs 46 months, respectively). Furthermore, OS seems to be strictly correlated with number of variants detected in plasma. Indeed, a number of variants greater than 3 determined an OS reduction from 62 to 46 months, giving thus a poorer prognosis [44]. Therefore, it seems that mutational load itself may be a good prognostic marker.

ctDNA Value in Real-Time Monitoring of the Disease

The translation in clinical practice of liquid biopsies is strictly requested in all those cases in which a disease progression monitoring is needed (Fig. 12.1). Indeed, on November 2015 the FDA-approved osimertinib as new treatment option for patients with metastatic EGFR T790M-positive NSCLC patients who failed prior EGFR-TKIs [48, 49]. Patients' selection is strictly based on the identification of T790M mutation, and for the first time the molecular analysis can be performed either through tissue re-biopsy or in plasma samples [50, 51]. The noninvasive potential of ctDNA has been deeply studied by Oxnard in many studies specifically focused on the molecular biology of NSCLC. In 2014, one of the first studies performed by its group highlighted the possibility to anticipate clinical evidence of progression through early molecular evidences. Indeed, the analysis of ctDNA through ddPCR, in serial plasma sampling, allowed the detection of resistance mutations (T790M) weeks and sometimes months prior to radiological progression [52].

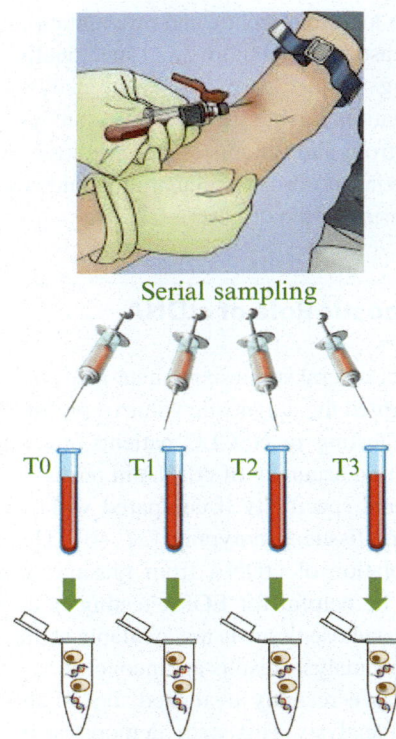

Fig. 12.1 Serial monitoring of NSCLC patients during treatment. Serial blood withdrawal can be obtained at different time points (T0, T1, T2 and T3) to detect CTCs, ctDNA, and exosomes; the dynamic changes of these different components of liquid biopsy may be useful for clinical management of lung cancer patients

Recently his group prospectively evaluated the sensitivity and specificity of plasma genotyping by ddPCR in 180 patients with advanced NSCLC, including 60 patients with acquired resistance to EGFR-TKI. Plasma genotyping by ddPCR exhibited 79% specificity and 77% sensitivity in the detection of T790M mutation, which are lower than those observed with EGFR-activating mutations at baseline. In addition Oxnard et al. showed that outcomes of T790M-positive patients included in the phase I AURA study were similar if T790M was detected in plasma or tumor tissue. Conversely both RR and PFS of T790M-negative patients on plasma were significantly higher than T790M-negative on tissue, and further tumor genotyping of plasma T790M-negative patients allowed to identify a subgroup of T790M-positive patients on tumor tissues who had better outcomes. According to these data, the authors suggest that plasma genotyping could represent the first step for the detection of T790M status at the time of PD. However, because of the low sensitivity (70%) of the current available technologies which are associated with a 30% false negative rate, patients with T790M-negative on plasma should repeat tumor tissue biopsy to further investigate the presence of such molecular alteration [53]. Clinical utility of ctDNA testing through NGS could be also proven in treatment monitoring, for the evaluation of tumor clone response to target treatment administration. Indeed, NGS analysis, as well as dPCR, provides also data concerning the mutations allele fraction. Therefore, it is possible to trace allele fraction modifications over time during a given targeted treatment and correlate these data with treatment response but also to predict relapse and disease progression [54]. In support of the high tumor heterogeneity, CAPP-Seq ctDNA studies performed by Chabon et al. on 41 patients harboring both EGFR-activating and EGFR-resistant T790M mutations on tumor tissue after progression to prior EGFR-TKI therapy revealed additional molecular alterations, including MET alteration or HER2 increased gene copy number (GCN) and/or single nucleotide variations [55]. Since the simultaneous presence of such a plethora of different molecular alterations has been associated with poorer outcomes to TKI therapies, ctDNA analysis could represent a valuable option in guiding clinicians in the choice of the proper treatment strategy. Notably it has been recently developed a novel targeted NGS approach for the detection of both driver mutations and rearrangements in ctDNA from advanced NSCLC patients [56]. This approach relies on the use of specific intronic probes that enable the detection of genome-level rearrangements that create chimeric gene fusions in ALK, ROS1, and RET. The assay and analysis software was able to identify mutation present at 0.1% even if the diagnostic performance was better, reaching 100% sensitivity and specificity, when mutations were present at an allelic frequency 0.4% or greater [56]. In addition to plasma, urine genotyping has also shown a high sensitivity in detecting T790M mutation status, ranging from 72% to 93%, in preliminary studies including few patients and is currently under investigation in trials including larger cohorts of patients [57].

Exosomes

The interest of the scientific community on the role of exosomes in NSCLC is growing, and as it happens with CTCs, exosomes are nowadays a pending subject to understand. Despite the misunderstanding of the exact exosome composition and function, this is becoming one of the most interesting fields of study in liquid biopsy. As aforementioned, exosomes contain a wide variety of material like miRNAs, proteins, and finally, messenger RNA that are surrounded by a lipid bilayer that confers stability. The exosomes differ from the other components of the liquid biopsy because they are actively released by the cells, earning a potential role in tumor progression.

The implementation of exosomes in clinical practice is several steps back as compared to ctDNA in NSCLC. This is mainly due to the lack of consensus in the best way of isolating exosomes from body fluids, but also to the high quantity of material needed to their study. For this reason, in this chapter we will talk about the principal advances in the study of exosomes in NSCLC that could lead to an implementation in the clinical practice in the following years.

The study of exosomal miRNAs is very promising, and new techniques have improved miRNA detection in NSCLC [58]. The new high-throughput technologies have allowed to identify differential miRNA expression between tumor-derived exosomes and exosomes derived from healthy volunteers. This has permitted the description of different miRNA profiles that can help for both tumor diagnosis and/or disease monitoring [59]. For example miRNA-373 and miRNA-512 seem to restrict both the growth and invasiveness of the tumor in normal conditions. However, in cancer patients these ncRNAs are epigenetically silenced, meaning a poor prognosis for the patients, while if the silencing disappears, the re-expression of the miRNAs inhibits the cell migration [60]. Regarding the treatment follow-up, the overexpression of miR-208a and miR-1246 seems to promote the resistance to chemotherapy in NSCLC patients. Similarly our group described that the overexpression of miR-221-3p and -222-3p in patients treated with third-generation TKI (osimertinib) is associated with better prognosis [58, 61, 62].

The sequencing of the exosomes transcriptome is a novel field of study, and thus, the information available are still limited. Through RNA sequencing it was also possible to detect EGFR mutations inside exosomes [63]. Accordingly we have recently detected the EML4-ALK translocation within exosomes derived from plasma of NSCLC patients [64].

The high-throughput technologies for exosomes proteomic analysis may allow to identify the primary tumor and analyze its molecular profile to better understand it. Regarding this, Yamashita et al. demonstrated that the presence of EGFR protein was significantly higher in the membrane of exosomes isolated from NSCLC patients compared to healthy donors [65]. Some other proteins have been described to be important prognostic biomarkers; for example, Sandfeld-Paulsen described CD171 on the membrane of the exosomes as a marker for positive overall survival in NSCLC [66], and also FAM3C have been described to be a good prognostic factor in squamous cell carcinoma patients [67]. The exosomes may be also helpful to the tumor diagnosis. Indeed, the same group has described different markers to discriminate the subtype of tumor, including also multi-marker models with a better discrimination curve [68].

A peculiar feature of the exosomes is their ability to be specifically phagocytized by cancer cells. This could lead to the use of exosomes as drug delivery components. It has been already demonstrated that in lung cancer mice models,

Paclitaxel encapsulated in the exosomes could be an effective treatment option [69]. Moreover, two clinical trials using this innovative approach of drug delivery have been performed. The first approach is a Phase I trial using dendritic cell-derived exosomes (DEX) immunotherapy; the second one is a Phase II trial where a vaccination with DEX carrying IL-15Ra and NKG2D in association with cyclophosphamide after platinum-based chemotherapy. The main objective of both studies was to measure the toxicity and the feasibility to produce autologous DEX. The results from both studies are eagerly awaited also because it has been shown that DEXs were also able to activate both the adaptive and the innate immune system [70, 71].

How the Future of Liquid Biopsy Looks Like: Platelets as a Source of Tumor-RNA

Rearrangements of ALK, ROS1, and RET genes are now important as much as EGFR-activating mutations because in this subgroup of patients very effective targeted treatment can be used. Nevertheless, it is important to point out that for this kind of analysis RNA is requested instead of DNA. This may represent a problem because circulating RNA undergoes degradation very quickly unless plasma samples are rapidly processed after withdrawal. Several research groups are trying to overcome this inconvenient. Indeed recent studies have shown that platelets can engulf tumor-related RNA preserving it from degradation, and thus permitting to identify primary tumor profiles with very high accuracy, and, in many cases, discriminate if the patients are metastatic or not [72, 73]. In 2016 Nilsson et al. have first shown that EML4-ALK translocation can be detected through RT-PCR from platelet-derived RNA with 65% sensitivity and 100% specificity [74] (Table 12.1).

Table 12.1 Summary of the useful components described along the chapter and their clinical utility

Liquid Biopsy Component	Detection	Utility	References
Circulating Tumor Cells	CTCs enumeration	↓Prognosis	[23, 26]
	EGFR	Diagnosis/Recurrence	[27]
	ALK-EML4	Diagnosis	[29–31]
Circulating Tumor DNA	EGFR	Diagnosis/Recurrence	[37–42]
	TP53	Diagnosis	[43]
	KRAS	Diagnosis	[43]
	T790M	↑Prognosis	[46, 47]
	[ctDNA] ng/mL	↓Prognosis	[44]
	T790M	Follow-up	[52]
Exosomes	miR -373, -512	↑Prognosis	[60]
	miR -208a, -2223p	↓Prognosis	[61, 62]
	miR -221-3p, -223-3p	↑Prognosis	[58]
	EGFR	Diagnosis	[63]
	EML4-ALK	Diagnosis	[64]
	CD171	↑Prognosis	[66]
	FAM3C	↑Prognosis	[67]
Platelets	EML4-ALK	Diagnosis	[74]

Conclusions

In conclusion, the incorporation of ctDNA analysis can definitely improve lung cancer patients' management because it can provide a better molecular stratification even when tissue cannot be obtained due to ethical and safety reasons. Although the implementation of both exosomes and CTCs in clinical practice is several steps back, the new advances and discoveries makes them, together with the ctDNA, a very promising tool. Liquid biopsy analysis can be used in different moments starting from diagnosis to relapse, earning multiple clinical meanings. In fact, at diagnosis, it can help in obtaining a better patients' stratification with both prognostic and predictive value, rather than during treatment, and it can be a valuable and simple test to follow tumor response and moreover to identify resistance mechanisms. Therefore it is clear that liquid biopsy has already improved NSCLC patients' management as it offers a noninvasive but valid method to detect actionable mutations.

References

1. Jemal A, Bray F, Center MM, Ferlay J, Ward E, Forman D. Global cancer statistics. CA Cancer J Clin [Internet]. 2011;61. Available from: http://dx.doi.org/10.3322/caac.20107.
2. Passiglia F, Bronte G, Castiglia M, Listi A, Calo V, Toia F, et al. Prognostic and predictive biomarkers for targeted therapy in NSCLC: for whom the bell tolls? Expert Opin Biol Ther England. 2015;15(11):1553–66.
3. Mok TS, Wu Y-L, Ahn M-J, Garassino MC, Kim HR, Ramalingam SS, et al. Osimertinib or platinum-pemetrexed in EGFR T790M-positive lung cancer. N Engl J Med. 2017 Feb 16;376(7):629-40.
4. Drizou M, Kotteas EA, Syrigos N. Treating patients with ALK-rearranged non-small-cell lung cancer: mechanisms of resistance and strategies to overcome it. Clin Transl Oncol. Italy; 2017.
5. Ho C-C, Liao W-Y, Lin C-A, Shih J-Y, Yu C-J, Chih-Hsin Yang J. Acquired BRAF V600E mutation as resistant mechanism after treatment with osimertinib. J Thorac Oncol. United States; 2016.
6. Kobayashi Y, Azuma K, Nagai H, Kim YH, Togashi Y, Sesumi Y, et al. Characterization of EGFR T790M, L792F, and C797S mutations as mechanisms of acquired resistance to afatinib in lung cancer. Mol Cancer Ther. United States; 2016.

7. Paik S, Shak S, Tang G, Kim C, Baker J, Cronin M, et al. A multigene assay to predict recurrence of tamoxifen-treated, node-negative breast cancer. N Engl J Med [Internet]. Massachusetts Medical Society; 2004;351(27):2817–26. Available from: http://dx.doi.org/10.1056/NEJMoa041588.

8. Allegra CJ, Jessup JM, Somerfield MR, Hamilton SR, Hammond EH, Hayes DF, et al. American society of clinical oncology provisional clinical opinion: testing for KRAS gene mutations in patients with metastatic colorectal carcinoma to predict response to anti–epidermal growth factor receptor monoclonal antibody therapy. J Clin Oncol [Internet]. American Society of Clinical Oncology; 2009;27(12):2091–6. Available from: http://ascopubs.org/doi/abs/10.1200/JCO.2009.21.9170.

9. Kuiper JL, Heideman DAM, Thunnissen E, Paul MA, van Wijk AW, Postmus PE, et al. Incidence of T790M mutation in (sequential) rebiopsies in EGFR-mutated NSCLC-patients. Lung Cancer. Ireland. 2014; 85(1):19–24.

10. Rolfo C, Castiglia M, Hong D, Alessandro R, Mertens I, Baggerman G, et al. Liquid biopsies in lung cancer: The new ambrosia of researchers. Biochim Biophys Acta. Elsevier B.V. 2014;1846(2):539–46.

11. Hanahan D, Weinberg RA. Hallmarks of cancer: the next generation. Cell [Internet]. 2014;144(5):646–74. Available from: http://www.sciencedirect.com/science/article/pii/S0092867411001279

12. Feng H, Wang X, Zhang Z, Tang C, Ye H, Jones L, et al. Identification of genetic mutations in human lung cancer by targeted sequencing. Cancer Inform [Internet]. Libertas Academica. 2015;14:83–93. Available from: http://www.ncbi.nlm.nih.gov/pmc/articles/PMC4489668/

13. Soda M, Choi YL, Enomoto M, Takada S, Yamashita Y, Ishikawa S, et al. Identification of the transforming EML4-ALK fusion gene in non-small-cell lung cancer. Nature [Internet]. Nature Publishing Group; 2007;448(7153):561–6. Available from: http://dx.doi.org/10.1038/nature05945.

14. Qian H, Gao F, Wang H, Ma F. The efficacy and safety of crizotinib in the treatment of anaplastic lymphoma kinase-positive non-small cell lung cancer: a meta-analysis of clinical trials. BMC Cancer. England. 2014;14:683.

15. Reck M, van Zandwijk N, Gridelli C, Baliko Z, Rischin D, Allan S, et al. Erlotinib in advanced non-small cell lung cancer: efficacy and safety findings of the global phase IV tarceva lung cancer survival treatment study. J Thorac Oncol [Internet]. 2010;5(10):1616–1622. Available from: http://www.sciencedirect.com/science/article/pii/S1556086415318098.

16. Rolfo C, Giovannetti E, Hong DS, Bivona T, Raez LE, Bronte G, et al. Novel therapeutic strategies for patients with NSCLC that do not respond to treatment with EGFR inhibitors. Cancer Treat Rev. Netherlands. 2014;40(8):990–1004.

17. Choi YL, Soda M, Yamashita Y, Ueno T, Takashima J, Nakajima T, et al. EML4-ALK mutations in lung cancer that confer resistance to ALK inhibitors. N Engl J Med. United States. 2010;363(18):1734–9.

18. Scheffler M, Merkelbach-Bruse S, Bos M, Fassunke J, Gardizi M, Michels S, et al. Spatial tumor heterogeneity in lung cancer with acquired epidermal growth factor receptor-tyrosine kinase inhibitor resistance: targeting high-level MET-amplification and EGFR T790M mutation occurring at different sites in the same patient. J Thorac Oncol. United States. 2015;10(6):e40–3.

19. Zhao Q, Wang Z-T, Sun J-L, Han D, An D-Z, Zhang D-K, et al. Intratumoral heterogeneity of subcutaneous nodules in a never-smoker woman of lung squamous cell carcinoma detected on 18F–fluorodeoxyglucose positron emission tomography and computed tomography: a case report. Medicine (Baltimore). United States. 2015;94(21):e851.

20. Massihnia D, Perez A, Bazan V, Bronte G, Castiglia M, Fanale D, et al. A headlight on liquid biopsies: a challenging tool for breast cancer management. Tumour Biol. Netherlands. 2016;37(4):4263–73.

21. Piotrowska Z, Niederst MJ, Karlovich CA, Wakelee HA, Neal JW, Mino-Kenudson M, et al. Heterogeneity underlies the emergence of EGFRT790 wild-type clones following treatment of T790M-positive cancers with a third-generation EGFR inhibitor. Cancer Discov. United States. 2015;5(7):713–22.

22. Yu N, Zhou J, Cui F, Tang X. Circulating tumor cells in lung cancer: detection methods and clinical applications. Lung [Internet]. 2015;193(2):157–71. Available from: http://dx.doi.org/10.1007/s00408-015-9697-7

23. Tanaka F, Yoneda K, Kondo N, Hashimoto M, Takuwa T, Matsumoto S, et al. Circulating tumor cell as a diagnostic marker in primary lung cancer. Clin Cancer Res. United States. 2009;15(22):6980–6.

24. Wendel M, Bazhenova L, Boshuizen R, Kolatkar A, Honnatti M, Cho EH, et al. Fluid biopsy for circulating tumor cell identification in patients with early-and late-stage non-small cell lung cancer: a glimpse into lung cancer biology. Phys Biol. England. 2012;9(1):16005.

25. Ge M, Shi D, Wu Q, Wang M, Li L. Fluctuation of circulating tumor cells in patients with lung cancer by real-time fluorescent quantitative-PCR approach before and after radiotherapy. J Cancer Res Ther. India. 2005;1(4):221–6.

26. Krebs MG, Sloane R, Priest L, Lancashire L, Hou J-M, Greystoke A, et al. Evaluation and prognostic significance of circulating tumor cells in patients with non–small-cell lung cancer. J Clin Oncol [Internet]. American Society of Clinical Oncology. 2011;29(12):1556–63. Available from: http://ascopubs.org/doi/abs/10.1200/JCO.2010.28.7045

27. Maheswaran S, Sequist LV, Nagrath S, Ulkus L, Brannigan B, Collura CV, et al. Detection of mutations in EGFR in circulating lung-cancer cells. N Engl

J Med [Internet]. Massachusetts Medical Society. 2008;359(4):366–77. Available from: http://dx.doi.org/10.1056/NEJMoa0800668

28. Punnoose EA, Atwal S, Liu W, Raja R, Fine BM, Hughes BGM, et al. Evaluation of circulating tumor cells and circulating tumor DNA in non-small cell lung cancer: association with clinical endpoints in a phase II clinical trial of pertuzumab and erlotinib. Clin Cancer Res. United States. 2012;18(8):2391–401.

29. Tan CL, Lim TH, Lim TK, Tan DS-W, Chua YW, Ang MK, et al. Concordance of anaplastic lymphoma kinase (ALK) gene rearrangements between circulating tumor cells and tumor in non-small cell lung cancer. Oncotarget. United States. 2016;7(17):23251–62.

30. Ilie M, Long E, Butori C, Hofman V, Coelle C, Mauro V, et al. ALK-gene rearrangement: a comparative analysis on circulating tumour cells and tumour tissue from patients with lung adenocarcinoma. Ann Oncol Off J Eur Soc Med Oncol. England. 2012;23(11):2907–13.

31. Pailler E, Adam J, Barthelemy A, Oulhen M, Auger N, Valent A, et al. Detection of circulating tumor cells harboring a unique ALK rearrangement in ALK-positive non-small-cell lung cancer. J Clin Oncol. United States. 2013;31(18):2273–81.

32. He W, Xu D, Wang Z, Xiang X, Tang B, Li S, et al. Detecting ALK-rearrangement of CTC enriched by nanovelcro chip in advanced NSCLC patients. Oncotarget. United Sterts; 2016.

33. Perez-Callejo D, Romero A, Provencio M, Torrente M. Liquid biopsy based biomarkers in non-small cell lung cancer for diagnosis and treatment monitoring. Transl lung cancer Res. China; 2016;5(5):455–465.

34. Sorber L, Zwaenepoel K, Deschoolmeester V, Van Schil PEY, Van Meerbeeck J, Lardon F, et al. Circulating cell-free nucleic acids and platelets as a liquid biopsy in the provision of personalized therapy for lung cancer patients. Lung Cancer. Ireland; 2016.

35. Meldrum C, Doyle MA, Tothill RW. Next-generation sequencing for cancer diagnostics: a practical perspective. Clin Biochem Rev. Australia. 2011;32(4):177–95.

36. Behjati S, Tarpey PS. What is next generation sequencing? Arch Dis Child Educ Pract Ed [Internet]. BMA House, Tavistock Square, London, WC1H 9JR: BMJ Publishing Group; 2013;98(6):236–8. Available from: http://www.ncbi.nlm.nih.gov/pmc/articles/PMC3841808/.

37. Qian X, Liu J, Sun Y, Wang M, Lei H, Luo G, et al. Circulating cell-free DNA has a high degree of specificity to detect exon 19 deletions and the single-point substitution mutation L858R in non-small cell lung cancer. Oncotarget. United States. 2016;7(20):29154–65.

38. Luo J, Shen L, Zheng D. Diagnostic value of circulating free DNA for the detection of EGFR mutation status in NSCLC: a systematic review and meta-analysis. Sci Rep. England. 2014;4:6269.

39. Wu Y, Liu H, Shi X, Song Y. Can EGFR mutations in plasma or serum be predictive markers of non-small-cell lung cancer? A meta-analysis. Lung Cancer. Ireland. 2015;88(3):246–53.

40. Qiu M, Wang J, Xu Y, Ding X, Li M, Jiang F, et al. Circulating tumor DNA is effective for the detection of EGFR mutation in non-small cell lung cancer: a meta-analysis. Cancer Epidemiol Biomarkers Prev. United States. 2015;24(1):206–12.

41. Sacher AG, Paweletz C, Dahlberg SE, Alden RS, O'Connell A, Feeney N, et al. Prospective validation of rapid plasma genotyping for the detection of EGFR and KRAS mutations in advanced lung cancer. JAMA Oncol. United States. 2016;2(8):1014–22.

42. Reck M, Hagiwara K, Han B, Tjulandin S, Grohe C, Yokoi T, et al. ctDNA determination of EGFR mutation status in European and Japanese patients with advanced NSCLC: the ASSESS study. J Thorac Oncol. United States. 2016;11(10):1682–9.

43. Villaflor V, Won B, Nagy R, Banks K, Lanman RB, Talasaz A, et al. Biopsy-free circulating tumor DNA assay identifies actionable mutations in lung cancer. Oncotarget. United States. 2016;7(41):66880–91.

44. Thompson JC, Yee SS, Troxel AB, Savitch SL, Fan R, Balli D, et al. Detection of therapeutically targetable driver and resistance mutations in lung cancer patients by next-generation sequencing of cell-free circulating tumor DNA. Clin Cancer Res. United States. 2016;22(23):5772–82.

45. Chen K-Z, Lou F, Yang F, Zhang J-B, Ye H, Chen W, et al. Circulating tumor DNA detection in early-stage non-small cell lung cancer patients by targeted sequencing. Sci Rep. England. 2016;6:31985.

46. Dietz S, Schirmer U, Merce C, von Bubnoff N, Dahl E, Meister M, et al. Low input whole-exome sequencing to determine the representation of the tumor exome in circulating DNA of non-small cell lung cancer patients. PLoS One. United States. 2016;11(8):e0161012.

47. Wang W, Song Z, Zhang Y. A comparison of ddPCR and ARMS for detecting EGFR T790M status in ctDNA from advanced NSCLC patients with acquired EGFR-TKI resistance. Cancer Med. United States. 2016.

48. Khozin S, Weinstock C, Blumenthal GM, Cheng J, He K, Zhuang L, et al. Osimertinib for the treatment of metastatic epidermal growth factor T970M positive non-small cell lung cancer. Clin Cancer Res. United States. 2016.

49. Janne PA, Yang JC-H, Kim D-W, Planchard D, Ohe Y, Ramalingam SS, et al. AZD9291 in EGFR inhibitor-resistant non-small-cell lung cancer. N Engl J Med. United States. 2015;372(18):1689–99.

50. Thress KS, Brant R, Carr TH, Dearden S, Jenkins S, Brown H, et al. EGFR mutation detection in ctDNA from NSCLC patient plasma: a cross-platform comparison of leading technologies to support the clinical development of AZD9291. Lung Cancer. Ireland. 2015;90(3):509–15.

51. Greig SL. Osimertinib: first global approval. Drugs. New Zealand. 2016;76(2):263–73.

52. Oxnard GR, Paweletz CP, Kuang Y, Mach SL, O'Connell A, Messineo MM, et al. Noninvasive detection of response and resistance in EGFR-mutant lung cancer using quantitative next-generation genotyping of cell-free plasma DNA. Clin Cancer Res. 2014;20:1698–705.

53. Oxnard GR, Thress KS, Alden RS, Lawrance R, Paweletz CP, Cantarini M, et al. Association between plasma genotyping and outcomes of treatment with osimertinib (AZD9291) in advanced non-small-cell lung cancer. J Clin Oncol. United States. 2016; 34(28):3375–82.

54. Frenel JS, Carreira S, Goodall J, Roda D, Perez-Lopez R, Tunariu N, et al. Serial next-generation sequencing of circulating cell-free DNA evaluating tumor clone response to molecularly targeted drug administration. Clin Cancer Res. United States. 2015;21(20):4586–96.

55. Chabon JJ, Simmons AD, Lovejoy AF, Esfahani MS, Newman AM, Haringsma HJ, et al. Corrigendum: circulating tumour DNA profiling reveals heterogeneity of EGFR inhibitor resistance mechanisms in lung cancer patients. Nat Commun. England. 2016;7:13513.

56. Paweletz CP, Sacher AG, Raymond CK, Alden RS, O'Connell A, Mach SL, et al. Bias-corrected targeted next-generation sequencing for rapid, multiplexed detection of actionable alterations in cell-free DNA from advanced lung cancer patients. Clin Cancer Res. United States. 2016;22(4):915–22.

57. Reckamp KL, Melnikova VO, Karlovich C, Sequist LV, Camidge DR, Wakelee H, et al. A highly sensitive and quantitative test platform for detection of NSCLC EGFR mutations in urine and plasma. J Thorac Oncol. United States. 2016;11(10):1690–700.

58. Giallombardo M, Chacártegui Borrás J, Castiglia M, Van Der Steen N, Mertens I, Pauwels P, et al. Exosomal miRNA analysis in non-small cell lung cancer (NSCLC) patients' plasma through qPCR: a feasible liquid biopsy tool. J Vis Exp. 2016;111: e53900. Available from: http://www.jove.com/video/ 53900

59. Reclusa P, Sirera R, Araujo A, Giallombardo M, Valentino A, Sorber L, et al. Exosomes genetic cargo in lung cancer: a truly Pandora's box. Transl lung cancer Res. China. 2016;5(5):483–91.

60. Adi Harel S, Bossel Ben-Moshe N, Aylon Y, Bublik DR, Moskovits N, Toperoff G, et al. Reactivation of epigenetically silenced miR-512 and miR-373 sensitizes lung cancer cells to cisplatin and restricts tumor growth. Cell Death Differ. England. 2015;22(8): 1328–40.

61. Yuan D, Xu J, Wang J, Pan Y, Fu J, Bai Y, et al. Extracellular miR-1246 promotes lung cancer cell proliferation and enhances radioresistance by directly targeting DR5. Oncotarget. 2016;7(22):32707–22.

62. Tang Y, Cui Y, Li Z, Jiao Z, Zhang Y, He Y, et al. Radiation-induced miR-208a increases the proliferation and radioresistance by targeting p21 in human lung cancer cells. J Exp Clin Cancer Res. England. 2016;35:7.

63. Krug AK, Karlovich C, Koestler T, Brinkmann K, Spiel A, Emenegger J, et al. Abstract B136: plasma EGFR mutation detection using a combined exosomal RNA and circulating tumor DNA approach in patients with acquired resistance to first-generation EGFR-TKIs. Am Assoc Cancer Res [Internet]. Molecular Cancer Therapeutics. 2016;14(12 Supplement 2):B136–.B136. Available from: http://mct.aacrjournals.org/content/14/12_Supplement_2/B136.

64. Rolfo C, Laes JF, Reclusa P, Valentino A, Lienard M, Gil-Bazo I, et al. P2.01-093 Exo-ALK proof of concept: exosomal analysis of ALK alterations in advanced NSCLC patients. J Thorac Oncol [Internet]. Elsevier. 2017;12(1):S844–5. Available from: http:// dx.doi.org/10.1016/j.jtho.2016.11.1145

65. Yamashita T, Kamada H, Kanasaki S, Maeda Y, Nagano K, Abe Y, et al. Epidermal growth factor receptor localized to exosome membranes as a possible biomarker for lung cancer diagnosis. Pharmazie. Germany. 2013;68(12):969–73.

66. Sandfeld-Paulsen B, Aggerholm-Pedersen N, Bæk R, Jakobsen KR, Meldgaard P, Folkersen BH, et al. Exosomal proteins as prognostic biomarkers in non-small cell lung cancer. Mol Oncol [Internet]. 2016;10(10):1595–602. Available from: http://www. sciencedirect.com/science/article/pii/S1574789 116301235

67. Wang LZ, Soo RA, Thuya WL, Wang TT, Guo T, Lau JA, Wong FC, Wong ALA, Lee SC, Sze SK, Goh BC. Exosomal protein FAM3C as a potential novel biomarker for non-small cell lung cancer. J Clin Oncol 32, 2014 (suppl; abstr e22162).

68. Sandfeld-Paulsen B, Jakobsen KR, Baek R, Folkersen BH, Rasmussen TR, Meldgaard P, et al. Exosomal proteins as diagnostic biomarkers in lung cancer. J Thorac Oncol. 2016;11:1701–10.

69. Kim MS, Haney MJ, Zhao Y, Mahajan V, Deygen I, Klyachko NL, et al. Development of exosome-encapsulated paclitaxel to overcome MDR in cancer cells. Nanomedicine Nanotechnology, Biol Med [Internet]. 2016;12(3):655–64. Available from: http:// www.sciencedirect.com/science/article/pii/ S1549963415002026

70. Viaud S, Thery C, Ploix S, Tursz T, Lapierre V, Lantz O, et al. Dendritic cell-derived exosomes for cancer immunotherapy: what's next? Cancer Res. United States. 2010;70(4):1281–5.

71. Morse MA, Garst J, Osada T, Khan S, Hobeika A, Clay TM, et al. A phase I study of dexosome immunotherapy in patients with advanced non-small cell lung cancer. J Transl Med [Internet]. 2005;3(1):1–8. Available from: http://dx.doi.org/10.1186/1479-5876-3-9

72. Nilsson RJA, Balaj L, Hulleman E, van Rijn S, Pegtel DM, Walraven M, et al. Blood platelets contain tumor-derived RNA biomarkers. Blood. United States. 2011;118(13):3680–3.

73. Best MG, Sol N, Kooi I, Tannous J, Westerman BA, Rustenburg F, et al. RNA-Seq of tumor-educated platelets enables blood-based pan-cancer, multiclass, and molecular pathway cancer diagnostics. Cancer Cell. United States. 2015;28(5): 666–76.

74. Nilsson RJA, Karachaliou N, Berenguer J, Gimenez-Capitan A, Schellen P, Teixido C, et al. Rearranged EML4-ALK fusion transcripts sequester in circulating blood platelets and enable blood-based crizotinib response monitoring in non-small-cell lung cancer. Oncotarget. United States. 2016;7(1):1066–75.

Liquid Biopsy in Colorectal Cancer

13

A. Galvano, M. Peeters, A.B. Di Stefano,
M. Castiglia, and Antonio Russo

Introduction

In the last years, the new knowledge on the tumor molecular biology has allowed to understand the mechanisms underlying the tumor carcinogenesis, identifying some genes (e.g., RAS, BRAF, PI3K) whose mutation status is associated with a different prognosis [1]. The same has been shown in case of high degree of microsatellite instability (MSI-H) detection. The mixture of all these new parameters within different classifications allowed to hypothesize four molecular subtypes of colorectal cancer (CRC) with different characteristics and biological behavior: CMS1 (characterized by microsatellite instability 15%), CMS2 (standard and characterized by the overexpression of WNT and MYC signal-dependent path-

ways, 35%), CMS3 (with metabolic dysregulation, 15%), and finally CMS4 (mesenchymal type, with overexpression of factors derived from mesenchyme-regulating angiogenesis and stromal invasion, 25%). The remaining portion (about 10%) can be defined by mixed characteristic. Therefore, liquid biopsy, studying features of circulating tumor cells (CTCs), cell-free DNA (cfDNA), exosomes, and microRNAs (miRNAs), could represent in the next future an interesting tool useful to help oncologists in the management of CRC patients (Fig. 13.1).

Circulating Tumor Cells (CTCs)

Among the main elements that constitute a liquid biopsy, there are CTCs. These cells are released into the bloodstream from the primary tumor although they often present some relevant differences with the primary tumor. To capture them from the blood is necessary, however, to use a series of new techniques and cellular markers that allow the enrichment and the CTC selection. As aforementioned, the first step is to enrich CTCs from whole blood in order to allow an easier identification. Generally, the newest tools exploited biological and physical characteristics of the cell surface (expression of specific proteins, size, shape, density, electrical charge). Subsequently, various strategies can be employed to select the cells, including the functional test

A. Galvano • A.B. Di Stefano • M. Castiglia
Department of Surgical, Oncological and Oral
Sciences, Section of Medical Oncology, University of
Palermo, Via del Vespro 129, 90127 Palermo, Italy

M. Peeters
Department of Oncology, Antwerp University
Hospital, Wilrijkstraat 10, 2650 Edegem, Belgium

A. Russo, MD, PhD (✉)
Department of Surgical, Oncological and Oral
Sciences, Section of Medical Oncology, University of
Palermo, Via del Vespro 129, 90127 Palermo, Italy

Institute for Cancer Research and Molecular
Medicine and Center of Biotechnology, College of
Science and Biotechnology, Philadelphia, PA, USA
e-mail: antonio.russo@usa.net

© Springer International Publishing AG 2017
A. Giordano et al. (eds.), *Liquid Biopsy in Cancer Patients*, Current Clinical Pathology,
DOI 10.1007/978-3-319-55661-1_13

Fig. 13.1 Possible implications of liquid biopsy in colorectal cancer (CRC) management

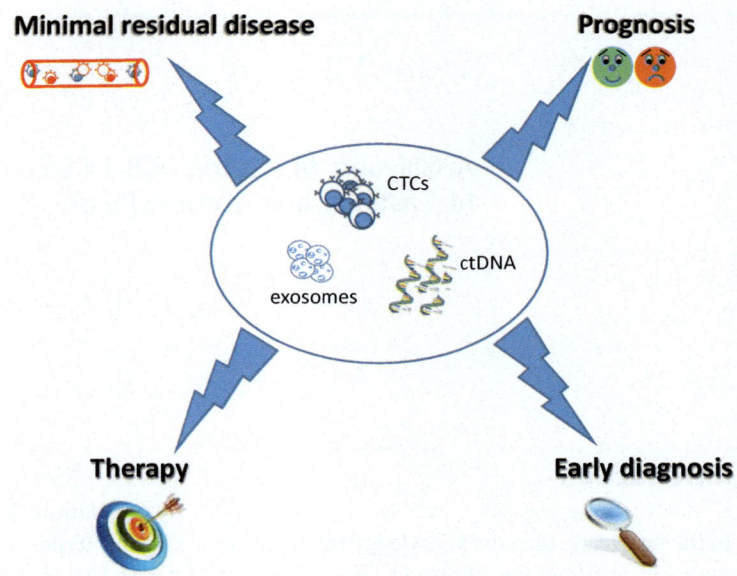

Minimal residual disease

Prognosis

CTCs

exosomes

ctDNA

Therapy

Early diagnosis

with the use of the cellular, immunological, and molecular assays. The completion of these new technologies and the not yet complete comprehension of the biological mechanisms and the functioning of CTCs have not allowed introducing their use in routinely clinical practice. The potential role of CTCs in oncology could be predictive and/or prognostic. In the first case, the CTCs may be useful in selecting the better therapeutic option in both adjuvant and metastatic settings through the identification of specific molecular targets; in the second case they could help to estimate the risk of recurrence in patients who underwent to curative surgery, defining prognosis. Starting from this last concept, it is crucial to remember that up to now the most important predictors of recurrence of CRC are TNM stage and residual disease. In the absence of macroscopic and microscopic residual tumor (R0), the 5-year survival rates range from approximately 75% of stage I to less than 10% of stage IV also presenting heterogeneity within the same disease (N1 >50%; N2 >35%). As for the R1/R2 surgery, the survival rate at 5 years is less than 5%. While the postoperative treatment of stage I does not require any kind of intervention, stage III requires chemotherapy or chemo/RT combination treatment. Postoperative stage II (pT3/pT4, N0, M0) intervention is not

uniquely defined by the main international guidelines. The layering stage II low/high risk currently originates from the evaluation of some parameters conventionally defined as independent prognostic factors. Among these, the main ones are represented by the depth of invasion (pT); the vascular, neural, and lymphatic invasion; the number of lymph nodes examined (pN); the grading (G); and the preoperative values of the tumor marker CEA.

The use of CTCs could be crucial in assessing the risk of recurrence, especially in situations of heightened uncertainty, as it is possible to determine the stage II where the risk of recurrence at 5 years still stands at around 30%. In this sense, the CTCs were evaluated in different experimental conditions. The main technical problem can be attributed to the low number of CTCs in the blood that requires the use of high specific and sensitive methods to discover them. Wang et al. [2] were able to identify CTCs in CRC through the detection of CEA mRNA using RT-PCR. Uen et al. [3] using a panel of mRNA markers that included cytokeratin-19 (CK-19), cytokeratin-20 (CK-20), carcinoembryonic antigen (CEA), and human telomerase reverse transcription (hTERT) mRNA were able to identify CTCs in the peripheral blood of 194 patients with stage II CRC who were subjected to surgery with curative intent. Of these patients, approximately 30% showed the expression of all markers. After a median follow-up of 40 months, approximately 30% of them had recurrent disease, showing that all the four mRNA markers had independent prognostic significance ($p < 0.001$), allowing the identification of high-risk patients' cohort. In another experience the same research group concluded that the persistence of CTCs could be a negative prognostic marker for overall survival (OS) and disease-free survival (DFS) in patients subjected to surgery [4], as later confirmed by CY Lu et al. [5] in a cohort of patients with stage I–III colorectal cancer too. All these results demonstrate why the peripheral CTCs could be a promising biomarker for prognosis in patients with II and III Dukes stage, able to select patients at high risk of recurrence [6]. In addition, another fundamental clinical impact of CTCs could be the ability to predict which patients with stage III CRC are more likely at risk of relapse at the end of adjuvant treatment containing oxaliplatin [7]. The same explorative research was carried out in the metastatic setting (mCRC). The number of CTCs discovered by the CellSearch system in the peripheral blood of patients affected by mCRC resulted in an independent prognostic factor affecting PFS and OS. Therefore, further analysis showed that the use of this parameter before and after the use of chemotherapy plus targeted agent could provide additional information on the biological aggressiveness of the disease. The RAS mutation detection in CTCs might in the near future help to define in advance the potential metastatic behavior and also to select patients who will show resistance and therefore can benefit from other treatment options. It has been proven that patients with mCRC receiving chemotherapy with a FOLFOX or FOLFIRI + cetuximab (anti-EGFR moAb) regimen had a PFS and OS longer if blood CTCs were KRAS wild-type carriers [8] assuming a possible use in clinical practice of this tool. Other experiences have shown that of CTCs may select patients with poor survival despite the response showed at the conventional radiological imaging [9]. The CTCs also seem appropriate in determining the favorite site of metastasis. The evidence recorded in surgical patients who under-

went liver resection has suggested that the detection of CTCs would seem greater in the hepatic, pulmonary, and mesenteric circulations than in the systemic circulation thus carving out a possible role in determining cell tropism [10, 11]. Even the enumeration of CTCs may have a decisive role in this context. Matsusaka S. et al. have recorded that a CTC count greater or equal to three cells per 10 mL of peripheral blood identifies a cohort of patients with a shorter PFS and OS [12], and this result is in agreement with what has been shown by de Albuquerque A. et al. about a significant correlation between the increase in CTCs and the occurrence of radiographically detectable metastases [13]. In a recent study, Shi et al. by using magnetic-activated cell sorting (MACS) and fluorescence-activated cell sorting (FACS) associated with real-time quantitative PCR (RT-qPCR) have speculated whether the number of CTCs found in 55 patients with mCRC before and after cryotherapy can represent a true diagnostic and prognostic marker of cryotherapy efficacy ($p < 0.01$) [14]. But not always the CTCs have been shown to be reliable in identifying patients at high risk of relapse. S Lalmahomed et al. have recently shown that preoperative recognition of CTCs in the peripheral blood of liver-limited CRC patients was not able to select high-risk patients after radical surgery [15]. Despite the sometimes conflicting data, a meta-analysis of 2013 by Groot Koerkamp et al. performed on approximately 1500 patients enrolled in 16 clinical trials of mCRC patients suggested the negative prognostic value on PFS and OS of the CTCs (HR 2.7 and HR 2.47, respectively) [16].

Circulating Tumor DNA (ctDNA)

The circulating cell-free DNA (cfDNA) can be detected either in healthy subjects (e.g., suffering from inflammatory diseases or infections) or from cancer patients. Nevertheless, in the latter case, its concentration may be related to biological characteristics such as tumor size and tumor growth rate, although several authors have assumed a role in the pathogenesis of distant metastases. There are numerous techniques to identify the cfDNA. Among these, more recently, the most used are represented by the quantitative real-time PCR (qPCR), digital polymerase chain reaction (dPCR), and the so-called next-generation sequencing (NGS) techniques generating a high rate of heterogeneity that make it more difficult to compare the results of different clinical trials. The importance of cfDNA, especially of the tumor DNA (ctDNA) component, has been demonstrated in a number of works, which also took into consideration colorectal tumors in several clinically relevant aspects [17, 18]. One of these is the monitoring of the minimal residual disease. As mentioned in the previous paragraph, the CRC radically operated still maintains a significant risk of recurrence especially within the first 5 years for stages II and III of Dukes at around 30% and 50%, respectively, probably caused by the presence of micrometastatic spread. It would seem that even the simple detection of ctDNA may constitute a valid instrument able to help clinicians to identify groups of patients classified as high risk of recurrence to design an appropriate adjuvant strategy, especially regarding the management of stage II that is the most controversial in CRC. In this light, the droplet digital PCR (ddPCR) would appear to be an effective technique with high sensitivity and specificity in predicting the risk of recurrence after radical surgery or after adjuvant strategy [19]. In a study by Tie J et al., it is reported that in 78 patients with stage II diagnosed CRC, the persistence of ctDNA in radically resected patients is associated with disease recurrence, suggesting ctDNA as a possible valid biomarker of tumor recurrence [20]. The addition of targeted agents to conventional chemotherapy has been an important breaking point in the treatment of solid tumors, including CRC, in which they have considerably increased mOS in several large cohort studies. Panitumumab and cetuximab are two monoclonal antibodies that are very effective in the treatment of mCRC only if patients are reported to be wild-type for RAS mutations (both K- and N-RAS genes). The first experiences in this setting had shown that the detection of a mutation of exon 2 of the KRAS (codons 12,13)

present in approximately 40–45% of cases conferred resistance to treatment with this class of drugs. Subsequent retrospective evaluations have also concluded that other mutations in KRAS and other genes from the same family were responsible for a further 17% of resistance to these moAbs molecules (KRAS exons 3,4; NRAS exons 2,3,4) and that probably also some BRAF mutations. Therefore, it has become mandatory to evaluate the mutational status of these genes in order to predict the clinical efficacy and the primary resistance. Routinely, this evaluation is performed on the tissue sample. A possible role of the cfDNA might be to predict in advance and in a less invasive way the response to these targeted agents and the emergence of any resistance, before it can be identified with imaging techniques, thus avoiding unnecessary and potentially toxic treatments to patients. Innovations in the field of molecular biology are leading to a continuous evolution of treatment strategies for CRC treatment, and this phenomenon is largely attributable to the potentially "driver" role that is assigned to a new gene on which next-generation drugs are targeted. The gene study requires neoplastic tissue for further genetic analysis, but in some conditions, the impossibility of a re-biopsy (because it is technically not feasible or because the patient is deemed unfit for invasive procedure) could lead to situations of "undertreatment" that could be avoided with the introduction of liquid biopsy in clinical practice. In particular, Thierry et al. demonstrated that the concordance of KRAS and BRAF mutational status between tissue and plasma samples, using qPCR-based technologies, was around 96% [21]. The previous results agree with what was reported by Kidess et al. regarding the identification of the tumor and plasma ctDNA using the SCODA (sequence-specific synchronous coefficient of drag alteration) assay [22]. Several authors have speculated on how ctDNA can also be used for assessing treatment response in combination with conventional radiology techniques, demonstrating that a decrease in tumor burden corresponds to a great decrease of ctDNA, even in the early cycles of chemotherapy [23]. The same role has been suggested by Spindler et al., which reported that an increase in ctDNA levels during treatment with cetuximab was able to anticipate the radiological disease progression [24]. There are, however, limitations to the use of the ctDNA in this field since increased levels could also be a consequence of benign disease (such as inflammation). Further investigations have tested the use of ctDNA in predicting the emergence of resistance during anti-EGFR treatment. It has been observed that there are different molecular mechanisms responsible for primary or secondary resistance to cetuximab or panitumumab in mCRC that take into account both KRAS mutations as previously reported and the involvement of other genes, such as PTEN, able to bypass the signal from EGFR and to activate the PI3K/AKT/mTOR pathway and other mechanisms that include the amplification of HER2, the activation of IGF-1R, and MET amplification. Undoubtedly, however, the main secondary resistance mechanism is dependent on the RAS mutations that arise during treatment with anti-EGFR after selective pressure (about 40% of cases). Identifying the occurrence of these conditions through the use of ctDNA has led several authors to speculate that ctDNA can somehow anticipate the appearance of radiographic progression [25–27]. The cfDNA could also serve as a new parameter in addition to the more well-known prognostic factors (nodes status, CEA levels, microsatellite stability status, KRAS/BRAF mutation status, resectability of metastatic disease, poor tumor grade, and hepatic tumor burden) to determine the prognosis of patients especially in difficult cases in order to make a decision regarding the chemotherapeutic treatment. Several studies show that high ctDNA levels correlate with lower mPFS and mOS [28]. In particular, Messaoudi SE et al. have evaluated 97 cases of mCRC demonstrating that the ctDNA may be an independent prognostic factor ($p = 0.034$) and that the mutation load and the level of ctDNA fragmentation in KRAS/BRAF mutant patients inversely correlate with OS, highlighting differences up to 10 months [29]. Also using qPCR to compare levels of KRAS mutation found in the primary tumor and plasma could be assumed as an independent factor for PFS ($p = 0.002$) and OS ($p = 0.001$) [30]. CfDNA

assessment could play a decisive role in cancer strategy in the next future, becoming a permanent part of a standard care protocol. A noble goal would be also the use ctDNA testing for early diagnosis of CRC. Most common screening methods used in clinical practice, such as colonoscopy, are indeed invasive and expensive procedures even if they ensure a good level of early diagnosis. Several studies have therefore investigated if it might be possible to detect mutations in the main genes involved in CRC pathogenesis directly from stool or blood, and nevertheless the results are still inconsistent. Today, the use of the liquid biopsy and in particular of ctDNA would also appear to be promising in this setting, since its levels could be positively correlated with the CRC (ROC: 0.709) in patients with the positive occult blood, although the method is still not able to intercept the precancerous lesions [31].

Exosomes and microRNAs (MiRNAs)

The study of exosomes is a recent further step forward in the road toward the identification of an ideal neoplastic marker. Exosomes have morph structural peculiarities; they are stable at room temperature, and their number increases in low-pH medium that is typical of cancer microenvironment [32, 33]. Exosomes are able to carry biological signals from the primary tumor, thus, fostering tumor diffusion. In particular, exosomes seem to modulate angiogenesis balance of the stromal cells favoring the engraftment of pre-metastatic niche. At the molecular level, exosomes contain information able to modulate cancer-mediated growth pathways by promoting cell-cell communication [34–42]. The data about exosomes in CRC are still very limited. The few published experiences have allowed to divide exosomes in a subgroup carrying protein typical of basolateral colonic epithelium region (A33 +) and a subgroup carrying protein of the apical one (EpCAM +). Furthermore, thanks to their ability to interact with the MHC II complex, exosomes exert a role in the immune surveillance of the intestinal mucosa [43]. It has been reported that exosomes derived from CRC cell lines contain a

Table 13.1 Role of liquid biopsy in CRC

	Prognostic	Predictive	Minimal residual disease	Early diagnosis
CTCs	Yes [12–14, 16]	Yes [8]	Yes [3–7]	No
cfDNA	Yes [28–30]	Yes [23–27]	Yes [19–20]	Yes [31]
miRNAs	Yes [48–49]	Yes [50]	No	No

greater number of miRNAs involved in proliferation and angiogenesis mechanisms compared to exosomes isolated from healthy cells. Accordingly, some factors involved in metastatic dissemination (MET, S100A8, S100A9, TNC) are higher in exosomes isolated from metastatic cell lines [38]. The main question remains: how can a researcher identify the specifically cancer-derived exosomes? A group of Japanese researchers led by Y. Yoshioka have experienced a new technique (called ExoScreen) able to isolate exosomes from peripheral blood with high degree of sensitivity and specificity, selecting cancer-specific exosomes using CD147 antigen [44]. MicroRNAs (miRNAs) are among the components that can be identified within the exosomes [45]. MiRNAs contained in CRC-derived exosomes could serve as potential biomarkers modulating the oncogenic properties of the target cells [46, 47]. MiR-21, for example, has proved to be a valid potential serum marker expressed in large amounts of exosomes because of its relation to CRC. MiR-21 is generally upregulated in several other malignancies and in case of inflammation. Subsequent studies have suggested that miR-23a and miR-1246 could be considered potential serum biomarkers for CRC due to their high sensitivity rates (95% and 92%, respectively) [48]. Also in a further experience, Chiba M et al., using CD81 antigen, were able to isolate exosomes from three different CRC cell lines, which contain three upregulated miRNAs involved in the metastatic process (miR-21, miR-221, and miR-192) [49]. The evaluation of miRNAs could ultimately play a role as predictors of response to chemotherapy treatments as shown by Senfter et al. They showed that exosomes secreted by resistant cells contain low levels of miR-200 family. Interestingly, this downregulation was correlated with an increased aggressiveness and invasiveness at both blood and lymphatic levels [50] (Table 13.1).

References

1. Rizzo S, et al. Prognostic vs predictive molecular biomarkers in colorectal cancer: is KRAS and BRAF wild type status required for anti-EGFR therapy? Cancer Treat Rev. 2010;36(Suppl 3):S56–61.
2. Wang JY, et al. Molecular detection of circulating tumor cells in the peripheral blood of patients with colorectal cancer using RT-PCR: significance of the prediction of postoperative metastasis. World J Surg. 2006;30:1007–13.
3. Uen YH, et al. Prognostic significance of multiple molecular markers for patients with stage II colorectal cancer undergoing curative resection. Ann Surg. 2007;246:1040–6.
4. Uen YH, et al. Persistent presence of postoperative circulating tumor cells is a poor prognostic factor for patients with stage I-III colorectal cancer after curative resection. Ann Surg Oncol. 2008;15:2120–8.
5. Lu CY, et al. Molecular detection of persistent postoperative circulating tumour cells in stages II and III colon cancer patients via multiple blood sampling: prognostic significance of detection for early relapse. Br J Cancer. 2011;104:1178–84.
6. Iinuma H, et al. Clinical significance of circulating tumor cells, including cancer stem-like cells, in peripheral blood for recurrence and prognosis in patients with Dukes' stage B and C colorectal cancer. J Clin Oncol. 2011;29:1547–55.
7. Lu CY, et al. Circulating tumor cells as a surrogate marker for determining clinical outcome to mFOLFOX chemotherapy in patients with stage III colon cancer. Br J Cancer. 2013;108:791–7.
8. Yen LC, et al. Detection of KRAS oncogene in peripheral blood as a predictor of the response to cetuximab plus chemotherapy in patients with metastatic colorectal cancer. Clin Cancer Res. 2009;15:4508–13.
9. Barbazán J, et al. A multimarker panel for circulating tumor cells detection predicts patient outcome and therapy response in metastatic colorectal cancer. Int J Cancer. 2014;135:2633–43.

10. Jiao LR, et al. Unique localization of circulating tumor cells in patients with hepatic metastases. J Clin Oncol. 2009;27:6160–5.
11. Rahbari NN, et al. Compartmental differences of circulating tumor cells in colorectal cancer. Ann Surg Oncol. 2012;19:2195–202.
12. Matsusaka S, et al. Circulating tumor cells as a surrogate marker for determining response to chemotherapy in Japanese patients with metastatic colorectal cancer. Cancer Sci. 2011;102:1188–92.
13. de Albuquerque A, et al. Prognostic and predictive value of circulating tumor cell analysis in colorectal cancer patients. J Transl Med. 2012;10:222.
14. Shi J, et al. Analysis of circulating tumor cells in colorectal cancer liver metastasis patients before and after cryosurgery. Cancer Biol Ther. 2016;17:935–42.
15. Lalmahomed ZS, et al. Prognostic value of circulating tumour cells for early recurrence after resection of colorectal liver metastases. Br J Cancer. 2015;112:556–61.
16. Groot Koerkamp B, Rahbari NN, Büchler MW, Koch M, Weitz J. Circulating tumor cells and prognosis of patients with resectable colorectal liver metastases or widespread metastatic colorectal cancer: a meta-analysis. Ann Surg Oncol. 2013;20:2156–65.
17. Bazan V, et al. Molecular detection of TP53, Ki-Ras and p16INK4A promoter methylation in plasma of patients with colorectal cancer and its association with prognosis. Results of a 3-year GOIM (Gruppo Oncologico dell'Italia Meridionale) prospective study. Ann Oncol. 2006;17(Suppl 7):vii84–90.
18. Andreyev HJ, et al. Mutant K-ras2 in serum. Gut. 2003;52:915–6.
19. Reinert T, et al. Analysis of circulating tumour DNA to monitor disease burden following colorectal cancer surgery. Gut. 2016;65:625–34.
20. Tie J, et al. Circulating tumor DNA (ctDNA) as a marker of recurrence risk in stage II colon cancer (CC). J Clin Oncol. 2014;32:5s.
21. Thierry AR, et al. Clinical validation of the detection of KRAS and BRAF mutations from circulating tumor DNA. Nat Med. 2014;20:430–5.
22. Kidess E, et al. Mutation profiling of tumor DNA from plasma and tumor tissue of colorectal cancer patients with a novel, high-sensitivity multiplexed mutation detection platform. Oncotarget. 2015;6:2549–61.
23. Tie J, et al. Circulating tumor DNA as an early marker of therapeutic response in patients with metastatic colorectal cancer. Ann Oncol. 2015;26:1715–22.
24. Spindler KL, Pallisgaard N, Vogelius I, Jakobsen A. Quantitative cell-free DNA, KRAS, and BRAF mutations in plasma from patients with metastatic colorectal cancer during treatment with cetuximab and irinotecan. Clin Cancer Res. 2012;18:1177–85.
25. Bardelli A, et al. Amplification of the MET receptor drives resistance to anti-EGFR therapies in colorectal cancer. Cancer Discov. 2013;3:658–73.
26. Morelli MP, et al. Characterizing the patterns of clonal selection in circulating tumor DNA from patients with colorectal cancer refractory to anti-EGFR treatment. Ann Oncol. 2015;26:731–6.
27. Spindler KL, Pallisgaard N, Andersen RF, Jakobsen A. Changes in mutational status during third-line treatment for metastatic colorectal cancer--results of consecutive measurement of cell free DNA, KRAS and BRAF in the plasma. Int J Cancer. 2014a;135:2215–22.
28. Spindler KL, et al. Cell-free DNA in healthy individuals, noncancerous disease and strong prognostic value in colorectal cancer. Int J Cancer. 2014b;135:2984–91.
29. El Messaoudi S, et al. Circulating DNA as a strong multimarker prognostic tool for metastatic colorectal cancer patient management care. Clin Cancer Res. 2016;22:3067–77.
30. Spindler KL, et al. Clinical utility of KRAS status in circulating plasma DNA compared to archival tumour tissue from patients with metastatic colorectal cancer treated with anti-epidermal growth factor receptor therapy. Eur J Cancer. 2015;51:2678–85.
31. Perrone F, et al. Circulating free DNA in a screening program for early colorectal cancer detection. Tumori. 2014;100:115–21.
32. Parolini I, et al. Microenvironmental pH is a key factor for exosome traffic in tumor cells. J Biol Chem. 2009;284:34211–22.
33. Ge Q, et al. miRNA in plasma exosome is stable under different storage conditions. Molecules. 2014;19:1568–75.
34. Zhou W, et al. Cancer-secreted miR-105 destroys vascular endothelial barriers to promote metastasis. Cancer Cell. 2014;25:501–15.
35. Kucharzewska P, et al. Exosomes reflect the hypoxic status of glioma cells and mediate hypoxia-dependent activation of vascular cells during tumor development. Proc Natl Acad Sci U S A. 2013;110:7312–7.
36. Ekström EJ, et al. WNT5A induces release of exosomes containing pro-angiogenic and immunosuppressive factors from malignant melanoma cells. Mol Cancer. 2014;13:88.
37. Skog J, et al. Glioblastoma microvesicles transport RNA and proteins that promote tumour growth and provide diagnostic biomarkers. Nat Cell Biol. 2008;10:1470–6.
38. Ji H, et al. Proteome profiling of exosomes derived from human primary and metastatic colorectal cancer cells reveal differential expression of key metastatic factors and signal transduction components. Proteomics. 2013;13:1672–86.
39. Al-Nedawi K, et al. Intercellular transfer of the oncogenic receptor EGFRvIII by microvesicles derived from tumour cells. Nat Cell Biol. 2008;10:619–24.
40. Lokody I. Genetics: exosomally derived miR-105 destroys tight junctions. Nat Rev Cancer. 2014;14:386–7.

41. Chowdhury R, et al. Cancer exosomes trigger mesenchymal stem cell differentiation into pro-angiogenic and pro-invasive myofibroblasts. Oncotarget. 2015;6: 715–31.

42. Maitland NJ. Carcinoma-derived exosomes modify microenvironment. Oncotarget. 2015;6:1344–5.

43. Tauro BJ, et al. Two distinct populations of exosomes are released from LIM1863 colon carcinoma cell-derived organoids. Mol Cell Proteomics. 2013;12:587–98.

44. Yoshioka Y, et al. Ultra-sensitive liquid biopsy of circulating extracellular vesicles using ExoScreen. Nat Commun. 2014;5:3591.

45. Gallo A, Tandon M, Alevizos I, Illei GG. The majority of microRNAs detectable in serum and saliva is concentrated in exosomes. PLoS One. 2012;7:e30679.

46. Caruso S, et al. MicroRNAs in colorectal cancer stem cells: new regulators of cancer stemness? Oncogenesis. 2012;1:e32.

47. Corsini LR, et al. The role of microRNAs in cancer: diagnostic and prognostic biomarkers and targets of therapies. Expert Opin Ther Targets. 2012;16(Suppl 2):S103–9.

48. Ogata-Kawata H, et al. Circulating exosomal microRNAs as biomarkers of colon cancer. PLoS One. 2014;9:e92921.

49. Chiba M, Kimura M, Asari S. Exosomes secreted from human colorectal cancer cell lines contain mRNAs, microRNAs and natural antisense RNAs, that can transfer into the human hepatoma HepG2 and lung cancer A549 cell lines. Oncol Rep. 2012;28: 1551–8.

50. Senfter D, et al. Loss of miR-200 family in 5-fluorouracil resistant colon cancer drives lymphendothelial invasiveness in vitro. Hum Mol Genet. 2015;24:3689–98.

Diagnostic and Prognostic Performance of Liquid Biopsy in Hepatocellular Carcinoma

14

Ismail Labgaa, Amanda J. Craig, and Augusto Villanueva

Introduction

Recent epidemiological data rank liver cancer 5th in terms of worldwide new cancer cases in males [1]. In the United States (US), its 5-year survival rate only reaches 16%, displaying the lowest rate after pancreatic cancer [2]. During the last 2 decades, mortality due to liver cancer has more than doubled, being now the second cause of cancer-related death worldwide [3]. As a result, liver cancer has alarmingly become the leading cause of increasing cancer-related mortality in the United States during the

I. Labgaa, MD
Division of Liver Diseases, Liver Cancer Program, Department of Medicine, Tisch Cancer Institute, Icahn School of Medicine at Mount Sinai, New York, NY, USA

Division of Visceral Surgery, University Hospital of Lausanne (CHUV), Lausanne, Switzerland

A.J. Craig, BS
Division of Liver Diseases, Liver Cancer Program, Department of Medicine, Tisch Cancer Institute, Icahn School of Medicine at Mount Sinai, New York, NY, USA

A. Villanueva, MD, PhD (✉)
Division of Liver Diseases, Liver Cancer Program, Department of Medicine, Tisch Cancer Institute, Icahn School of Medicine at Mount Sinai, New York, NY, USA

Division of Hematology/Medical Oncology, Department of Medicine, Icahn School of Medicine at Mount Sinai, New York, NY, USA
e-mail: augusto.villanueva@mssm.edu

last 20 years [4]. Hepatocellular carcinoma (HCC) is the most frequent form of primary liver cancer, and unlike most solid tumors, it typically arises in a chronically damaged organ (i.e., cirrhotic liver). The leading etiologies for the underlying liver disease are viral hepatitis – hepatitis B (HBV) and/or hepatitis C virus (HCV) – or excessive alcohol consumption. Of note, nonalcoholic steatohepatitis (NASH) has increasingly become a major cause of liver disease, resulting in an aberrant accumulation of fat in the hepatocytes, mostly in patients with diabetes, overweight, and metabolic syndrome [5]. The raising prevalence of NASH in Western countries is particularly worrisome considering its association with the risk of HCC development [6].

According to American (AASLD) and European Associations for the Study of the Liver (EASL), clinical practice guidelines (CPG), surgery (i.e., resection and transplantation) and thermal ablation are potentially curative treatments for patients at early stages (Barcelona Clinic Liver Cancer (BCLC) stage A) [7, 8]. The therapeutic arsenal for patients at advanced stages (BCLC-C) is restricted to a single FDA-approved systemic drug, namely, sorafenib [9]. Since its approval in 2007, a number of phase 3 clinical trials testing other molecular therapies have failed to improve survival, highlighting the need to develop new strategies to improve HCC outcomes. Recently, another phase 3 clinical trial showed how regorafenib was able to increase survival in HCC patients in second line [10].

CPG endorsed the BCLC staging algorithm for patient stratification and treatment allocation [11]. The BCLC incorporates clinical variables related to tumor burden, liver dysfunction, and patient symptoms, but it doesn't consider tumor molecular readouts. Although many molecular-based prognostic predictors have been identified including gene signatures [12, 13], none has yet reached the clinical arena. In addition, HCC has the distinctive feature of allowing for a noninvasive diagnosis using imaging techniques under certain conditions [7, 8]. As a consequence, diagnostic biopsy is obtained in less than 20% of HCC patients, thus substantially reducing the access to tissue for molecular analysis. This is particularly detrimental for patients at advanced stages, where identification of oncogenic addiction loops may be pivotal to select optimal responders to molecular therapies. This approach was proved highly effective in other malignan-

cies like lung cancer where ALK rearrangements are a strong predictor of response to crizotinib [14]. In addition to the potential low risk of complications (e.g., bleeding, seeding), prediction derived from tissue biopsy for large HCC may underestimate the landscape of candidate molecular drivers due to intra-tumoral heterogeneity. There are very few studies on this topic, but a recent study revealed significant genetic heterogeneity in 121 tumors from 21 patients [15].

Recent next-generation sequencing analysis including close to 1000 samples has provided a comprehensive mutational landscape of HCC [16–18]. In the meantime, reports on liquid biopsy in HCC are still relatively limited [19]. The identification of genomic aberrations from the tumor via liquid biopsy is thus still lagging behind molecular analysis from tissue samples (Fig. 14.1).

Herein, we provide an overview of the potential role of liquid biopsy in two well-defined

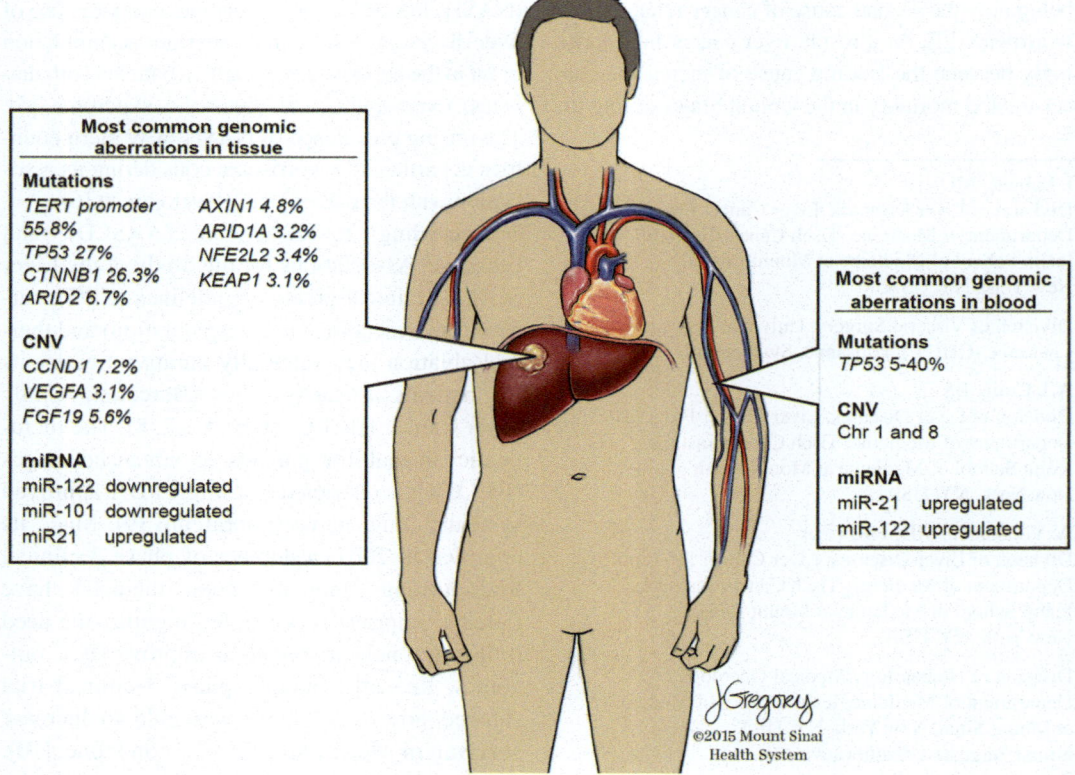

Fig. 14.1 Summary of the most common genomic aberrations in HCC, reported in both tissue and blood

Table 14.1 The diagnostic role of liquid biopsy in HCC

Tumor by-product	Etiology	Early stage (%)[a]	Number of HCC patients	Biomarkers	Technique	Reference
CTC	HBV (85%)	NA	85	CTC enumeration	IMS	[20]
ctDNA	NA	NA	25	p53 mutation	PCR	[21]
	HBV (51%), HCV (24%)	NA	50	Methylation of RASSF1A, P16	Methylation-specific PCR	[22]
	HBV (85%)	NA	72	Methylation of four genes (APC, GSTP1, RASSF1A, SFRP1)	Methylation-specific PCR	[23]
	NA	NA	151	Methylation of four genes (RGS10, ST8SIA6, RUNX2 and VIM)	MCTA-seq[b]	[24]
miRNA	HBV	NA	70	miR-122	qRT-PCR	[25]
	HCV (68%)	63	136	miR-21	qRT-PCR	[26]
	HBV	45	337	miRNA classifier (miR-29a, miR-29C, miR-133a, miR-143, miR-145, miR-192, and miR-505)	qRT-PCR	[27]

IMS immunomagnetic separation, *NA* nonavailable
[a]Early stage defined by BCLC 0-A
[b]Methylated CpG tandems amplification and sequencing

clinical scenarios in HCC, as a diagnostic (Table 14.1) and a prognostic (Table 14.2) tool. We will systematically explore the potential clinical performance of each tumor by-product detected in the blood of HCC patients including circulating DNA (ctDNA), circulating tumor cells (CTCs), and circulating-free RNA (cfRNA).

Liquid Biopsy as a Potential Diagnostic Tool in HCC

Current CPG consensually recommend surveillance every 6 months for patients at high risk for HCC development (i.e., cirrhotic patients, non-cirrhotic HBV patients with active hepatitis of family history of HCC, and non-cirrhotic patients with chronic HCV and advanced liver fibrosis) [7]. Following standard recommendations, this subset of patients should undergo abdominal ultrasound every 6 months. Once a liver nodule is detected on ultrasound, computed tomography (CT) or magnetic resonance imaging (MRI) are thus the gold standard imaging for HCC diagnosis. While their

sensitivity is close to 100% for large lesions (>2 cm), it drastically drops for smaller lesions (<1 cm) [38]. In terms of laboratory tests, alpha-fetoprotein (AFP) is widely used in clinical practice to help HCC diagnosis. However, its role remains limited since its performance as an early detection tool is suboptimal as underscored in the European and American guidelines [7, 8]. In this context, liquid biopsy, as an early detection tool, may offer interesting perspectives that could fulfil the gap.

Circulating Tumor Cells (CTCs)

Most cancer-related deaths follow hematogenous dissemination of malignant cells to distant organs [39], which typically occurs in the late course of the disease. Technologies to isolate CTCs include two major parts: enrichment (isolation) and detection (identification) (Table 14.3). Enrichment approaches mostly rely on physical or biological properties of CTCs, such as size, shape, or surface markers. In HCC, immunological enrichment, targeting cancer cell markers, is

Table 14.2 The prognostic value of liquid biopsy in HCC

Tumor by-product	Number of HCC patients	Etiology	Validation (Yes/No)	Biomarker	Technique	Outcomes	Reference
CTC	44	NA	No	CTC and microemboli detection	Isolation by cells size	Tumor invasion, portal vein thrombosis, and survival	[28]
	85	HBV (85%)	No	ASGPR	IMS	Tumor size, portal vein thrombus, differentiation status, TNM stage, and Milan criteria	[20]
	123	HBV	Yes	EpCAM	CellSearch®	Recurrence	[29]
	82	HBV	No	CSC	Flow cytometry	Intra- and extrahepatic recurrence, survival	[30]
	96	HBV	No	CSC	IMS	Tumor grade, size, BCLC stage, and recurrence	[31]
	60	HBV	Yes	ICAM-1	Flow cytometry	Survival	[32]
	59	HBV (85%)	Yes	pERK/pAkt CTCs	IMS	Progression-free survival	[33]
ctDNA	72	HBV (85%)	No	Methylation RASSF1A	Methylation-specific PCR	Overall survival	[23]
	46	HCV/HBV	No	Presence of ctDNA	Targeted sequencing and exome sequencing	Tumor progression, vascular invasion, recurrence	[34]
miRNA	122	NA	No	miR-122	qRT-PCR	Overall survival	[35]
	195	HCV (15%) Alcohol abuse (33%) HBV (17%)	No	miR-1	qRT-PCR	Overall survival	[36]
	113	NA	Yes	Vps4A		TNM stage, tumor size, recurrence free survival	[37]

NA non available

Table 14.3 Technical details for CTCs isolation in HCC

Enrichment		HCC patients (n)	Detection	Number of CTCs recovered	Reference
Technique	Marker				
IMS	CD45 – EpCAM +	55	HepPar1+, hTERT+, AFP+	1–5/2 mL	[40]
IMS	CD45-	11	CD45-, DAPI+, ASGPR1+, EpCAM+, pan-CK+ or Vim + or N-cad+	Not reported	[41]
IMS	CD45-	59	EpCAM+, CK+, CD45-, DAPI+	7–35/7.5 mL	[42]
CellSearch®	CD45- EpCAM+	123	EpCAM+, CD45-, CK+, CD133+, ABCG2+, CD90+, beta-cat+, vim+, cad+	1–34/7.5 mL	[29]
IMS	CD45-	6	EpCAM+, AFP+, CK+, DAPI+	4–37/7.5 mL	[43]
CellSearch®	CD45-, EpCAM+	20	EpCAM+, CK+, DAPI+, CD45- WGA vs PMBC banked	1/7.5 mL	[44]
IMS	ASGPR+	85	HepPar1+, DAPI+, CD45- TP53-, Her2+	3–40/5 mL	[20]
IMS	ASGPR+	27	CPS1+, HepPar1+, CK+, CD45-, DAPI+	7–61/5 mL	[45]

IMS immunomagnetic separation

the most commonly used technique. As an example, CellSearch® targeting EpCAM is the most widely used method and the first FDA-approved system for CTC isolation. This technique allowed exploring the impact of CTCs in HCC and further identified a subset of CTCs with stem cell-like features [29]. Of note, there is some debate regarding the use of EpCAM-based enrichment in HCC, since only 30% of HCC cells overexpress this marker [46]. Attempting to overpass this limitation, a variety of different technological approaches has been explored to accurately isolate CTCs in HCC patients. A recent study reported data of a new isolation technique based on immunomagnetic bead selection, using the ligand of asialoglycoprotein receptor (ASGPR). In a cohort of 85 HCC patients, 20 healthy patients, 16 cirrhotic patients, and 14 controls with non-HCC cancers, CTCs were detected in 69 HCC patients (81%) but in none of the patients from the control groups [20]. More recently, a novel technology for CTC isolation has been reported which included the use of an Image-Stream flow cytometer. This allowed to detect multiple biomarkers and to generate high-resolution images, which resulted in isolated cells with a high specificity [43]. Interestingly, authors were able to validate this method in different types of cancers, including HCC. Although data on CTCs are promising, further investigations are needed to clarify whether they may be used for early HCC detection. Based on the fact that CTC detection is more frequent in patients at advanced stages, its potential role as a surveillance tool for early detection is questionable.

Circulating DNA (ctDNA)

Similar to other tumors, release of DNA to the bloodstream by HCC cells seems to follow two patterns: passive and/or active. The former is mainly caused by necrosis and apoptosis and seems to be the main source of ctDNA, while the latter is explained by newly synthesized DNA, released into the bloodstream by tumor cells [47]. The fragments of DNA generated by apoptosis have a typical length of ~150 bp (coincidental

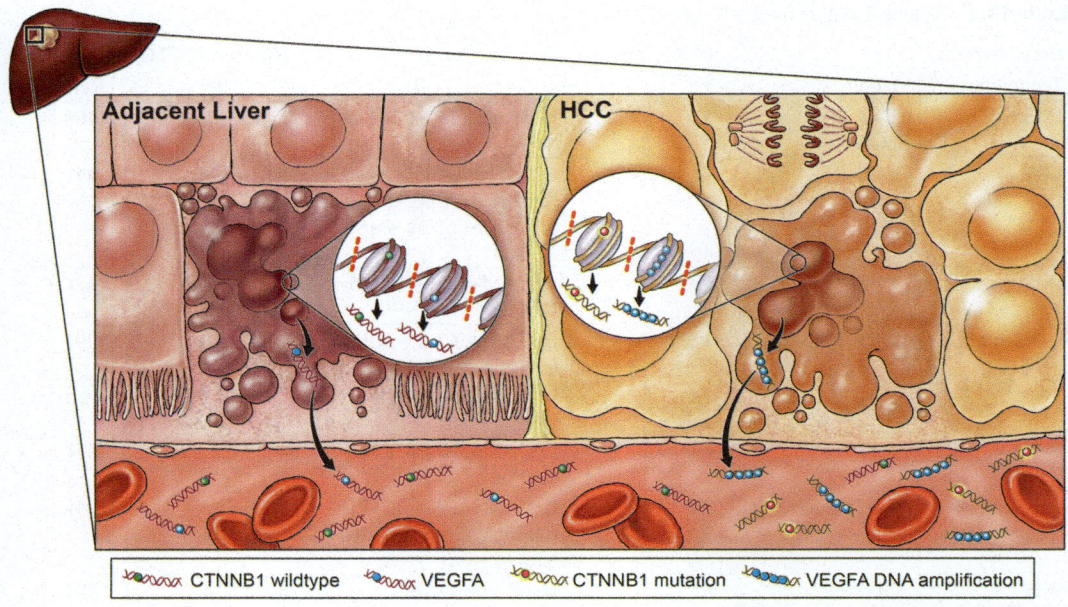

CTNNB1 wildtype   VEGFA   CTNNB1 mutation   VEGFA DNA amplification

J Gregory ©2015 Mount Sinai Health System

Fig. 14.2 Normal and HCC apoptotic cells releasing DNA into the blood supply. The DNA released by the HCC into blood, the so-called circulating tumor DNA (ctDNA), is characterized by genomic aberrations, like CTNNB1 mutation or VEGFA amplification in this case

with the DNA size encapsulated by a nucleosome), and they are generally shorter than the ones caused by necrosis. In HCC, a recent paper was able to infer the length of ctDNA in a cohort of 90 HBV-HCC patients showing shorter fragments (~166 bp) in DNA derived from tumor compared to non-tumoral circulating DNA. This further suggested that apoptosis was a dominant mechanism of ctDNA release (Fig. 14.2) [48]. By looking at a specific pattern of DNA aberrations in the plasma, authors developed a score highly correlated with the presence of HCC. Interestingly, patients initially labeled as controls (i.e., HBV carriers) but with an abnormal ctDNA profile were soon after diagnosed with HCC, reflecting the potential capacity of ctDNA as a surveillance tool [49]. Following a similar approach but using genome-wide methylation sequencing in a cohort of pregnant women, HCC patients, and transplant recipients, the same group was able to infer the contribution of each component (i.e., placenta, tumor, graft) to the circulating DNA pool [50]. A thorough catalogue of specific DNA alterations such as point mutations or high-level DNA

amplifications detected on ctDNA from HCC patients is not yet available. More importantly, its correlation with tissue findings is also lacking (Fig. 14.1). Regarding mutations, *TP53* is the most commonly mutated gene in HCC for which mutated forms have been detected in ctDNA, with a frequency ranging from 5% to 40% [21, 51]. *TP53* mutations are highly prevalent in the context of aflatoxin B1 dietary exposure or chronic HBV infection, like in certain regions of Africa and East Asia, respectively [51]. Nevertheless, its use as a potential diagnostic tool is limited due to low specificity. Hence, a diagnostic tool relying only on *TP53* plasmatic mutations could lead to a high rate of false-negative tests.

For diagnostic purposes, methylation changes have been explored as potential surrogate markers of HCC development. The diagnostic value of the aberrant hypermethylation of three genes (i.e., *RASSF1A*, *P16*, and *P15*) was evaluated in the plasma of 50 HCC patients. Combining the methylation status of these genes with other clinical variables such as age, viral status, smoking, and alcohol intake, authors reported 84% sensitivity and 94% specificity for HCC detection [22]. Moreover, a signature of four aberrantly methylated genes (*APC*, *GSTP1*, *RASSF1A*, and *SFRP1*) for HCC diagnosis in a cohort of 72 patients showed sensitivity and specificity of 93% and 82%, respectively [23]. Aberrant hypermethylation of CpG sites in plasma of HCC patients was also used to detect small HCC (≤3 cm), in a cohort of patients with HCC (*n* = 36), cirrhosis (*n* = 17), and healthy controls (*n* = 38). Authors developed two classifiers able to achieve a sensitivity and specificity of 94% and 89% for HCC diagnosis, respectively [24].

Circulating-Free RNA (cfRNA)

Circulating RNA, also called cell-free RNA is mostly encapsulated and released in small vesicles. The so-called exosomes account for an important fraction of the vesicles carrying cfRNA. Exosomes are small enclosed vesicles (30–100 nm) released into body fluids by exocytosis and transporting cell-specific proteins and nucleic acids such as mRNA, microRNA (miRNA), and other noncoding RNA [52]. While mRNA circulates in exosomes, free miRNA may be found in plasma and serum, associated with proteins [53]. There is limited data whether exosomes may be used for HCC diagnosis [52]. Conversely, numerous circulating miRNAs have been investigated for the ability to identify HCC at early stage. Although several miRNAs displayed a good performance in distinguishing HCC patients from healthy controls, most showed a relatively poor specificity, being unable to accurately discriminate HCC patients from other patients with chronic liver injury, such as viral hepatitis, alcohol-related liver disease, or nonalcoholic fatty liver disease (NAFLD). MiR-122 and miR-21 appear as appealing candidates [25, 26]. Indeed, a study revealed that miR-122 was significantly increased in HCC patients, compared to healthy controls, showing a sensitivity and specificity of 81.6% and 83.3%, respectively [25]. Similarly, miR-21 was higher in HCC patients than in chronic hepatitis and healthy

volunteers. When differentiating HCC patients from healthy ones, the ROC analysis yielded in an AUC of 0.953 with high sensitivity (87.3%) and specificity (92%), whereas these numbers dropped when analyzing the performance to discriminate HCC patients from patients with chronic hepatitis, leading to an AUC of 0.773 and sensitivity and specificity of 61% and 83%, respectively [26]. In a recent study, Lin et al. developed a miRNA classifier (C_{mi}) integrating Seven differentially expressed miRNA (miR-29a, miR-29c, miR-133a, miR-143, miR-145, miR-192, and miR-505), which showed a higher performance than AFP to distinguish patients with HCC from healthy controls [27]. Such approaches may be valuable to noninvasively detect preclinical HCC, providing a chance to identify tumors at an earlier stage where patients are still candidates for curative treatments.

The Prognostic and Predictive Performance of Liquid Biopsy in HCC

Once HCC is diagnosed, current recommendations follow the BCLC algorithm as a guide for therapeutic decision-making. There are still some clinical situations where outcome prediction could improve therapeutic decision. An instance is the prediction of tumor recurrence after transplant for patients within Milan criteria or considering transplant for patients exceeding Milan criteria but who have good outcomes. These clinical examples underscore that it is sometimes difficult to adequately capture prognosis in HCC, solely with clinical variables. As a result, the integration of tumor readouts could presumably refine current practice, and liquid biopsy could be a powerful and noninvasive mean to obtain this data.

Circulating Tumor Cells (CTCs)

The presence of metastatic dissemination to distant organs is probably the worse prognostic factor in cancer. This results from the spread and seed of malignant cells through the blood or lymphatic circulations [39, 54]. Identification of CTCs may thus be regarded as bona fide markers of potential disease dissemination. Interestingly, different studies showed that the release of CTCs may even occur during surgery for patients at early stages and that even the surgical procedure itself could facilitate to the release of CTCs [55, 56]. It is also well established that metastasis needs not only the presence of malignant cells on the circulation but also a favorable microenvironment for them to graft and grow, the so-called "seed and soil" theory in metastasis formation [57]. The majority of studies exploring the relevance of CTCs in HCC included surgical patients and investigated the correlation of CTCs with outcomes after resection. One of the pioneer study in the field revealed that the presence of CTCs was associated with shorter survival. Furthermore, they were able to identify *CTNNB1* mutations in a subset of CTCs [28]. In a cohort of 85 HCC patients, a report showed that the presence of CTCs correlated with other clinical variables such as tumor size, vascular invasion, TNM stage, and Milan criteria [20]. Hypothesizing that circulating cancer stem cells (CSC) may display a more aggressive pattern and thus being of particular relevance to predict outcome, several studies explored their role in HCC. As mentioned previously, a study showed CTC isolation by targeting EpCAM+ in a cohort of 123 HCC patients and further demonstrated that EpCAM+ CTCs expressed cancer stem cell markers (i.e., CD133 and ABCG2), epithelial-mesenchymal transition, activation of Wnt pathway, and high tumorigenic and low apoptotic potential [29]. Interestingly, patients with CTCs showing CSC-like features were at a higher risk of recurrence after resection [29–31], as well as reduced overall survival [30, 32]. The poor prognosis associated with the presence of CTCs was confirmed by a recent meta-analysis, which also established its association with poor prognostic factors such as vascular invasion, AFP levels, and tumor stage [58]. A more recent study assessed the impact of CTCs in a cohort of 109 HCC patients at advanced stage who received sorafenib [33].

Authors first provided a new system to measure phosphorylation of the drug's predicted targets (i.e., pERK and pAkt) and showed a concordant expression of these genes in tissue and CTCs. They were further able to identify a subset of patients with pERK$^+$/pAkt$^-$ CTCs, who show better response to sorafenib. Indeed, patients with $\geq$40% of pERK$^+$/pAkt$^-$ had a significant prolonged PFS compared to those with <40% of pERK$^+$/pAkt$^-$.

Circulating DNA (ctDNA)

Nucleic acids (DNA and RNA) extracted from HCC tissue proved to be a useful resource for molecular analysis and for the development of new prognostic tools, such as gene expression or methylation signatures [12, 59]. Conversely, the prognostic value of ctDNA is still under scrutiny. In addition to diagnostic properties, the study that explored the potential diagnostic role of aberrant methylation of three genes also found hypermethylation of *RASSF1A* significantly associated with patient's survival [23]. More recently, a comprehensive study applied targeted sequencing in a cohort of patients undergoing resection and transplant and exosome sequencing in one patient who received transarterial chemoembolization (TACE) [34]. Authors were able to show that 83% of mutations detected in tissue were also present in ctDNA. Moreover, the presence of ctDNA was a predictor of vascular invasion and recurrence, especially for early extrahepatic recurrence. Surprisingly, none of the common mutations reported in HCC tissue (>10%) were detected in ctDNA in this cohort.

Circulating-Free RNA (cfRNA)

Deregulated miRNA may play a critical role in hepatocarcinogenesis, and the degree of their abnormal expression may be used as a prognostic marker in HCC patients. For example, miR-122 – which already demonstrated interest for diagnostic purposes (see above) – correlated with tumor size and was independently associated with overall survival (OS) in a cohort of 122 HCC patients [35]. Consistently, miR-1 was also independently associated with overall survival although no correlation with other clinical variables was observed [36]. A recent study highlighted how Vps4A played a key role in regulating the secretion and the uptake of miRNAs through exosome biogenesis [37]. Their findings further suggested that Vps4A is a tumor suppressor in HCC, since its downregulation was associated with tumor progression and metastasis.

Conclusion

Liver cancer is an aggressive type of tumor with a particularly worrisome epidemiological progression. Although substantial improvements have allowed defining its molecular subclasses, no oncogene addiction loop has yet been identified. The limited access to tissue, justified by the fact few patients are candidate for surgery and that tissue biopsy is not mandatory for diagnosis, underscores the need to develop new approaches to access genomic information from the tumor. Preliminary results on liquid biopsy remain very limited in HCC, albeit promising. To date, miRNA displayed appealing diagnostic performances. Underlying dissemination and thus arising at more advanced stages, CTCs are likely to play a major role as prognostic surrogates. Finally, ctDNA seems to be a polyvalent biomarker, offering interesting options for both diagnosis and prognosis. In the future, the diagnostic and prognostic role of liquid biopsy may have a radical leverage effect on the decision-making for HCC treatment.

Acknowledgments The authors would like to thank Jill Gregory for her design support with Figs. 14.1 and 14.2. IL is supported by Foundation Roberto & Gianna Gonella, SICPA Foundation, and the Swiss National Science Foundation (SNF). AV is the recipient of the American Association for the Study of Liver Diseases (AASLD) Foundation Alan Hofmann Clinical and Translational Award. AV is supported by the U.S. Department of Defense (CA150272P3) and the Tisch Cancer Institute.

Disclosure The authors report no conflicts of interest.

References

1. Torre LA, Bray F, Siegel RL, Ferlay J, Lortet-Tieulent J, Jemal A. Global cancer statistics, 2012. CA Cancer J Clin. 2015;65(2):87–108.
2. DeSantis CE, Lin CC, Mariotto AB, Siegel RL, Stein KD, Kramer JL, et al. Cancer treatment and survivorship statistics, 2014. CA Cancer J Clin. 2014;64(4):252–71.
3. Murray CJ, Vos T, Lozano R, Naghavi M, Flaxman AD, Michaud C, et al. Disability-adjusted life years (DALYs) for 291 diseases and injuries in 21 regions, 1990–2010: a systematic analysis for the Global Burden of Disease Study 2010. Lancet. 2012;380(9859):2197–223.
4. Llovet JM, Villanueva A, Lachenmayer A, Finn RS. Advances in targeted therapies for hepatocellular carcinoma in the genomic era. Nat Rev Clin Oncol. 2015;12(8):436.
5. Calle EE, Rodriguez C, Walker-Thurmond K, Thun MJ. Overweight, obesity, and mortality from cancer in a prospectively studied cohort of U.S. adults. N Engl J Med. 2003;348(17):1625–38.
6. White DL, Kanwal F, El-Serag HB. Association between nonalcoholic fatty liver disease and risk for hepatocellular cancer, based on systematic review. Clin Gastroenterol Hepatol. 2012;10(12):1342–59.e2.
7. European Association For The Study Of The L, European Organisation For R, Treatment Of C. EASL-EORTC clinical practice guidelines: management of hepatocellular carcinoma. J Hepatol. 2012;56(4):908–43.
8. Bruix J, Sherman M, American Association for the Study of Liver D. Management of hepatocellular carcinoma: an update. Hepatology. 2011;53(3):1020–2.
9. Llovet JM, Ricci S, Mazzaferro V, Hilgard P, Gane E, Blanc JF, et al. Sorafenib in advanced hepatocellular carcinoma. N Engl J Med. 2008;359(4):378–90.
10. Bruix J, Qin S, Merle P, Granito A, Huang YH, Bodoky G, Pracht M, Yokosuka O, Rosmorduc O, Breder V, Gerolami R, Masi G, Ross PJ, Song T, Bronowicki JP, Ollivier-Hourmand I, Kudo M, Cheng AL, Llovet JM, Finn RS, LeBerre MA, Baumhauer A, Meinhardt G, Han G; RESORCE Investigators. Regorafenib for patients with hepatocellular carcinoma who progressed on sorafenib treatment (RESORCE): a randomised, double-blind, placebo-controlled, phase 3 trial. Lancet. 2017 Jan 7;389(10064):56–66.
11. Forner A, Llovet JM, Bruix J. Hepatocellular carcinoma. Lancet. 2012;379(9822):1245–55.
12. Villanueva A, Portela A, Sayols S, Battiston C, Hoshida Y, Mendez-Gonzalez J, et al. DNA methylation-based prognosis and epidrivers in hepatocellular carcinoma. Hepatology. 2015;61(6):1945–56.
13. Villanueva A, Hoshida Y, Battiston C, Tovar V, Sia D, Alsinet C, et al. Combining clinical, pathology, and gene expression data to predict recurrence of hepatocellular carcinoma. Gastroenterology. 2011;140(5):1501–12.e2.

14. Shaw AT, Kim DW, Nakagawa K, Seto T, Crino L, Ahn MJ, et al. Crizotinib versus chemotherapy in advanced ALK-positive lung cancer. N Engl J Med. 2013;368(25):2385–94.

15. Friemel J, Rechsteiner MP, Frick L, Boehm F, Struckmann K, Sigg M, et al. Intratumor heterogeneity in hepatocellular carcinoma. Clin Cancer Res. 2015;21(8):1951–61.

16. Schulze K, Imbeaud S, Letouze E, Alexandrov LB, Calderaro J, Rebouissou S, et al. Exome sequencing of hepatocellular carcinomas identifies new mutational signatures and potential therapeutic targets. Nat Genet. 2015;47(5):505–11.

17. Villanueva A, Llovet JM. Liver cancer in 2013: mutational landscape of HCC–the end of the beginning. Nat Rev Clin Oncol. 2014;11(2):73–4.

18. Zucman-Rossi J, Villanueva A, Nault JC, Llovet JM. Genetic landscape and biomarkers of hepatocellular carcinoma. Gastroenterology. 2015;149(5):1226–39.e4.

19. Labgaa I, Villanueva A. Liquid biopsy in liver cancer. Discov Med. 2015;19(105):263–73.

20. Xu W, Cao L, Chen L, Li J, Zhang XF, Qian HH, et al. Isolation of circulating tumor cells in patients with hepatocellular carcinoma using a novel cell separation strategy. Clin Cancer Res. 2011;17(11):3783–93.

21. Jackson PE, Qian GS, Friesen MD, Zhu YR, Lu P, Wang JB, et al. Specific p53 mutations detected in plasma and tumors of hepatocellular carcinoma patients by electrospray ionization mass spectrometry. Cancer Res. 2001;61(1):33–5.

22. Zhang YJ, Wu HC, Shen J, Ahsan H, Tsai WY, Yang HI, et al. Predicting hepatocellular carcinoma by detection of aberrant promoter methylation in serum DNA. Clin Cancer Res. 2007;13(8):2378–84.

23. Huang ZH, Hu Y, Hua D, Wu YY, Song MX, Cheng ZH. Quantitative analysis of multiple methylated genes in plasma for the diagnosis and prognosis of hepatocellular carcinoma. Exp Mol Pathol. 2011;91(3):702–7.

24. Wen L, Li J, Guo H, Liu X, Zheng S, Zhang D, et al. Genome-scale detection of hypermethylated CpG islands in circulating cell-free DNA of hepatocellular carcinoma patients. Cell Res. 2015;25(11):1250–64.

25. Qi P, Cheng SQ, Wang H, Li N, Chen YF, Gao CF. Serum microRNAs as biomarkers for hepatocellular carcinoma in Chinese patients with chronic hepatitis B virus infection. PLoS One. 2011;6(12):e28486.

26. Tomimaru Y, Eguchi H, Nagano H, Wada H, Kobayashi S, Marubashi S, et al. Circulating microRNA-21 as a novel biomarker for hepatocellular carcinoma. J Hepatol. 2012;56(1):167–75.

27. Lin XJ, Chong Y, Guo ZW, Xie C, Yang XJ, Zhang Q, et al. A serum microRNA classifier for early detection of hepatocellular carcinoma: a multicentre, retrospective, longitudinal biomarker identification study with a nested case-control study. Lancet Oncol. 2015;16(7):804–15.

28. Vona G, Estepa L, Beroud C, Damotte D, Capron F, Nalpas B, et al. Impact of cytomorphological detection of circulating tumor cells in patients with liver cancer. Hepatology. 2004;39(3):792–7.

29. Sun YF, Xu Y, Yang XR, Guo W, Zhang X, Qiu SJ, et al. Circulating stem cell-like epithelial cell adhesion molecule-positive tumor cells indicate poor prognosis of hepatocellular carcinoma after curative resection. Hepatology. 2013;57(4):1458–68.

30. Fan ST, Yang ZF, Ho DW, Ng MN, Yu WC, Wong J. Prediction of posthepatectomy recurrence of hepatocellular carcinoma by circulating cancer stem cells: a prospective study. Ann Surg. 2011;254(4):569–76.

31. Cheng SW, Tsai HW, Lin YJ, Cheng PN, Chang YC, Yen CJ, et al. Lin28B is an oncofetal circulating cancer stem cell-like marker associated with recurrence of hepatocellular carcinoma. PLoS One. 2013;8(11):e80053.

32. Liu S, Li N, Yu X, Xiao X, Cheng K, Hu J, et al. Expression of intercellular adhesion molecule 1 by hepatocellular carcinoma stem cells and circulating tumor cells. Gastroenterology. 2013;144(5):1031–41.e10.

33. Li J, Shi L, Zhang X, Sun B, Yang Y, Ge N, et al. pERK/pAkt phenotyping in circulating tumor cells as a biomarker for sorafenib efficacy in patients with advanced hepatocellular carcinoma. Oncotarget. 2015;7(3):2646–59.

34. Ono A, Fujimoto A, Yamamoto Y, Akamatsu S, Hiraga N, Imamura M, et al. Circulating tumor DNA analysis for liver cancers and its usefulness as a liquid biopsy. Cell Mol Gastroenterol Hepatol. 2015;1:516–34.

35. Xu Y, Bu X, Dai C, Shang C. High serum microRNA-122 level is independently associated with higher overall survival rate in hepatocellular carcinoma patients. Tumour Biol. 2015;36(6):4773–6.

36. Koberle V, Kronenberger B, Pleli T, Trojan J, Imelmann E, Peveling-Oberhag J, et al. Serum microRNA-1 and microRNA-122 are prognostic markers in patients with hepatocellular carcinoma. Eur J Cancer. 2013;49(16):3442–9.

37. Wei JX, Lv LH, Wan YL, Cao Y, Li GL, Lin HM, et al. Vps4A functions as a tumor suppressor by regulating the secretion and uptake of exosomal microRNAs in human hepatoma cells. Hepatology. 2015;61(4):1284–94.

38. Ronot M, Vilgrain V. Hepatocellular carcinoma: diagnostic criteria by imaging techniques. Best Pract Res Clin Gastroenterol. 2014;28(5):795–812.

39. Pantel K, Brakenhoff RH, Brandt B. Detection, clinical relevance and specific biological properties of disseminating tumour cells. Nat Rev Cancer. 2008;8(5):329–40.

40. Waguri N, Suda T, Nomoto M, Kawai H, Mita Y, Kuroiwa T, et al. Sensitive and specific detection of circulating cancer cells in patients with hepatocellular carcinoma; detection of human telomerase reverse transcriptase messenger RNA after immunomagnetic separation. Clin Cancer Res. 2003;9(8):3004–11.

41. Nel I, Baba HA, Ertle J, Weber F, Sitek B, Eisenacher M, et al. Individual profiling of circulating tumor cell

composition and therapeutic outcome in patients with hepatocellular carcinoma. Transl Oncol. 2013;6(4): 420–8.

42. Schulze K, Gasch C, Staufer K, Nashan B, Lohse AW, Pantel K, et al. Presence of EpCAM-positive circulating tumor cells as biomarker for systemic disease strongly correlates to survival in patients with hepatocellular carcinoma. Int J Cancer. 2013;133(9):2165–71.

43. Dent BM, Ogle LF, O'Donnell RL, Hayes N, Malik U, Curtin NJ, et al. High-resolution imaging for the detection and characterisation of circulating tumour cells from patients with oesophageal, hepatocellular, thyroid and ovarian cancers. Int J Cancer. 2016;138(1):206–16.

44. Kelley RK, Magbanua MJ, Butler TM, Collisson EA, Hwang J, Sidiropoulos N, et al. Circulating tumor cells in hepatocellular carcinoma: a pilot study of detection, enumeration, and next-generation sequencing in cases and controls. BMC Cancer. 2015;15:206.

45. Li J, Chen L, Zhang X, Zhang Y, Liu H, Sun B, et al. Detection of circulating tumor cells in hepatocellular carcinoma using antibodies against asialoglycoprotein receptor, carbamoyl phosphate synthetase 1 and pan-cytokeratin. PLoS One. 2014;9(4):e96185.

46. Yamashita T, Forgues M, Wang W, Kim JW, Ye Q, Jia H, et al. EpCAM and alpha-fetoprotein expression defines novel prognostic subtypes of hepatocellular carcinoma. Cancer Res. 2008;68(5):1451–61.

47. Schwarzenbach H, Hoon DS, Pantel K. Cell-free nucleic acids as biomarkers in cancer patients. Nat Rev Cancer. 2011;11(6):426–37.

48. Chiang DY, Villanueva A, Hoshida Y, Peix J, Newell P, Minguez B, et al. Focal gains of VEGFA and molecular classification of hepatocellular carcinoma. Cancer Res. 2008;68(16):6779–88.

49. Jiang P, Chan CW, Chan KC, Cheng SH, Wong J, Wong VW, et al. Lengthening and shortening of plasma DNA in hepatocellular carcinoma patients. Proc Natl Acad Sci U S A. 2015;112(11):E1317–25.

50. Sun K, Jiang P, Chan KC, Wong J, Cheng YK, Liang RH, et al. Plasma DNA tissue mapping by genome-wide methylation sequencing for noninvasive prenatal, cancer, and transplantation assessments. Proc Natl Acad Sci U S A. 2015;112(40):E5503–12.

51. Hosny G, Farahat N, Tayel H, Hainaut P. Ser-249 TP53 and CTNNB1 mutations in circulating free DNA of Egyptian patients with hepatocellular carcinoma versus chronic liver diseases. Cancer Lett. 2008;264(2):201–8.

52. Masyuk AI, Masyuk TV, Larusso NF. Exosomes in the pathogenesis, diagnostics and therapeutics of liver diseases. J Hepatol. 2013;59(3):621–5.

53. Enache LS, Enache EL, Ramiere C, Diaz O, Bancu L, Sin A, et al. Circulating RNA molecules as biomarkers in liver disease. Int J Mol Sci. 2014;15(10): 17644–66.

54. Eccles SA, Welch DR. Metastasis: recent discoveries and novel treatment strategies. Lancet. 2007;369(9574):1742–57.

55. Liu CL, Fan ST, Cheung ST, Lo CM, Ng IO, Wong J. Anterior approach versus conventional approach right hepatic resection for large hepatocellular carcinoma: a prospective randomized controlled study. Ann Surg. 2006;244(2):194–203.

56. Toso C, Mentha G, Majno P. Liver transplantation for hepatocellular carcinoma: five steps to prevent recurrence. Am J Transplant. 2011;11(10):2031–5.

57. Fidler IJ. The pathogenesis of cancer metastasis: the 'seed and soil' hypothesis revisited. Nat Rev Cancer. 2003;3(6):453–8.

58. Fan JL, Yang YF, Yuan CH, Chen H, Wang FB. Circulating cumor cells for predicting the prognostic of patients with hepatocellular carcinoma: a meta analysis. Cell Physiol Biochem. 2015;37(2):629–40.

59. Hoshida Y, Moeini A, Alsinet C, Kojima K, Villanueva A. Gene signatures in the management of hepatocellular carcinoma. Semin Oncol. 2012;39(4):473–85.

Liquid Biopsy in Esophageal, Gastric, and Pancreatic Cancers

15

E. Giovannetti, D. Massihnia, N. Barraco, A. Listì,
L. Incorvaia, M. Castiglia, and Antonio Russo

Esophageal Cancer

Esophageal carcinoma (EC) is one of the most common tumors in the world [1] and the sixth most common cause of cancer-related death, with the 5-year overall survival not greater than 20% [2–4]. EC is mainly diagnosed at advanced stages and this is due to the lack of specific screening methods [5]. Generally, it is divided into two main subtypes: esophageal adenocarcinoma and esophageal squamous-cell carcinoma (ESCC). ESCC is the most common esophageal cancer, particularly in Asian countries, and it is one of the most aggressive carcinomas of the gastrointestinal tract [6]. The major risks associated with the onset of the ESCC are tobacco and alcohol abuse, gastroesophageal reflux disease, diet, obesity, and body composition. The risk factors are different between developed and underdeveloped nations. Several studies have shown that the lack of an adequate vitamin intake may be one of the causes of EC. In the era of personalized treatment, standard chemotherapy is still the main therapeutic approach for EC, but several combination therapies of preoperative chemotherapy or chemoradiotherapy followed by surgery have been developed and experimented [7]. Moreover, there are few drugs approved by the FDA for the treatment of esophageal cancer, although with limited response [2]. Nevertheless, it seems that HER2 receptor plays an important role in gastroesophageal cancer, and several studies have shown a significant response with trastuzumab compared with chemotherapy alone in this tumor setting [8].

One of the first steps in the development of EC is the transition from normal esophageal epithelium to columnar and secretory epithelium, a process often associated with chronic inflammatory events triggered by gastroesophageal reflux [9]. This condition is commonly called Barrett esophagus (BE). However, it was demonstrated that there is a correlation between genetics and EC. Indeed, the use of massive parallel sequencing technology has identified specific genomic alterations in ESCC [10].

Nowadays, endoscopic biopsies are the main tool to evaluate the histological grade of EC. However, there are many problems for tissue

E. Giovannetti
Department of Medical Oncology, VU University
Medical Center, Cancer Center Amsterdam,
CCA room 1.52, De Boelelaan 1117, 1081, HV,
Amsterdam, The Netherlands

Cancer Pharmacology Lab, AIRC Start Up Unit,
University of Pisa, Pisa, Italy
e-mail: e.giovannetti@vumc.nl

D. Massihnia • N. Barraco • A. Listì • L. Incorvaia
M. Castiglia • A. Russo, MD, PhD (✉)
Department of Surgical, Oncological and Oral
Sciences, Section of Medical Oncology, University of
Palermo, Via del Vespro 129, 90127 Palermo, Italy
e-mail: antonio.russo@usa.net

© Springer International Publishing AG 2017
A. Giordano et al. (eds.), *Liquid Biopsy in Cancer Patients*, Current Clinical Pathology,
DOI 10.1007/978-3-319-55661-1_15

biopsy, together with possible surgical complications, tumor diffusion, and incorrect and/or negative results. Furthermore, in many cases there is no sufficient material from primary tumors as well as from metastasis [11]. Therefore, it is necessary to identify new biomarkers for EC patients' follow-up.

CTCs in Esophageal Cancer

Circulating tumor cells (CTCs) represent an important tool to obtain important information prior to various treatments, including surgery, chemotherapy, and chemoradiation therapy [12]. CTCs are rare and have been found in the peripheral blood of cancer patients. Their presence is correlated with poor prognosis and they are considered indicators of treatment efficacy. In EC, CTC analysis may be helpful for better patients' stratification. In the study published by Kubish et al. in 2015, the prognostic value of CTCs in patients with advanced gastric and gastroesophageal adenocarcinomas is investigated [13]. The presence of CTCs was evaluated before systemic treatment initiation and at follow-up, using immunomagnetic-based technique for CTC enrichment. In particular mucin 1 (MUC1) and epithelial cell adhesion molecule (EpCAM) were used as CTC membrane markers, and real time was performed to evaluate specific tumor-associated genes (KRT19, MUC1, EPCAM, CEACAM5, and BIRC5). The patients were stratified in different groups based on CTC detection: CTC negative with all marker genes negative and CTC positive with at least one of the marker genes positive. Interestingly, it was reported that patients who were CTC positive had a shorter median progression-free survival and overall survival than patients lacking CTCs. Nevertheless, alterations in the profile marker during chemotherapy were not predictive of clinical outcome or response to therapy. The data of this study suggest that the presence of CTC may have a role in the prediction of patients' outcome [13]. Moreover, it was reported that changes in CTC numbers reflect tumor progression and predict treatment efficacy in ESCC [14]. Another

study has highlighted the role of CTCs as prognostic factor in ESCC, the study included 90 patients who received chemotherapy or chemoradiotherapy, and the CellSearch system was used for CTC enumeration [12]. CTCs were detected in nearly 30% of patients at baseline but follow-up samples were available only in 71 out of 90 patients. The OS was shown to be significantly shorter in patients with than without CTCs at baseline. CTC positivity after treatment in progressive disease patients was significantly higher than that reported in patients showing partial response. Moreover, patients with a change in CTC status from positive to negative had a good prognosis as well as patients without baseline CTCs. These results highlight the role of CTCs as promising indicator of tumor prognosis but also as surrogate marker for chemotherapy or chemoradiation efficacy in ESCC [12].

ctDNA in Esophageal Cancer

As well as CTCs, ctDNA is a valid biomarker also in EC patients. Indeed it has been recently proven that ctDNA can be used to analyze the molecular alterations harbored in EC. In the study from Lou et al., ctDNA was used to monitor tumor dynamics changes over time. Interestingly, they have evaluated, through next-generation sequencing, several samples including tumor, tumor-adjacent, and normal tissue, as well as presurgery and postsurgery plasma. The reported results are very exciting; indeed, exome sequencing of eight patients was identified between 29 and 134 somatic mutations in ESCCs, many of which were confirmed in ctDNA. Moreover, the comparison between presurgery and postsurgery plasma has shown that mutations decreased or disappeared after surgery. These results demonstrate that ctDNA can be used to evaluate treatment efficacy [15]. Cell-free DNA levels (cfDNA) were also reported to be modified after esophagectomy. In a cohort of 81 patients who underwent esophagectomy, cfDNA levels were evaluated through real-time PCR; according to the results obtained, patients could be divided in two groups defined as lower cfDNA or higher cfDNA. The mean cfDNA concentration was 5918 copies/mL in lower and 53,311 copies/mL in higher cfDNA groups. Moreover, higher cfDNA levels were associated with tumor relapse and poorer disease-free survival [16].

Circulating miRNA and Exosomes in Esophageal Cancer

Circulating microRNAs (miRNAs) and exosomes are emerging as novel noninvasive biomarkers. Zhang et al., profiled miRNAs in serum of patients with EAC using sequencing technologies [17]. The analysis demonstrated that 195 miRNAs are deregulated between EAC patients and healthy controls. In particular 96 were upregulated whereas 99 were downregulated. Subsequently, they also confirmed that miR-25-3p and miR-151a-3p were significantly elevated, while the concentrations of miR-100-5p and miR-375 were significantly decreased in EAC patients compared with healthy controls indicating that the profile of these four miRNAs may potentially serve as a serum biomarker to identify patients with EAC [17]. MiRNA may also be involved in neoplastic/metaplastic progression, and they might be useful for progression risk prediction as well as for monitoring of BE patients. Some miRNAs (miR-143, miR-145, miR-194, miR-203, miR-205, and miR-215) appear to have a key role in metaplasia and neoplastic progression. Caruso et al. have recently evaluated the expression levels of these miRNA, comparing tissue vs. serum samples, in 30 patients diagnosed with esophagitis, columnar-lined esophagus (CLO), or BE [18]. The analysis showed that miR-143, miR-145, miR-194, and miR-215 levels were significantly higher, while miR-203 and miR-205 were lower in BE tissues compared with their corresponding normal tissues. Analysis on circulating miRNA levels confirmed that miR-194 and miR-215 were significantly upregulated in both BE and CLO compared to esophagitis, while miR-143 was significantly upregulated only in the Barrett group. Therefore, miRNA might also be used for patients' follow-up even when a pre-

cancerous lesion is present. Another study investigated the association between circulating plasma miRNAs and tumor diagnosis or prognosis in ESCC patients. Plasma levels of miR-16, miR-21, miR-22, miR-126, miR-148b, miR-185, miR-221, miR-223, and miR-375 were evaluated by qRT-PCR assays from ESCC patients prior to treatment initiation. Levels of four of the selected miRNAs (miR-16, miR-21, miR-185, and miR-375) were found to be significantly higher in ESCC patients than in controls. Moreover, Kaplan-Meier survival analysis showed that high plasma levels of miR-16 and miR-21 correlate with shortened PFS and OS in ESCC patients [19].

Exosomes play important roles in cancer progression. Masumoto et al. have evaluated the concentration of exosomes isolated from patients with ESCC [20]. They showed that exosome quantification provides diagnostic and prognostic information. Indeed, exosome levels were higher in EC patients than nonmalignant patients, and their enumeration was an independent prognostic marker.

Gastric Cancer

Gastric cancer (GC) is the fifth most common cancer, its incidence is one million new cases each year, and it is the third cause of cancer-related mortality in both sexes worldwide [21, 22]. GC displays the highest incidence rates in developed countries as Eastern Asia followed by Central and Eastern Europe than in North America and Western Africa [22]. The majority of GCs are adenocarcinomas, including sporadic, familiar, or hereditary syndrome-associated tumors [23]. Histologically, according to the Lauren criteria, gastric adenocarcinoma is classified into intestinal or diffuse subtypes. Male gender, *Helicobacter pylori* infection, diet, lifestyle, tobacco and alcohol use, obesity, gastritis, reflux and Barrett esophagus, partial gastrectomy, and Ménétrier's disease are all considered potential risk factors for the intestinal subtype of GC [24]. Conversely, the causes of diffuse subtype are researched in the genetic aberrations [25]. Indeed, the risk of developing GC is related to the occurrence of both genetic and epigenetic aberrations, including activation of oncogenes, inactivation of tumor suppressor genes, deregulation of growth factors/receptors, mutations of DNA repair genes, and silencing of tumor suppressors by CpG island methylation. Consequently, the molecular pathways regulating the main functional biological processes are altered, resulting in the high heterogeneity of this cancer type [26]. To date, the TNM classification can be used to predict patients' prognosis. However, the current TNM classification system does not adequately reflect the tumor biological behavior and thus the prognosis of GC patients [27]. Clinically, gastric carcinoma is subdivided in early/localized or advanced/metastatic stage, in order to define the best treatment strategy. The early-stage tumor has a better prognosis than the advanced disease [28]. The treatment of early gastric carcinoma depends exclusively by various pathological factors. In light of these, it's necessary to evaluate the benefit of neoadjuvant therapy before resection [29, 30]. Conversely, in advanced stage, the choice of the chemotherapy and/or target therapy depends by molecular factors. As previously reported, it has been shown that a subgroup of gastric adenocarcinoma is characterized by HER2 gene amplification [31, 32]. Indeed, HER2-positive advanced gastric carcinoma benefits from the addition of a humanized monoclonal antibody against HER2, trastuzumab (Herceptin), in combination with chemotherapy (capecitabine or 5-fluorouracil and cisplatin). This combination has been shown to improve overall survival, progression-free survival, and response rate. Based on these impressive results, all the international guidelines currently recommend to investigate the status of HER at diagnosis, in order to decide the best treatment for each patient [33]. Therefore, biomarker identification is imperative for deciding the best treatment option.

In the last decades, the incidence of GC has gradually decreased [34, 35]. This result was the demonstration of small steps forward. Diagnostic techniques and perioperative management have only partially allowed the early detection of the disease and have not been able to completely break down mortality. Moreover, the biological pathways that regulate initiation, progression, metastasis, and pharmacological resistance are also poorly understood.

To date, the tissue biopsy after surgical or endoscopic procedure is the gold standard for both histological and genetic analysis of GC. These surgical methods are invasive and represent a snapshot of the heterogeneity of gastric cancer, especially in metastatic cases [36, 37]. The researchers have identified circulating tumor cells (CTCs) and cell-free nucleic acids (cfNAs) that could represent a "liquid biopsy" to detect GC at an early stage or during the therapy. In this scenario, the identification of CTCs and cfNAs as new potential diagnostic, prognostic, and predictive molecular biomarkers in GC, together with aberrant proteins, autoantibodies, extracellular vesicles (EVs), and tumor-derived metabolites, represents a new challenge for current translational research [38]. Indeed, these circulating molecules obtained from the bloodstream may offer a complete picture of the tumor characteristics.

Circulating Tumor Cells (CTCs) in GC

New biomarkers for the GC detection in early stage represent the key point of scientific research. The CTCs were detected in peripheral blood of GC patients as already found in another tumor histotypes. In GC patients, the concentration of peripheral blood CTCs is very low [39]. So, the researchers developed alternative methods for isolation and enrichment to exceed the problem of low concentrations [40]. Furthermore, it would be necessary to analyze the isolated cells with the use of equally sensitive techniques.

The isolation and enrichment of CTCs from bloodstream of GC patients can occur through two main methods that have been previously explained. After their isolation, the real-time PCR or quantitative real-time PCR (qRT PCR) is used for CTC characterization, but their sensitivity in early stage of GC is still limited. Other researchers have developed a sensitive assay, based on a high-throughput colorimetric membrane array, which is able to detect multiple membrane markers such as human telomerase reverse transcriptase (TERT). Moreover, this method was shown to be more sensitive compared to real-time PCR for CTC analysis [41, 42].

There are still limited studies looking at the clinical impact of the CTC evaluation in GC. A prospective study on 52 advanced GC patients has shown that low CTC levels (<4 CTCs enumerated at baseline and 4 weeks after initiation of chemotherapy) were associated with higher OS and PFS. Conversely, high CTC levels (>4 CTCs enumerated at baseline and 4 weeks after initiation of chemotherapy) were associated with lower OS and PFS [43]. Several evidences have shown that the CTCs isolated in the bloodstream of cancer patients could be a useful tool for early detection of GC, for predicting metastasis and prognosis and for monitoring the effects of therapy [43, 44].

Circulating-Free Nucleic Acids (cfNAs) in GC

In GC, the detection of genetic and epigenetic aberration by the isolation and analysis of circulating free nucleic acids represents an innovative approach to evaluate the disease in early stage or during the treatment. Generally, these molecules are the mirror of deregulated DNA, RNA, and noncoding RNA (ncRNA) in tumor tissue and in circulating plasma/serum. Recently, higher levels of ctDNA, RNA, and noncoding RNA levels have been detected in plasma and serum of GC patients compared to healthy volunteers. Leon et al. first described the reduction of ctDNA levels in the serum of cancer patients during the radiotherapy. Recently, the next-generation sequencing approach allowed the identification of aberrant translocations in ctDNA of cancer patients confirming the result in the correspondent tissue samples.

Several studies on plasma of GC patients have shown higher levels of cfDNAs than healthy controls. Studies on rare circulating cfDNA are very few. Comparing different diseases, high levels of cfDNAs have been detected not only in cancer but also in inflammatory diseases and cardiovascular disorders, suggesting that it is not a peculiar feature of the tumor. qPCR methods have been used to evaluate the overexpression and activation of some oncogenes, including MYC and HER2, that are generally deregulated in GC. Higher levels of MYC have been shown both in the blood and in the tissue samples of GC patients compared with healthy volunteers [45]. The amplification of HER2 has been associated with 7–32% of GC patients. The status of HER2 has resulted in aggressiveness and poor survival of patients. To date, no studies have shown the correlation between the status of HER2 in plasma/serum cfDNA and the effects on chemotherapy in GC. The results of amplification of HER2, which have been reported in GC tissue samples, were not associated with the level of GC plasma [46]. More sensitive techniques will be needed for the routine use of these genetic investigations. Furthermore, gene hypermethylation has been detected in plasma/serum GC as diagnostic and prognostic marker.

The analysis performed on the serum of GC patients has also shown hypermethylation of several genes such as *MYC* and *HER2*. The hypermethylation of promoter region of *RPRM*, *XAF1*, *KCNA4*, and *CYP26B1* genes in GC produced the silencing of these genes. *RPRM* encodes reprimo, which is a regulator dependent by TP53. The hypermethylation of its promoter causes the silencing of this gene observed in GC cfDNA [47]. Conversely, XAF1 gene is downregulated in GC serum after hypermethylation of its promoter. It is a negative regulator of the inhibition of apoptosis. The percentages of downregulation are similar between tissue and serum and may represent possible markers of methylation to identify changes of DNA [48].

Compared to DNA, mRNA transcripts and noncoding RNAs are more easily subjected to degradation; thus, their analysis from plasma in cancer patients is not simple. Nevertheless, several evidences have shown that both mRNA and ncRNAs can be packed inside extracellular vesicles (exosome, macro- and microvesicles) and thus protected by RNase activity.

Long Noncoding RNA (lncRNA) in GC

The long noncoding RNAs (lncRNAs) belong to a class of regulatory RNA that does not code for proteins. The lncRNAs are generated through a molecular pathway similar to that used for protein-coding genes [49]. They play essential biological functions including chromatin modification and transcriptional and posttranscriptional processing [50, 51]. lncRNAs have been arbitrary defined according to their size, as transcribed RNA molecules greater than 200 nt in length in their mature form. In contrast to the small ncRNAs (siRNAs, miRNAs, and piRNAs), which are highly conserved in commonly studied species, and act as negative regulator of gene expression, lncRNAs are modestly conserved and regulate gene expression through mechanisms that are mostly poorly understood [52, 53]. lncRNAs are emerging as essential regulators of genetic and epigenetic networks, and their deregulation may underlie the carcinogenesis processes. In GC, the analysis on fresh tissue samples has shown upregulation of H19, HOX antisense intergenic RNA, and MALAT1, and this aberrant expression has been associated with tumor aggressiveness and metastasis and poor patients' survival. The same results have been confirmed on plasma. H19, HOX antisense intergenic RNA, and MALAT1 genes have been detected in the blood of GC patients. In particular, H19 lncRNA showed higher expression levels in GC patients compared to healthy controls. However, the expression levels of H19 decreased after surgery [54]. lncRNAs could be good candidates as diagnostic and predictive "circulating biomarkers" in this disease. Interestingly, the lncRNAs could vehicles information both in the neighboring areas but also to distant sites; another interesting feature of lncRNA is the capability to pack miRNA with ribonucleoproteins or with mRNA target. Moreover, the lncRNAs can act as precursor of microRNAs. Indeed, they can serve as a source of microRNAs after processing [55, 56]. High expression level of miR-451 and miR-486 in tissue and serum of GC patients has been recently reported, but they decreased after surgery. These data suggested that microRNAs play a key role in the molecular pathway regulating GC development, acting either as oncomiR or as tumor suppressor. A list of circulating miRNAs isolated in the blood of GC patients acting as oncomiRs includes miR-17-5p, miR-18a, miR-20a, miR-200c, miR-21, miR-218, miR-221, miR-222, miR-25, miR-27a, miR-376c, and miR-744, while miR-122, miR-195-5p, miR-203, miR-218, and miR-375 act as tumor suppressor. These miRNAs can be used as diagnostic biomarker to identify GC patients [57].

Initially, the researchers attempted to confirm the data obtained in the tumor tissue. They were not always been able to confirm the result. The CTC and CfNAs are able to contribute in the study of molecular pathway that regulates the tumor, although many mechanisms must be explored.

Pancreatic Cancer

Pancreatic cancer is one of the most lethal solid tumors. Despite extensive preclinical and clinical research, the prognosis of this disease has not significantly improved, with a 5-year survival rate around 7%. The reason for this poor outcome can be partially explained by (i) the lack of reliable biomarkers for screening and diagnosis at the earlier stages and (ii) by the tumor resistance to most of the currently available chemotherapy regimens. This resistance has been attributed to both the desmoplastic tumor microenvironment and to the strong inter- and intra-tumor heterogeneity in terms of complexity of genetic aberrations and the resulting signaling pathway activities, as well as to resistance mechanisms that quickly adapt the tumor to drugs [58].

Pancreatic cancer is most often observed in the old population as it results from developed genetic defects over many years. The median age of the diagnosis is 71 years, with the 75% of patients diagnosed between the ages of 55 and 84 years. Age is therefore the main risk factor for pancreatic cancer. Chronic pancreatitis represents another important risk factor for the development of PDAC. Several other factors involved with increased risk of developing PDAC include family history, substance abuse (e.g., smoking and heavy alcohol), chronic pancreatitis, and metabolic syndrome (e.g., diabetes and obesity). Conversely, alcohol consumption does not seem to be a risk factor unless the alcohol abuse results in pancreatitis. About 95% of pancreatic cancers are ductal adenocarcinomas (PDAC) [59].

Unlike several common cancers, such as lung and breast cancer, there are not yet established treatment strategies based on molecular profiling for PDAC. Similarly, molecular signatures cannot improve staging or prognostication. However, different studies performed in the last years have shown a signature of common genetic abnormalities in PDAC, which highlights potential molecular targets and reveals signaling pathways that are important for the PDAC tumorigenesis and development. The main "driver" oncogene is KRAS, which is genetically activated in more than 95% of PDACs. Unfortunately, targeted therapy against this gene has not been successful [60].

Mutated KRAS activates multiple signaling pathways including BRAF/MAP-K, to affect cell proliferation; PI3K/mammalian target of rapamycin, to promote cell growth and survival; and phospholipase C/PKC/Ca11, to induce calcium and second messenger signaling. The other high-frequency mutation genes (CDKN2A, TP53, and SMAD4) are classified as tumor suppressor genes. These genes are often deactivated through a mutation in one allele, combined with genetic loss (i.e., loss of heterozygosity) in the corresponding chromosome region of the second allele as a result of chromosomal instability. Areas where genetic losses most frequently occur are nonrandom in the PDAC genome, because they usually happen at loci containing the aforementioned tumor suppressor genes, such as 9p (CDKN2A), 19p (TP53), and 18q (SMAD4) [61]. More recently, deep genomic analyses revealed other biologically relevant events with clinical significance, and whole-genome sequencing subclassified PDAC into different subtypes, on the basis of the differential expression of transcription factors and downstream targets with a key role in lineage specification and differentiation in pancreas growth and regeneration [62]. In particular, the most recent classification includes

four subtypes. The *squamous subtype* comprises gene networks involved in inflammation, hypoxia response, metabolic reprogramming, TGF-β signaling, MYC pathway initiation, autophagy, and upregulated expression of TP63ΔN and its target genes. This subtype has also been associated with mutations in TP53 and KDM6A, while *the pancreatic progenitor* subtype especially expresses genes included in initial pancreatic development, such as FOXA2/FOXA3, PDX1, and MNX1. Conversely, *the aberrantly differentiated endocrine exocrine (ADEX)* is defined by transcriptional networks that are relevant in later stages of pancreatic development and differentiation and is a subclass of pancreatic progenitor tumors. This subtype displays upregulations of genes that control networks involved in KRAS activation, exocrine (NR5A2 and RBPJL), and endocrine differentiation (NEUROD1 and NKX2-2). Finally, the *immunogenic subtype* shares most of the characteristics of the pancreatic progenitor class, but is linked with evidence of a substantial immune infiltrate. Immunogenic tumors contain indeed upregulated immune networks including pathways involved in acquired immune suppression.

Management of the patient with PDAC is based on the stage of the disease. Patients with local disease (stages I and II) are assessed for resection and offered surgical therapy if they are considered medically fit for pancreatectomy, and the tumor is considered resectable on the basis of available imaging data. Localized PDAs are categorized as resectable, borderline resectable, or locally advanced and usually reflect the possibility of having a complete resection. However, surgical resection is only possible in a small subset of patients, i.e., less than 20% of all the PDAC cases. Most patients are indeed diagnosed with advanced-stage disease, characterized by infiltration of lymph nodes and vasculature, as well as metastasis to 2–3 distant organs such as the liver, lungs, and peritoneum. The median survival of patients undergoing curative resection is significantly longer than for those with unresectable pancreatic cancer. This implies that improvement for screening in people within groups at risk, such people with familial pancreatic cancer,

BRCA1 mutations, premalignant cysts, and new-onset diabetes, would be the key to initiate earlier detection and better survival rates.

Liquid Biopsy in Pancreatic Cancer

Tissue biopsy is the gold standard for the diagnosis of pancreatic cancer [43, 63]. However, there are many problems for tissue biopsy, together with possible surgical complications, tumor diffusion, and incorrect and/or negative results. Furthermore, in many cases there is no sufficient material from primary tumors as well as from metastasis in the patients with advanced disease [11].

Nowadays, liquid biopsies represent an attractive minimally invasive methodology for the management of the oncological patient, becoming thus an attractive tool for scientists and clinicians. Liquid biopsy includes circulating tumor cells (CTCs), circulating tumor DNA (ctDNA), circulating microRNAs, circulating proteins, and extracellular vesicles [64]. CTCs and ctDNA are the most commonly studied targets in liquid biopsy and may acquire a different role for cancer management, in order to assess risk factors and early diagnosis, but also for prognostic information, response to treatment, drug resistance, analysis of tumoral heterogeneity, recurrence, and metastasis [65] (See Fig. 15.1).

Circulating Tumor Cells (CTCs)

Several studies investigated CTCs in patients with pancreatic cancer as a biomarker for early diagnosis, treatment monitoring, and predicting prognosis. Currently, no accurate early diagnostic tools are available; as a consequence, pancreatic cancers are diagnosed at an advanced stage, when they cannot be resected [66]. The most common screening for the detection of pancreatic cancer is by radiological imaging, but this method can be inconclusive, and there are different technical complications. Therefore, CTCs may be necessary for an early detection of pancreatic tumors. Indeed, Rhim et al. evaluated CTC as pre-diagnostic biomarker. The technique used in this study was a microfluidic technology, and they tested 11 patients with pancreatic cancer at all stages, 21 patients with benign disease, and 19 healthy subjects. They showed that CTCs were differently detected among the three groups, with the highest percentage of positive results in the pancreatic cancer group (73%); accordingly, none of the healthy subjects were found to be CTC positive. Nevertheless, 33% of patients with benign disease were also found positive, demonstrating that in this case the analysis was not completely able to discriminate benign from malignant lesions [67]. Allard et al. have evaluated the CTCs in 964 patients with 12 different metastatic carcinomas, including 16 patients with pancreatic cancer. In fact, they demonstrated that the detection of CTCs in patients with pancreatic cancer is more difficult with respect to other tumors, but different results were obtained in another study, in which all 15 pancreatic cancer patients analyzed had detectable CTCs [40]. Based on these studies, the researchers concluded that detection of CTCs could be considered a valid tool for diagnosis of pancreatic cancer but technique standardization is still required.

CTC enumeration cannot be used in clinical practice for the evaluation of prognosis and for treatment monitoring in pancreatic cancer patients. Nevertheless, there are several studies that have focused on the study of the prognostic and predictive role of CTCs. Soeth et al. demonstrated that CTC detection in 52 out of 154 subjects with pancreatic cancer predicted a shorter OS and same results were reported also for PFS [68–70].

In the last decades, we have started to face the problem of tumor heterogeneity; indeed, it is a main hurdle in the battle to defeat cancer. In pancreatic cancer, as in other tumor types, heterogeneity in primary and metastatic tumors is mainly due to genomic instability [71]. Since CTCs are probably involved in tumor spread, the information that we may obtain from their analysis would be helpful in the dissection of tumor complexity and provide critical insights to discover new therapeutic targets. Nevertheless, there are not many studies that have investigated CTCs to better understand tumor heterogeneity in pancreatic cancer.

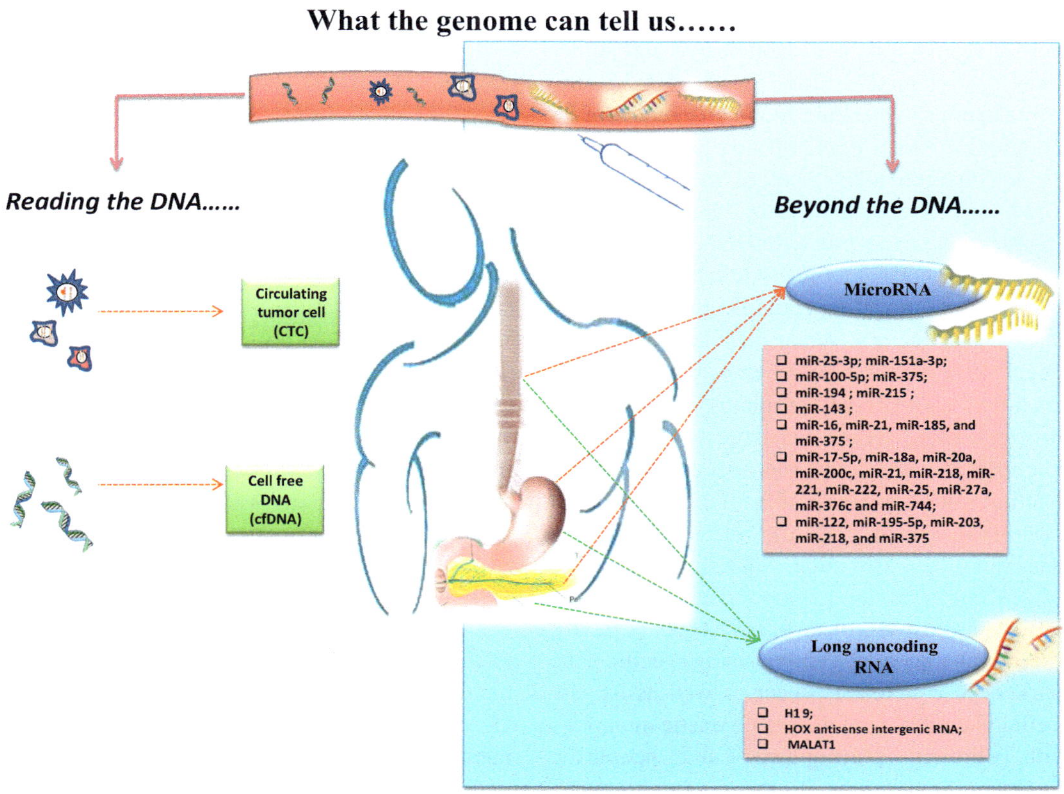

Fig. 15.1 Circulating tumor cells (CTCs), cell-free DNA (ctDNA), and noncoding RNAs could represent a "liquid biopsy" to detect esophageal, gastric, and pancreatic cancer. CTCs and ctDNA can be used to analyze the molecular alterations harbored in the plasma/serum of EC, GC, and PDAC patients. Modification beyond the DNA sequences can be studied to analyze the deregulation of noncoding RNAs: microRNA and long noncoding RNA. Higher levels of miR-25-3p and miR-151a-3p, miR-194 and miR-215, miR-143, miR-16, miR-21, miR-185 and miR-375, miR-17-5p, miR-18a, miR-20a, miR-200c, miR-21, miR-218, miR-221, miR-222, miR-25, miR-27a, miR-376c, and miR-744 have been detected in plasma and serum of some EC or GC or PDAC patients compared to healthy volunteers. miR-100-5p and miR-375, miR-122, miR-195-5p, miR-203, miR-218, and miR-375 were significantly decreased in EC or GC or PDAC patients compared with healthy control. In GC, H19, HOX antisense intergenic RNA, and MALAT1 genes have been detected in the blood of GC patients

Circulating Tumor DNA (ctDNA)

Several evidences suggest that detection and genetic characterization of ctDNA might provide an easily accessible source for prognostic and predictive information. Differential methodological approaches have been developed for the detection of ctDNA by identification of tumor-specific mutations, such as allele-specific PCR, BEAMing, droplet digital PCR, and various next-generation sequencing protocols [72]. The study of circulating cell-free DNA in the plasma/serum includes two major strategies: the measurement of the amount of cell-free DNA in the circulation and the detection of tumor-derived genetic aberrations such as point mutations, allelic imbalances, microsatellite instability, genetic polymorphisms, loss of heterozygosity, and methylation.

Initial Diagnosis More than 90% of the PDAC patients harbor mutations in the KRAS gene, which might be therefore a potential surrogate marker. Due to these high rate of KRAS mutation, it has been questioned whether the investigation of this alteration in PDAC could serve for early tumor detection. The results obtained from these investigations are inconclusive and sometimes discordant [73, 74]. Besides KRAS, the whole exome sequencing found an average of 26 mutations in tumor tissue of early pancreatic cancer, so, theoretically, many of these mutations could also be detected in the circulation. Therefore, a conceptual "ctDNA-Chip" could assay more genes at a time, while an appropriate mathematical modeling could be applied to evaluate several factors. When ctDNA is used as a diagnostic tool, the researchers should take into consideration different problems. Firstly, false positive can be a common issue of this genetic diagnosis as many mutations appeared in malignant but also in benign lesions. Furthermore, the tissue from which ctDNA is released is hard to determine because some mutations, such as KRAS and TP53, are hallmarks alterations present in the most common tumors types [75, 76]. These issues should be solved using specific gene markers of pancreatic cancer as well as by dissecting the relation of different genetic mutations with different preneoplastic and neoplastic lesions of the pancreas. However, these biomarkers should be always coupled with imaging techniques. For instance, the finding of cancer-associated mutations in KRAS or TP53 in ctDNA may prompt a clinician to do an imaging abdomen scan with the ability to detect a cancer in different anatomical locations and not just in the pancreas.

Treatment Monitoring Genetic variations in ctDNA reflect what is happening in tumor tissues [77]; thus, ctDNA could be used to track tumor development with higher specificity than the available tools. Remarkably, the half-time of ctDNA is only estimated to be about 2 h. Thus, the analysis of ctDNA could be used as a flexible method to monitor the tumor development dynamically. Different studies have shown that ctDNA in advanced colorectal cancer patients who underwent complete resection experienced a 99.0% of median reduction 2–10 days after the surgery. On the opposite, the patients with incomplete resection showed minor reduction or even amplified level of ctDNA. Interestingly, the undetectable level of ctDNA after surgery predicted

no recurrence "negative ctDNA" which is also a key indicator for long-term survival [78]. Detection of ctDNA after resection was an indicator for clinical relapse, also for pancreatic cancer, where ctDNA detected clinical recurrence 6.5 months earlier than CT imaging [79].

Prognostic Information The prognosis of pancreatic cancer is mainly given by histological characteristics, clinical presentations, and tumor stage, whereas the prognostic significance of ctDNA is still controversial [80]. However, some potential genetic aberrations appearing in early-stage pancreatic cancers have been found to be linked with disease development and survival, and more studies are warranted. In late-stage pancreatic cancer patients, ctDNA would also be helpful for prognostic purposes because they can provide thorough information on tumor characteristics. Several researches have explored the potential prognostic function of ctDNA focusing mainly on common point mutations, such as the KRAS gene mutations. About 98% of KRAS mutations in PDAC arise in position G12, and predominant substitution found at this position is G12D (51%), followed by G12V (30%) and G12R (12%). It has been verified that KRAS mutations in ctDNA could be found in about 50% and 90% of early-stage and late-stage pancreatic cancer patients, respectively, which clearly demonstrate the potential of this prognostic marker. A pilot study enrolling 45 pancreatic cancer patients at different disease stages showed that KRAS mutations in the plasma correlated with a significantly worse overall survival. In this study, KRAS mutation was found in 26% of patients of all stages by droplet digital PCR, and the majority mutation position was G12D [81]. Another research shows a higher sensitivity of KRAS mutation in serum (62.6%) by droplet digital PCR, and it predicted a worse prognosis. Moreover, G12V mutation in serum was found to be connected to a significantly lower survival compared with G12D/G12R/wild type.

Selection of Chemotherapy and Targeted Therapy Targeted therapy has become the standard therapy regimen for some cancers in the past 20 years, such as breast tumor, colorectal tumor, lung tumor, melanoma, etc. [82]. For pancreatic tumor, only erlotinib, an epidermal growth factor receptor inhibitor, is approved by FDA for clinical utilization. Nevertheless, the overall survival of gemcitabine plus erlotinib is 0.33 month longer than gemcitabine alone (median 6.24 months vs. 5.91 months), so erlotinib has not been accepted in the management of pancreatic cancer due to the limited survival benefit and cost-effect margin. A potential reason for the unsatisfactory efficacy of targeted therapy in pancreatic cancer was the lack of identification of genomic profiling due to the inadequate biopsy for molecular characterization. Chemotherapy is usually uniformly administered despite the chemotherapeutic sensitivity. However, some patients will never relapse even deprived of chemotherapy, and some patients will relapse soon even with a certain chemotherapy regimen. This condition involves for an accurate evaluation tool that could predict the individualized treatment response, therefore avoiding overtreatment or futile treatment. ctDNA exhibits excellent features to resolve the above issues. On one hand, ctDNA could clarify the molecular marker of tumor tissue with satisfactory sensitivity and specificity, which could help to select optimal treatment. Additionally, low level of ctDNA indicated a promising prognosis. Therefore, future trials should administer treatment regimen according to genetic status by ctDNA. Different studies have shown the potential of ctDNA in the cancer management. In a recent clinical study, it was demonstrated that EGFR deletion was detected in ctDNA 7 months earlier than tissue biopsy and the subsequent capecitabine and erlotinib lead to radiographic response. This event indicated that ctDNA could be used to guide targeted therapy, thus avoiding overtreatment and realizing precision medicine.

Exosomes

Most recently, the detection of *exosomes* has emerged as a new strategy to identify diagnostic, predictive, and prognostic markers of pancreatic cancer [83]. These extracellular vesicles are lipid bilayer membrane-enclosed nano-sized (30~100 nm) vesicles, secreted by virtually all cell types. Exosomes have also been confirmed in all bodily fluids, including blood, and have emerged as an important tool for intercellular communication through different functional biomolecules, including proteins, lipids, RNA, and DNA. Exosomes derived from pancreatic cancer enrich distinctive proteins and characteristics of mutated DNA and are becoming a very attractive marker of detection of early pancreatic cancer. Indeed, glypican-1 (GPC1) was identified as a specific marker of pancreatic cancer cell-derived exosomes, using flow cytometry from the serum of patients and mice with cancer [84]. These findings were confirmed in the serum of patients with pancreatic cancer, showing that GPC1+ exosomes can distinguish with absolute specificity and sensitivity healthy subjects and patients with a benign pancreatic disease from patients with early- and late-stage pancreatic cancer. Additionally, the levels of GPC1+ exosomes correlated with tumor burden and survival. This study clearly supports the role of tumor-derived exosomes as discriminatory biomarkers in blood and saliva.

References

1. Thrift AP. The epidemic of oesophageal carcinoma: where are we now? Cancer Epidemiol. 2016;41: 88–95.
2. Gaur P, Kim MP, Dunkin BJ. Esophageal cancer: recent advances in screening, targeted therapy, and management. J Carcinog. 2014;13:11.
3. Mao WM, Zheng WH, Ling ZQ. Epidemiologic risk factors for esophageal cancer development. Asian Pac J Cancer Prev. 2011;12(10):2461–6.
4. Engel LS, et al. Population attributable risks of esophageal and gastric cancers. J Natl Cancer Inst. 2003; 95(18):1404–13.
5. Chandra S, et al. Barrett's esophagus in 2012: updates in pathogenesis, treatment, and surveillance. Curr Gastroenterol Rep. 2013;15(5):322.
6. Arnold M, et al. Global burden of cancer attributable to high body-mass index in 2012: a population-based study. Lancet Oncol. 2015;16(1):36–46.
7. Ando N, et al. A randomized trial comparing postoperative adjuvant chemotherapy with cisplatin and 5-fluorouracil versus preoperative chemotherapy for localized advanced squamous cell carcinoma of the thoracic esophagus (JCOG9907). Ann Surg Oncol. 2012;19(1):68–74.

8. Bang YJ, et al. Trastuzumab in combination with chemotherapy versus chemotherapy alone for treatment of HER2-positive advanced gastric or gastro-oesophageal junction cancer (ToGA): a phase 3, open-label, randomised controlled trial. Lancet. 2010; 376(9742):687–97.

9. Tosh D, Slack JM. How cells change their phenotype. Nat Rev Mol Cell Biol. 2002;3(3):187–94.

10. Song Y, et al. Identification of genomic alterations in oesophageal squamous cell cancer. Nature. 2014; 509(7498):91–5.

11. Overman MJ, et al. Use of research biopsies in clinical trials: are risks and benefits adequately discussed? J Clin Oncol. 2013;31(1):17–22.

12. Matsushita D, et al. Clinical significance of circulating tumor cells in peripheral blood of patients with esophageal squamous cell carcinoma. Ann Surg Oncol. 2015;22(11):3674–80.

13. Kubisch I, et al. Prognostic role of a Multimarker analysis of circulating tumor cells in advanced gastric and gastroesophageal adenocarcinomas. Oncology. 2015;89(5):294–303.

14. Qiao YY, et al. Monitoring disease progression and treatment efficacy with circulating tumor cells in esophageal squamous cell carcinoma: a case report. World J Gastroenterol. 2015;21(25):7921–8.

15. Luo H, et al. Noninvasive diagnosis and monitoring of mutations by deep sequencing of circulating tumor DNA in esophageal squamous cell carcinoma. Biochem Biophys Res Commun. 2016;471(4):596–602.

16. Hsieh CC, et al. Circulating cell-free DNA levels could predict oncological outcomes of patients undergoing esophagectomy for esophageal squamous cell carcinoma. Int J Mol Sci. 2016;17(12). pii: E2131.

17. Zhang K, et al. Circulating miRNA profile in esophageal adenocarcinoma. Am J Cancer Res. 2016;6(11): 2713–21.

18. Cabibi D, et al. Analysis of tissue and circulating microRNA expression during metaplastic transformation of the esophagus. Oncotarget. 2016;7(30): 47821–30.

19. Li BX, et al. Circulating microRNAs in esophageal squamous cell carcinoma: association with locoregional staging and survival. Int J Clin Exp Med. 2015;8(5):7241–50.

20. Matsumoto Y, et al. Quantification of plasma exosome is a potential prognostic marker for esophageal squamous cell carcinoma. Oncol Rep. 2016;36(5): 2535–43.

21. Torre LA, et al. Global cancer statistics, 2012. CA Cancer J Clin. 2015;65(2):87–108.

22. Ferlay J, et al. Cancer incidence and mortality worldwide: sources, methods and major patterns in GLOBOCAN 2012. Int J Cancer. 2015;136(5): E359–86.

23. Röcken C. Gastric tumors and tumor precursors. Pathologe. 2017;38(2):75–86.

24. Arnold M, et al. Recent trends in incidence of five common cancers in 26 European countries since 1988: analysis of the European cancer observatory. Eur J Cancer. 2015;51(9):1164–87.

25. Hwang SW, et al. Preoperative staging of gastric cancer by endoscopic ultrasonography and multidetector-row computed tomography. J Gastroenterol Hepatol. 2010;25(3):512–8.

26. Yasui W, et al. Molecular pathobiology of gastric cancer. Scand J Surg. 2006;95(4):225–31.

27. Lauren P. The two histological main types of gastric carcinoma: diffuse and so-called intestinal-type carcinoma. An attempt at a histo-clinical classification. Acta Pathol Microbiol Scand. 1965;64:31–49.

28. Everett SM, Axon AT. Early gastric cancer in Europe. Gut. 1997;41(2):142–50.

29. Cunningham D, et al. Perioperative chemotherapy versus surgery alone for resectable gastroesophageal cancer. N Engl J Med. 2006;355(1):11–20.

30. Ychou M, et al. Perioperative chemotherapy compared with surgery alone for resectable gastroesophageal adenocarcinoma: an FNCLCC and FFCD multicenter phase III trial. J Clin Oncol. 2011; 29(13):1715–21.

31. Akiyama T, et al. The product of the human c-erbB-2 gene: a 185-kilodalton glycoprotein with tyrosine kinase activity. Science. 1986;232(4758):1644–6.

32. Popescu NC, King CR, Kraus MH. Localization of the human erbB-2 gene on normal and rearranged chromosomes 17 to bands q12-21.32. Genomics. 1989;4(3):362–6.

33. Okines AF, Cunningham D. Trastuzumab: a novel standard option for patients with HER-2-positive advanced gastric or gastro-oesophageal junction cancer. Therap Adv Gastroenterol. 2012;5(5):301–18.

34. Devesa SS, Blot WJ, Fraumeni JF. Changing patterns in the incidence of esophageal and gastric carcinoma in the United States. Cancer. 1998;83(10):2049–53.

35. Blot WJ, et al. Rising incidence of adenocarcinoma of the esophagus and gastric cardia. JAMA. 1991; 265(10):1287–9.

36. Alix-Panabières C, Pantel K. Circulating tumor cells: liquid biopsy of cancer. Clin Chem. 2013;59(1): 110–8.

37. van de Stolpe A, et al. Circulating tumor cell isolation and diagnostics: toward routine clinical use. Cancer Res. 2011;71(18):5955–60.

38. Schwarzenbach H, Hoon DS, Pantel K. Cell-free nucleic acids as biomarkers in cancer patients. Nat Rev Cancer. 2011;11(6):426–37.

39. Krebs MG, et al. Circulating tumour cells: their utility in cancer management and predicting outcomes. Ther Adv Med Oncol. 2010;2(6):351–65.

40. Allard WJ, et al. Tumor cells circulate in the peripheral blood of all major carcinomas but not in healthy subjects or patients with nonmalignant diseases. Clin Cancer Res. 2004;10(20):6897–904.

41. Tsujiura M, et al. Liquid biopsy of gastric cancer patients: circulating tumor cells and cell-free nucleic acids. World J Gastroenterol. 2014;20(12): 3265–86.

42. Wu CH, et al. Development of a high-throughput membrane-array method for molecular diagnosis of circulating tumor cells in patients with gastric cancers. Int J Cancer. 2006;119(2):373–9.

43. Crowley E, et al. Liquid biopsy: monitoring cancer-genetics in the blood. Nat Rev Clin Oncol. 2013;10(8):472–84.

44. Matsusaka S, et al. Circulating tumor cells as a surrogate marker for determining response to chemotherapy in patients with advanced gastric cancer. Cancer Sci. 2010;101(4):1067–71.

45. Park KU, et al. MYC quantitation in cell-free plasma DNA by real-time PCR for gastric cancer diagnosis. Clin Chem Lab Med. 2009;47(5):530–6.

46. Shoda K, et al. HER2 amplification detected in the circulating DNA of patients with gastric cancer: a retrospective pilot study. Gastric Cancer. 2015;18(4):698–710.

47. Ooki A, et al. DNA damage-inducible gene, reprimo functions as a tumor suppressor and is suppressed by promoter methylation in gastric cancer. Mol Cancer Res. 2013;11(11):1362–74.

48. Ling ZQ, et al. Circulating methylated XAF1 DNA indicates poor prognosis for gastric cancer. PLoS One. 2013;8(6):e67195.

49. Derrien T, et al. The GENCODE v7 catalog of human long noncoding RNAs: analysis of their gene structure, evolution, and expression. Genome Res. 2012;22(9):1775–89.

50. Yu B, Shan G. Functions of long noncoding RNAs in the nucleus. Nucleus. 2016;7(2):155–66.

51. Ponting CP, Oliver PL, Reik W. Evolution and functions of long noncoding RNAs. Cell. 2009;136(4):629–41.

52. Bernstein E, Allis CD. RNA meets chromatin. Genes Dev. 2005;19(14):1635–55.

53. Wilusz JE, Sunwoo H, Spector DL. Long noncoding RNAs: functional surprises from the RNA world. Genes Dev. 2009;23(13):1494–504.

54. Arita T, et al. Circulating long non-coding RNAs in plasma of patients with gastric cancer. Anticancer Res. 2013;33(8):3185–93.

55. Yoon JH, Abdelmohsen K, Gorospe M. Functional interactions among microRNAs and long noncoding RNAs. Semin Cell Dev Biol. 2014;34:9–14.

56. Angrand PO, et al. The role of long non-coding RNAs in genome formatting and expression. Front Genet. 2015;6:165.

57. Tsai MM, et al. Potential diagnostic, prognostic and therapeutic targets of MicroRNAs in human gastric cancer. Int J Mol Sci. 2016;17(6). pii: E945.

58. Massihnia D, et al. Phospho-Akt overexpression is prognostic and can be used to tailor the synergistic interaction of Akt inhibitors with gemcitabine in pancreatic cancer. J Hematol Oncol. 2017;10(1):9.

59. Yu DD, et al. Exosomes in development, metastasis and drug resistance of breast cancer. Cancer Sci. 2015;106(8):959–64.

60. Rishi A, et al. Pathological and molecular evaluation of pancreatic neoplasms. Semin Oncol. 2015;42(1):28–39.

61. Lewis AR, Valle JW, McNamara MG. Pancreatic cancer: are "liquid biopsies" ready for prime-time? World J Gastroenterol. 2016;22(32):7175–85.

62. Bailey P, et al. Genomic analyses identify molecular subtypes of pancreatic cancer. Nature. 2016;531(7592):47–52.

63. Gao Y, Zhu Y, Yuan Z. Circulating tumor cells and circulating tumor DNA provide new insights into pancreatic cancer. Int J Med Sci. 2016;13(12):902–13.

64. Best MG, et al. Liquid biopsies in patients with diffuse glioma. Acta Neuropathol. 2015;129(6):849–65.

65. Hayes DF, Paoletti C. Circulating tumour cells: insights into tumour heterogeneity. J Intern Med. 2013;274(2):137–43.

66. Ohmoto A, Rokutan H, Yachida S. Pancreatic neuroendocrine neoplasms: basic biology, current treatment strategies and prospects for the future. Int J Mol Sci. 2017;18(1). pii: E143.

67. Rhim AD, et al. Detection of circulating pancreas epithelial cells in patients with pancreatic cystic lesions. Gastroenterology. 2014;146(3):647–51.

68. Soeth E, et al. Detection of tumor cell dissemination in pancreatic ductal carcinoma patients by CK 20 RT-PCR indicates poor survival. J Cancer Res Clin Oncol. 2005;131(10):669–76.

69. de Albuquerque A, et al. Multimarker gene analysis of circulating tumor cells in pancreatic cancer patients: a feasibility study. Oncology. 2012;82(1):3–10.

70. Han L, Chen W, Zhao Q. Prognostic value of circulating tumor cells in patients with pancreatic cancer: a meta-analysis. Tumour Biol. 2014;35(3):2473–80.

71. Kling J. Beyond counting tumor cells. Nat Biotechnol. 2012;30(7):578–80.

72. Riva F, et al. Clinical applications of circulating tumor DNA and circulating tumor cells in pancreatic cancer. Mol Oncol. 2016;10(3):481–93.

73. Castells A, et al. K-ras mutations in DNA extracted from the plasma of patients with pancreatic carcinoma: diagnostic utility and prognostic significance. J Clin Oncol. 1999;17(2):578–84.

74. Uemura T, et al. Detection of K-ras mutations in the plasma DNA of pancreatic cancer patients. J Gastroenterol. 2004;39(1):56–60.

75. Chuang HC, et al. Pharmacological strategies to target oncogenic KRAS signaling in pancreatic cancer. Pharmacol Res. 2017;117:370–6.

76. Muller PA, Vousden KH. Mutant p53 in cancer: new functions and therapeutic opportunities. Cancer Cell. 2014;25(3):304–17.

77. Sundaresan TK, et al. Detection of T790M, the acquired resistance EGFR mutation, by tumor biopsy versus noninvasive blood-based analyses. Clin Cancer Res. 2016;22(5):1103–10.

78. Diehl F, et al. Circulating mutant DNA to assess tumor dynamics. Nat Med. 2008;14(9):985–90.

79. Wolfgang CL, et al. Recent progress in pancreatic cancer. CA Cancer J Clin. 2013;63(5):318–48.

80. Madic J, et al. Circulating tumor DNA and circulating tumor cells in metastatic triple negative breast cancer patients. Int J Cancer. 2015;136(9):2158–65.

81. Takai E, Yachida S. Circulating tumor DNA as a liquid biopsy target for detection of pancreatic cancer. World J Gastroenterol. 2016;22(38):8480–8.

82. Bahrami A, et al. Targeted stroma in pancreatic cancer: promises and failures of target therapies. J Cell Physiol. 2017. doi:10.1002/jcp.25798.

83. Nuzhat Z, et al. Tumour-derived exosomes as a signature of pancreatic cancer – liquid biopsies as indicators of tumour progression. Oncotarget. 2016. doi:10.18632/oncotarget.13973.

84. Melo SA, et al. Glypican-1 identifies cancer exosomes and detects early pancreatic cancer. Nature. 2015;523(7559):177–82.

Liquid Biopsy in Gastrointestinal Stromal Tumor

16

Daniele Fanale, Lorena Incorvaia, Marta Castiglia, Nadia Barraco, Giuseppe Badalamenti, Alex Le Cesne, and Antonio Russo

Introduction

Although gastrointestinal stromal tumors (GISTs) comprise fewer than 1% of all gastrointestinal (GI) tumors, they are the most common primary mesenchymal neoplasms of the GI tract [1]. Over the past 15 years, this group of tumors has emerged from a poorly understood neoplasm to a well-defined tumor entity.

Typically, GISTs are tumors highly resistant to conventional cytotoxic chemotherapy and, in the past, were typically managed surgically. Starting from 2000, the discovery of gain-of-function mutations involving *KIT* or *PDGFRα* (platelet-derived growth factor-α) genes and the development of tyrosine kinase inhibitors (TKIs), such as imatinib, revolutionized dramatically the management of GISTs. These TKIs are allowed to target the specific molecular events occurring in GIST cancer cells responsible for the pathogenesis and tumor progression, transforming GISTs from a chemotherapy-resistant disease with poor outcomes to a paradigm of targeted agent-responsive tumors.

Due to the almost continual emergence of new data about biological complexity of GISTs and more sophisticated whole-genome technologies, to date, the role of molecular biology is clinically important to drive therapeutic decision making.

Clinical, Pathological, and Molecular Features

GISTs can occur across the age spectrum but are more common in patients older than 40 years. They arise mostly in the stomach, followed by the small bowel and colon, but less commonly they are found in the esophagus, rectum, omentum, mesentery, or retroperitoneum. Clinical and radiologic features of GISTs vary depending on tumor size and organ of origin. They most commonly have an exophytic growth pattern and manifest as dominant masses outside the organ of origin. For this reason, the clinical manifestations

Daniele Fanale and Lorena Incorvaia contributed equally to this work.

D. Fanale • L. Incorvaia • M. Castiglia • N. Barraco
G. Badalamenti
Department of Surgical, Oncological and Oral Sciences, Section of Medical Oncology, University of Palermo, 90127 Palermo, Italy

A. Le Cesne
Department of Cancer Medicine, Gustave Roussy Cancer Campus, 114, rue Edouard Vaillant, 94800 Villejuif, France

A. Russo (✉)
Department of Surgical, Oncological and Oral Sciences, Section of Medical Oncology, University of Palermo, 90127 Palermo, Italy

Institute for Cancer Research and Molecular Medicineand Center of Biotechnology, College of Science and Biotechnology, Philadelphia, PA, USA
e-mail: antonio.russo@usa.net

© Springer International Publishing AG 2017
A. Giordano et al. (eds.), *Liquid Biopsy in Cancer Patients*, Current Clinical Pathology,
DOI 10.1007/978-3-319-55661-1_16

include often asymptomatic patients and nonspecific symptoms until the achievement of large
masses that can cause obstruction or massive
intraperitoneal bleeding secondary to rupture.
Unlike carcinoma, radiologic features of GISTs
are peculiar. GISTs may contain areas of hemor-
rhage, necrosis, or cyst formation that appear as
focal areas of low attenuation on computed tomo-
graphic images. Imaging features often change
during TKI treatment, such as central cystic
degenerative changes. Therefore, it is important
that radiologists and clinicians characterize and
detect the lesions and correctly evaluate the
tumor response.

For many years, GISTs were classified as
smooth muscle tumors and misclassified as leiomyomas, leiomyosarcomas, or leiomyoblastomas. To date, the hypothesis about GIST origin
suggests that they originate from a cell population in the gastrointestinal tract called interstitial
cells of Cajal (ICCs), which function as pacemaker cells that cause peristaltic contractions.
Histologically, depending on the cytomorphol-
ogy, spindle cell GISTs (70% of cases), GISTs
with epithelioid cell morphology (approximately
20% of cases), and GISTs with mixed morphology, both spindle and epithelioid cells (10% of
cases), can be recognized.

Two groundbreaking discoveries revolutionized the approach toward GISTs as entity:

- Approximately 95% of GISTs are immuno-
  histochemically positive for the tyrosine

kinase receptor KIT (CD117) [2]. Many
tumors previously diagnosed as leiomyomas,
leiomyoblastomas, or leiomyosarcomas have
been found to be positive for CD117 and are
now considered GISTs. Indeed, about 5% of
GISTs are negative for detectable KIT expression [3–5].

- The identification of KIT receptor mutations
  represents a pathogenic mechanism for GISTs
  [6]. Increasing experimental evidences
  revealed that the great majority of GISTs harbor mutually exclusive activating mutations in
  genes coding for the receptor tyrosine kinases
  KIT and PDGFRα (Fig. 16.1). There is also a
  small subgroup of GISTs, called wild type
  (WT), which does not harbor either *KIT* or
  PDGFRα mutations. Less commonly, GISTs
  have also been reported to harbor mutations
  elsewhere, including *BRAF*, *NF1*, and *SDH*
  complex genes.

KIT and PDGFRα are receptors for stem cell
factor (SCF) and platelet-derived growth factor
(PDGF), respectively. Under normal conditions,
in the absence of SCF, the receptors are maintained in an inactive state. The activation of the
receptors occurs via binding of their ligands,
resulting in signal transduction cascades that promote cell cycle activation, cell proliferation, survival, and apoptosis inhibition [7–9].

KIT and PDGFRα mutations in GISTs cause
ligand-independent constitutive activation of
the tyrosine kinase receptors [10], resulting in

Fig. 16.1 Activating
mutations in KIT
(75–80%) and PDGFRA
(5–10%)

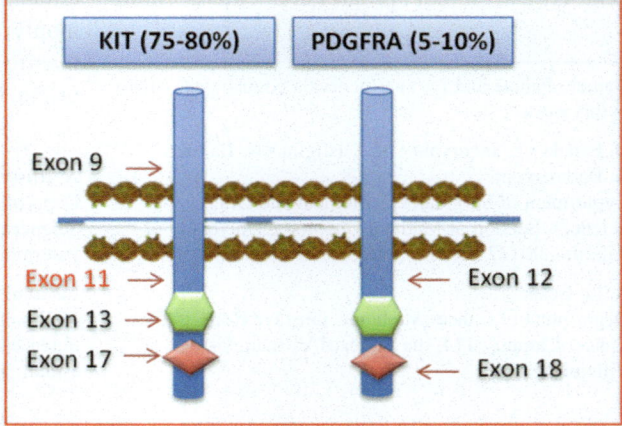

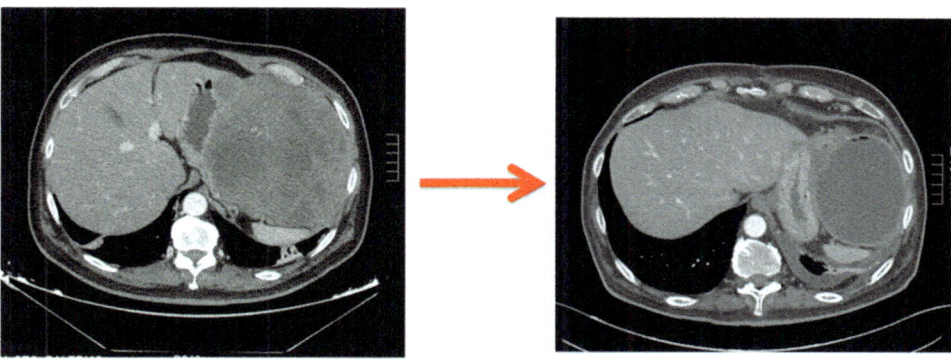

Fig. 16.2 CT scan of gastric GIST before (**a**) and after (**b**) 2 months of imatinib treatment

aberrant cell growth and tumor formation [11]. The most common mutations are harbored in *KIT* exon 11 [12]; other mutations have been demonstrated in *KIT* exons 9, 13, and 17. The knowledge of *KIT* and *PDGFRα* mutational status has led to the understanding of a potential correlation between site of mutations and clinical outcome: for example, patients with *KIT* exon 11 mutations show a poorer clinical outcome compared to patients with tumor WT or other mutations. These findings revealed the clinical significance of the mutational status and its role as prognostic factor. In addition, accumulating evidences showed its value as a predictive factor in advanced disease. The majority of GIST patients with advanced disease initially achieves disease control and clinical benefit from imatinib treatment (Fig. 16.2). However, approximately 10% of patients progresses within 6 months of starting therapy (defined as primary resistance to imatinib), and also 50–60% of the responding patients develops disease progression within 2 years (secondary or acquired resistance to imatinib) [13–15]. Several studies showed a stronger correlation between response to tyrosine kinase inhibitors and certain genotypes [16–19]. For example, patients with GISTs harboring *KIT* exon 11 mutations subjected to treatment with imatinib 400 mg/daily have a longer progression-free and overall survival compared to patients with wild-type *KIT* or mutated in exon 9 and *PDGFRα* D842V-mutated GISTs. The latter frequently show primary resistance [16, 19, 20]. Patients with *KIT* exon 9 mutations have a longer progression-free survival (PFS) with a higher dose level of imatinib, i.e., 800 mg/daily.

Mutations in exon 9 affect the extracellular KIT domain, mimicking the conformation change when SCF binds to the receptor, which induces higher degree of dimerization [21]. Since this mutation does not interfere with the kinase domain, exon 9-mutated *KIT* has the same kinase domain as that of wild-type *KIT*, in which decreased sensitivity to imatinib was observed in vitro compared to exon 11 KIT mutant [12]. Dose escalation is suggested for treatment of GISTs harboring these mutations [20]. KIT mutation is a clinically important therapeutic target in GISTs, and thanks to known relationship with tumor response, GISTs represent a model for molecular targeted therapy.

Standard biopsy is an invasive procedure, because it cannot be repeated during the medical treatment, and provides a static print of the mutational status, not detecting the numerous changes in tumor DNA over time.

The clinical potential role of the liquid biopsy in GIST was presented for the first time at the 2013 ASCO Annual Meeting. Detection of circulating tumor DNA (ctDNA) offers a wide spectrum of applications in GIST management. CtDNA correlates with the tumor burden, thus, after surgery may indicate the presence of minimal residual disease and patients with high risk of recurrence. In addition, during the clinical treatment, this approach could be used to identify early biomarkers of response and asses variations in whole genome, early identifying the development of secondary resistance.

Circulating Tumor Cells and Circulating Tumor DNA in GIST

The opportunity offered by liquid biopsy as a tool for patient monitoring over time is becoming very interesting also in GIST. Nevertheless, since the application of liquid biopsy in GISTs has only recently been reported, there are still few but very promising data on the application of both circulating tumor cells (CTCs) and circulating tumor DNA (ctDNA) as prognostic/diagnostic and predictive biomarkers.

The analysis of CTCs in GIST patients has been recently proven to have a prognostic and a predictive value. A cohort of 121 GIST patients and 54 non-GIST samples was enrolled in the study published in 2016 by Li et al. [22]. The approach used for the identification of GIST-specific CTCs was based on the evaluation of the DOG1 expression in peripheral blood mononuclear cells (PBMCs). The DOG1 expression levels were first compared between GIST and non-GIST samples, reporting an increased DOG1 expression in PBMC isolated from GIST patients. DOG1-positive PBMCs were more frequently detected in unresectable patients compared to resectable subjects. The DOG1 expression levels in PBMC were reported to be higher in locally advanced GIST patients compared to resectable GISTs (73.1% versus 54%, $p < 0.001$). Accordingly, large tumor size, mitotic count, and high-risk tumors correlate with a higher DOG1 expression. Moreover, the presence of CTCs significantly correlates with poor disease-free survival (16.3 versus 19.6 months, $p = 0.038$), providing important prognostic information after surgery. Indeed, all patients who turned positive after surgery experienced recurrence. Furthermore, in neoadjuvant setting, the decrease of DOG1-positive cells after imatinib administration was correlated with response.

From a technical point of view, the mutational analysis of KIT and PDGFRα is challenging due to the high heterogeneity and wide variability of tyrosine kinase mutations that could be identified. Therefore, "targeted methods" (such as real-time PCR, droplet digital PCR, and BEAMing), which are able to detect known mutation using specific probes, may be unable to identify other clinically relevant mutations. These limitations can be overcome by next-generation sequencing (NGS) analysis, which enables the sequencing of large genomic regions or several exons.

The possibility of using ctDNA as liquid biopsy in GISTs was reported for the first time at the 2013 ASCO Annual Meeting. As for other tumor types, such as non-small cell lung cancer, also in GIST, it is important to determine the genotype in TKI-refractory disease, even though re-biopsy is not always feasible and patients may not be compliant. Therefore, circulating plasma can be used as source of tumor DNA to characterize and evaluate the new mutational landscape after TKI treatment in GIST patients [23]. In the work presented at ASCO meeting in 2013, the authors have analyzed both archival tumor tissue ($n = 102$) and plasma samples ($n = 163$) in a subgroup of GIST patients enrolled in the phase III GRID trial. Looking at primary mutation in KIT gene, a 84% concordance between tissue and plasma was found, whereas secondary KIT mutations were more commonly detected in plasma (47%) than in tissue (12%) and correlated with shorter PFS in patients receiving placebo.

Subsequently, Maier et al. [24] developed a series of 25 different allele-specific L-polymerase chain reaction assays covering KIT and PDGFRα mutations in order to examine 291 plasma samples from 38 patients. Using this approach, mutations in KIT and PDGFRα were detectable in 15 out of 38 patients. Interestingly, the dynamic changes of the allele fraction in ctDNA have been shown to correlate with disease course. Indeed, patients with progressive disease or relapse were characterized by repeated positive test results or increase in ctDNA. Accordingly, a decrease of ctDNA or conversion from positive to negative was observed in patients responding to treatment [24]. Similarly, Yoo et al. [25] analyzed ctDNA isolated from serum in 30 patients using BEAMing (beads, emulsions, amplification, and magnetics) technology. In 17% of patients it was possible to identify the primary kinase mutation with 100% concordance with the results obtained from the corresponding tissue. The relatively low detection rate of primary mutations was probably due to the specific design of the BEAMing assay that aims mainly at the identification of secondary mutations.

Also in GISTs, as well as in other tumor types, the major mechanism of acquired resistance to imatinib is the development of secondary mutations that can be found in 50–70% of patients who experience disease progression [26]. Thus, it would be very useful to promptly identify resistance mutation and eventually modify treatment accordingly. Several data suggest that acquisition of secondary kinase mutations can be detected from ctDNA and correlate with treatment impairment and OS [24].

As previously mentioned, the mutational analysis of *KIT* and *PDGFRα* is challenging, due to the wide mutation variability. Thus, the use of "targeted methods" could not provide comprehensive data, losing the chance to identify other and rare mutations. NGS may overcome this technical limit by using focused gene panels designed to narrow down the coverage on clinically relevant targets so that each read is sequenced thousands of times, ensuring a high degree of sensitivity [27, 28]. The data on NGS analysis in ctDNA from GISTs patients are promising, but still few. There are only two studies reporting the analysis of ctDNA through NGS in a limited number of GIST patients. In the study by Wada et al. [29], NGS approach was used to analyze four patients who underwent resection of imatinib-resistant GIST. Plasma samples were obtained before and after surgery, and corresponding tissue sample was available for each patient. Imatinib-resistant lesions were characterized by secondary mutations mainly localized in KIT exon 13; the same genetic alterations were detectable in ctDNA with a mutant fraction ranging from 0.010% to 9.385%. Moreover, the concentration of ctDNA is affected by treatment and can be used as a surrogate biomarker of treatment response.

The identification of surgical resections R0 and R1 is still controversial in several tumor types, including GIST. Despite the use of the Fletcher-Miettinen classification, there are no other markers that can help in a better stratification of patients who underwent to curative resec-

tion. Thus, there is an attempt to use liquid biopsy, especially ctDNA, as surrogate biomarker in GISTs in order to distinguish between R0 and R1 patients [29, 30]. In the study performed by Kang et al. [23], plasma samples were collected from 25 patients before surgery, and paired plasma-tissue samples were analyzed through NGS panel covering exons 9, 11, 13, and 17 of *KIT* and exon 18 of *PDGFRα*. The reported concordance between plasma and tissue samples was 72% with allele frequencies ranging from 0.19% to 21.96%. Moreover, none of the patients reported to be wild type in tissue had detectable mutations in plasma, suggesting a good specificity of the assay.

The discovery of the so-called liquid biopsy has already brought a wind of change in molecular oncology. The number of "targetable" alterations is visibly growing and accordingly the number of available targeted drugs. In parallel, the request for an accurate and complete molecular characterization over "time" and "space" has become a clinical need for a proper treatment choice. As for other solid tumors, several new clinical trials for GISTs are now including liquid biopsy in their study design, and some of them are specifically designed to investigate the role of ctDNA in GIST patient management (NCT02331914; NCT02443948), proving a growing interest in this field. Indeed, liquid biopsy may be used in different moments during the disease course. CTCs may probably be useful for a better stratification of GIST patients, whereas ctDNA might be fundamental for monitoring treatment over time and for the reevaluation of the tumor molecular status after resistance onset (Fig. 16.3).

Potential Use of Circulating microRNAs as a Liquid Biopsy for GIST Patients

MicroRNAs (miRNAs) are a class of small non-coding RNA molecules, about 19–25 nucleotides in length, encoded by endogenous genes which negatively modulate about 30% of coding genes in the human genome, by binding a complementary

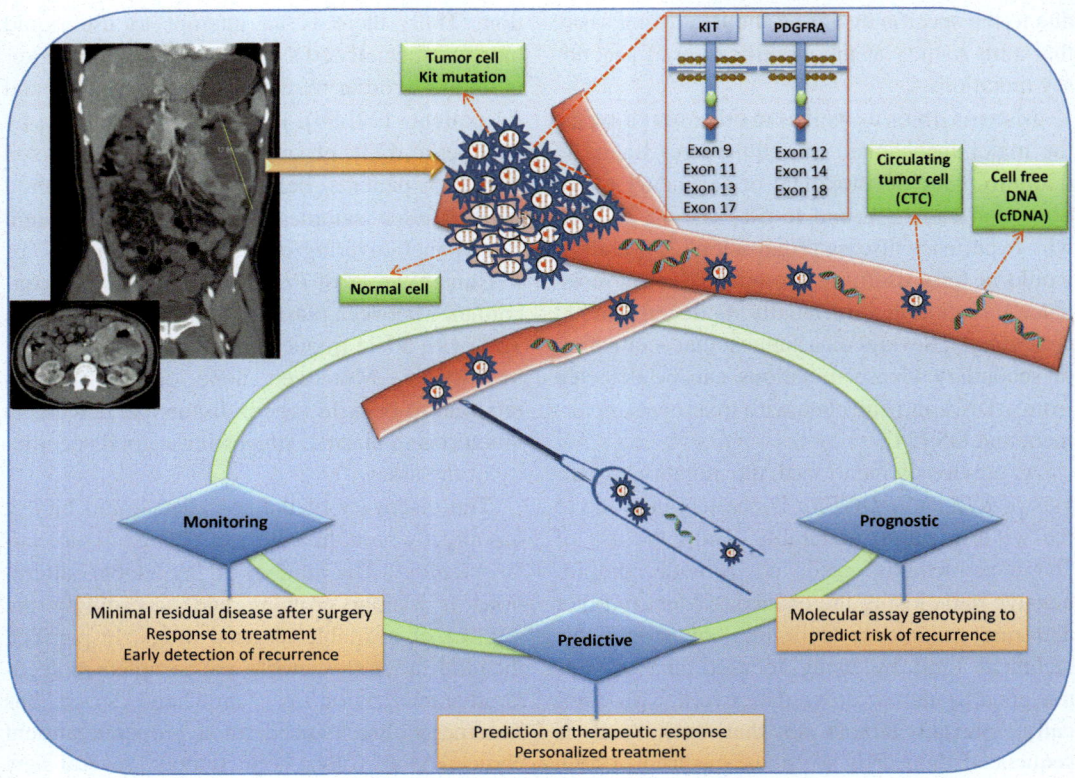

Fig. 16.3 Liquid biopsy in GIST: clinical application

sequence present in the 3'-untranslated region (UTR) of target mRNAs, resulting in direct mRNA cleavage or translational inhibition [31–33]. Experimental evidence showed that miRNAs may play a key role in the modulation of different biological processes, such as immune response, apoptosis, cell growth, angiogenesis, and regulation of several metabolic pathways [34–39], whose alteration may be crucial for the cancer onset and progression, metastasis development, and drug resistance [31, 40, 41]. In recent years, the role of miRNAs as novel potential biomarkers for diagnostic, prognostic, and predictive purposes has been investigated, in order to develop new therapeutic strategies for the treatment of several diseases [42, 43]. Therefore, the identification of miRNA signatures currently seems to be an interesting field to explore in oncology research, also thanks to recent advances in the development of miRNA-based antitumor therapeutic approaches.

Several studies highlighted the crucial role of miRNA expression variations in GIST biology, especially in tumorigenesis, prognosis, progression, metastasis, therapy response, and acquisition of primary and secondary resistance [44–48]. Over these years, the role of miRNAs in GIST was investigated mainly through expression analysis in cell lines and fresh or formalin-fixed paraffin-embedded (FFPE) tissue specimens. However, despite encouraging preliminary results, the introduction of miRNAs in clinical practice appears to be currently still far, due to the low number of analyzed cases and other limitations such as the use of unstandardized methodologies and poor reproducibility of data [44]. In recent years, several evidences suggested the possibility of using specific circulating miRNAs as liquid biopsy for GIST patients. Although an increasing number of researchers are focusing on the finding of new circulating miRNAs to use as potential noninvasive biomarkers for GIST, however, to date, studies concerning plasma/serum miRNAs or miRNAs from exosomes or animal models were not reported in literature. The molecular investigation of circulating and exosome miRNAs in peripheral blood of GIST patients could represent, in future, an important tool for identifying biomarkers useful for the diagnosis, progression risk prediction, prognosis, and response to treatment [49, 50].

Long Noncoding RNAs (lncRNAs) in GIST

A new, valid, and largely unexplored field of investigation is represented by a class of noncoding RNAs called long noncoding RNAs (lncRNAs). lncRNAs have been defined according to their size greater than 200 nt in length. lncRNAs belong to a class of regulatory RNA noncoding for proteins that, as it has been estimated, represent approximately 1.5% of the almost entirely transcribed eukaryotic genome [51, 52]. They contribute to oncogenesis in cancer as oncogenic and/or tumor suppressor factors [53]. They play essential biological functions, including chromatin modification, and transcriptional and posttranscriptional processing [54, 55]. In GIST, upregulation of HOTAIR has been associated with tumor aggressiveness and metastasis and poor patients' survival. Niinuma et al. [45] in 2012 described the upregulation of the HOTAIR expression in high-risk malignancy samples from frozen GIST tissues. An additional study by Lee et al. [56] has recently confirmed such evidences, showing that if the target gene subjected to silencing is a tumor suppressor such as PCDH10, the final result will be the failure of the mechanisms which control both tumor invasion and progression. Even if this is very interesting, these are the only published data currently available regarding expression of lncRNAs in GISTs. Further analyses are needed to confirm these data and evaluate the potential role of such lncRNAs, as prognostic/predictive molecular biomarkers. Furthermore, no evidence exists that these molecules have been obtained from the bloodstream. Nevertheless, lncRNAs may represent interesting candidates as prognostic and predictive "circulating biomarkers" in this disease.

References

1. Judson I, Demetri G. Advances in the treatment of gastrointestinal stromal tumours. Ann Oncol. 2007;18 Suppl 10:x20–4. doi:10.1093/annonc/mdm410 18/suppl_10/x20 [pii].
2. Kindblom LG, Remotti HE, Aldenborg F, Meis-Kindblom JM. Gastrointestinal pacemaker cell tumor (GIPACT): gastrointestinal stromal tumors show phenotypic characteristics of the interstitial cells of Cajal. Am J Pathol. 1998;152(5):1259–69.
3. Fletcher CD, Berman JJ, Corless C, Gorstein F, Lasota J, Longley BJ, et al. Diagnosis of gastrointestinal stromal tumors: a consensus approach. Hum Pathol. 2002;33(5):459–65. doi:S0046817702000151 [pii].
4. Medeiros F, Corless CL, Duensing A, Hornick JL, Oliveira AM, Heinrich MC, et al. KIT-negative gastrointestinal stromal tumors: proof of concept and therapeutic implications. Am J Surg Pathol. 2004;28(7):889–94. doi:00000478-200407000-00007 [pii].
5. Debiec-Rychter M, Wasag B, Stul M, De Wever I, Van Oosterom A, Hagemeijer A, et al. Gastrointestinal stromal tumours (GISTs) negative for KIT (CD117 antigen) immunoreactivity. J Pathol. 2004;202(4):430–8. doi:10.1002/path.1546.
6. Hirota S, Isozaki K, Moriyama Y, Hashimoto K, Nishida T, Ishiguro S, et al. Gain-of-function mutations of c-kit in human gastrointestinal stromal tumors. Science. 1998;279(5350):577–80.
7. Heldin CH. Dimerization of cell surface receptors in signal transduction. Cell. 1995;80(2):213–23. doi:0092-8674(95)90404-2 [pii].
8. Hubbard SR, Mohammadi M, Schlessinger J. Autoregulatory mechanisms in protein-tyrosine kinases. J Biol Chem. 1998;273(20):11987–90.
9. Roskoski R, Jr. Signaling by Kit protein-tyrosine kinase--the stem cell factor receptor. Biochem Biophys Res Commun. 2005;337(1):1–13. doi:10.1016/j.bbrc.2005.08.055 S0006-291X(05)01759-6 [pii].
10. Gajiwala KS, Wu JC, Christensen J, Deshmukh GD, Diehl W, DiNitto JP et al. KIT kinase mutants show unique mechanisms of drug resistance to imatinib and sunitinib in gastrointestinal stromal tumor patients. Proc Natl Acad Sci U S A 2009;106(5):1542–1547. doi:10.1073/pnas.0812413106 0812413106 [pii].
11. Corless CL, Fletcher JA, Heinrich MC. Biology of gastrointestinal stromal tumors. J Clin Oncol 2004;22(18):3813–3825. doi:10.1200/JCO.2004.05.140 22/18/3813 [pii].
12. Corless CL, Barnett CM, Heinrich MC. Gastrointestinal stromal tumours: origin and molecular oncology. Nat Rev Cancer 2011;11(12):865–878. doi:10.1038/nrc3143 nrc3143 [pii].

13. Blanke CD, Rankin C, Demetri GD, Ryan CW, von Mehren M, Benjamin RS et al. Phase III randomized, intergroup trial assessing imatinib mesylate at two dose levels in patients with unresectable or metastatic gastrointestinal stromal tumors expressing the kit receptor tyrosine kinase: S0033. J Clin Oncol 2008;26(4):626–632. doi:10.1200/JCO.2007.13.4452 26/4/626 [pii].

14. van Oosterom AT, Judson IR, Verweij J, Stroobants S, Dumez H, Donato di Paola E, et al. Update of phase I study of imatinib (STI571) in advanced soft tissue sarcomas and gastrointestinal stromal tumors: a report of the EORTC Soft Tissue and Bone Sarcoma Group. Eur J Cancer. 2002;38(Suppl 5):S83–7.

15. Verweij J, Casali PG, Zalcberg J, LeCesne A, Reichardt P, Blay JY et al. Progression-free survival in gastrointestinal stromal tumours with high-dose imatinib: randomised trial. Lancet 2004;364(9440):1127–1134. doi:10.1016/S0140-6736(04)17098-0 S0140673604170980 [pii].

16. Debiec-Rychter M, Sciot R, Le Cesne A, Schlemmer M, Hohenberger P, van Oosterom AT et al. KIT mutations and dose selection for imatinib in patients with advanced gastrointestinal stromal tumours. Eur J Cancer. 2006;42(8):1093–1103. doi:10.1016/j.ejca.2006.01.030 S0959-8049(06)00175-4 [pii].

17. Debiec-Rychter M, Dumez H, Judson I, Wasag B, Verweij J, Brown M et al. Use of c-KIT/PDGFRA mutational analysis to predict the clinical response to imatinib in patients with advanced gastrointestinal stromal tumours entered on phase I and II studies of the EORTC Soft Tissue and Bone Sarcoma Group. Eur J Cancer 2004;40(5):689–695. doi:10.1016/j.ejca.2003.11.025 S0959804904000048 [pii].

18. Heinrich MC, Corless CL, Demetri GD, Blanke CD, von Mehren M, Joensuu H et al. Kinase mutations and imatinib response in patients with metastatic gastrointestinal stromal tumor. J Clin Oncol 2003;21(23):4342–4349. doi:10.1200/JCO.2003.04.190 JCO.2003.04.190 [pii].

19. Heinrich MC, Owzar K, Corless CL, Hollis D, Borden EC, Fletcher CD et al. Correlation of kinase genotype and clinical outcome in the North American Intergroup Phase III Trial of imatinib mesylate for treatment of advanced gastrointestinal stromal tumor: CALGB 150105 Study by Cancer and Leukemia Group B and Southwest Oncology Group. J Clin Oncol 2008;26(33):5360–5367. doi:10.1200/JCO.2008.17.4284 JCO.2008.17.4284 [pii].

20. Comparison of two doses of imatinib for the treatment of unresectable or metastatic gastrointestinal stromal tumors: a meta-analysis of 1,640 patients. J Clin Oncol. 2010;28(7):1247–53. doi:10.1200/JCO.2009.24.2099 JCO.2009.24.2099 [pii].

21. Yuzawa S, Opatowsky Y, Zhang Z, Mandiyan V, Lax I, Schlessinger J. Structural basis for activation of the receptor tyrosine kinase KIT by stem cell factor. Cell. 2007;130(2):323–334. doi:10.1016/j.cell.2007.05.055 S0092-8674(07)00759-3 [pii].

22. Li Q, Zhi X, Zhou J, Tao R, Zhang J, Chen P et al. Circulating tumor cells as a prognostic and predictive marker in gastrointestinal stromal tumors: a prospective study. Oncotarget 2016;7(24):36645–36654. doi:10.18632/oncotarget.9128 9128 [pii].

23. Kang G, Bae BN, Sohn BS, Pyo JS, Kang GH, Kim KM. Detection of KIT and PDGFRA mutations in the plasma of patients with gastrointestinal stromal tumor. Target Oncol 2015;10(4):597–601. doi:10.1007/s11523-015-0361-1 10.1007/s11523-015-0361-1 [pii].

24. Maier J, Lange T, Kerle I, Specht K, Bruegel M, Wickenhauser C et al. Detection of mutant free circulating tumor DNA in the plasma of patients with gastrointestinal stromal tumor harboring activating mutations of CKIT or PDGFRA. Clin Cancer Res 2013;19(17):4854–4867. doi:10.1158/1078-0432.CCR-13-0765 1078-0432.CCR-13-0765 [pii].

25. Yoo C, Ryu MH, Na YS, Ryoo BY, Park SR, Kang YK. Analysis of serum protein biomarkers, circulating tumor DNA, and dovitinib activity in patients with tyrosine kinase inhibitor-refractory gastrointestinal stromal tumors. Ann Oncol. 2014;25(11):2272–7. doi:10.1093/annonc/mdu386.

26. Gounder MM, Maki RG. Molecular basis for primary and secondary tyrosine kinase inhibitor resistance in gastrointestinal stromal tumor. Cancer Chemother Pharmacol. 2011;67(Suppl 1):S25–43. doi:10.1007/s00280-010-1526-3.

27. Paweletz CP, Sacher AG, Raymond CK, Alden RS, O'Connell A, Mach SL et al. Bias-corrected targeted next-generation sequencing for rapid, multiplexed detection of actionable alterations in cell-free DNA from advanced lung cancer patients. Clin Cancer Res 2016;22(4):915–922. doi:10.1158/1078-0432.CCR-15-1627-T 1078-0432.CCR-15-1627-T [pii].

28. Couraud S, Vaca-Paniagua F, Villar S, Oliver J, Schuster T, Blanche H et al. Noninvasive diagnosis of actionable mutations by deep sequencing of circulating free DNA in lung cancer from never-smokers: a proof-of-concept study from BioCAST/IFCT-1002. Clin Cancer Res 2014;20(17):4613–4624. doi:10.1158/1078-0432.CCR-13-3063 1078-0432.CCR-13-3063 [pii].

29. Wada N, Kurokawa Y, Takahashi T, Hamakawa T, Hirota S, Naka T et al. Detecting secondary C-KIT mutations in the peripheral blood of patients with imatinib-resistant gastrointestinal stromal tumor. Oncology 2016;90(2):112–117. doi:10.1159/000442948 000442948 [pii].

30. Kang G, Sohn BS, Pyo JS, Kim JY, Lee B, Kim KM. Detecting Primary KIT Mutations in Presurgical Plasma of Patients with Gastrointestinal Stromal Tumor. Mol Diagn Ther. 2016;20(4):347–351. doi:10.1007/s40291-016-0203-6 10.1007/s40291-016-0203-6 [pii].

31. Raza U, Zhang JD, Sahin O. MicroRNAs: master regulators of drug resistance, stemness, and metastasis. J Mol Med (Berl). 2014;92(4):321–36. doi:10.1007/s00109-014-1129-2.

32. Bartel DP. MicroRNAs: genomics, biogenesis, mechanism, and function. Cell 2004;116(2):281–297. doi:S0092867404000455 [pii].

33. Bronte F, Bronte G, Fanale D, Caruso S, Bronte E, Bavetta MG et al. HepatomiRNoma: the proposal of a new network of targets for diagnosis, prognosis and therapy in hepatocellular carcinoma. Crit Rev Oncol Hematol 2016;97:312–321. doi:10.1016/j.critrevonc.2015.09.007 S1040-8428(15)30047-0 [pii].

34. Di Fiore R, Fanale D, Drago-Ferrante R, Chiaradonna F, Giuliano M, De Blasio A, et al. Genetic and molecular characterization of the human osteosarcoma 3AB-OS cancer stem cell line: a possible model for studying osteosarcoma origin and stemness. J Cell Physiol. 2013;228(6):1189–201. doi:10.1002/jcp.24272.

35. Caruso S, Bazan V, Rolfo C, Insalaco L, Fanale D, Bronte G et al. MicroRNAs in colorectal cancer stem cells: new regulators of cancer stemness? Oncogenesis 2012;1:e32. doi:10.1038/oncsis.2012.33 oncsis201233 [pii].

36. Amodeo V, Bazan V, Fanale D, Insalaco L, Caruso S, Cicero G, et al. Effects of anti-miR-182 on TSP-1 expression in human colon cancer cells: there is a sense in antisense? Expert Opin Ther Targets. 2013;17(11):1249–61. doi:10.1517/14728222.2013.832206.

37. Su Z, Yang Z, Xu Y, Chen Y, Yu Q. MicroRNAs in apoptosis, autophagy and necroptosis. Oncotarget. 2015;6(11):8474–8490. doi:10.18632/oncotarget.3523 3523 [pii].

38. Fanale D, Amodeo V, Bazan V, Insalaco L, Incorvaia L, Barraco N et al. Can the microRNA expression profile help to identify novel targets for zoledronic acid in breast cancer? Oncotarget. 2016;7(20):29321–29332. doi:10.18632/oncotarget.8722 8722 [pii].

39. Chen J, Deng S, Zhang S, Chen Z, Wu S, Cai X et al. The role of miRNAs in the differentiation of adipose-derived stem cells. Curr Stem Cell Res Ther 2014;9(3):268–279. doi:CSCRT-EPUB-59186 [pii].

40. Iorio MV, Croce CM. MicroRNAs in cancer: small molecules with a huge impact. J Clin Oncol 2009;27(34):5848–5856. doi:10.1200/JCO.2009.24.0317 JCO.2009.24.0317 [pii].

41. Rolfo C, Fanale D, Hong DS, Tsimberidou AM, Piha-Paul SA, Pauwels P et al. Impact of microRNAs in resistance to chemotherapy and novel targeted agents in non-small cell lung cancer. Curr Pharm Biotechnol 2014;15(5):475–485. doi:CPB-EPUB-60568 [pii].

42. Corsini LR, Bronte G, Terrasi M, Amodeo V, Fanale D, Fiorentino E, et al. The role of microRNAs in cancer: diagnostic and prognostic biomarkers and targets of therapies. Expert Opin Ther Targets. 2012;16(Suppl 2):S103–9. doi:10.1517/14728222.2011.650632.

43. Zarate R, Boni V, Bandres E, Garcia-Foncillas J. MiRNAs and LincRNAs: could they be considered as biomarkers in colorectal cancer? Int J Mol Sci 2012;13(1):840–865. doi:10.3390/ijms13010840 ijms-13-00840 [pii].

44. Nannini M, Ravegnini G, Angelini S, Astolfi A, Biasco G, Pantaleo MA. miRNA profiling in gastrointestinal stromal tumors: implication as diagnostic and prognostic markers. Epigenomics. 2015;7(6):1033–49. doi:10.2217/epi.15.52.

45. Niinuma T, Suzuki H, Nojima M, Nosho K, Yamamoto H, Takamaru H et al. Upregulation of miR-196a and HOTAIR drive malignant character in gastrointestinal stromal tumors. Cancer Res 2012;72(5):1126–1136. doi:10.1158/0008-5472.CAN-11-1803 0008-5472.CAN-11-1803 [pii].

46. Kim WK, Park M, Kim YK, Tae YK, Yang HK, Lee JM et al. MicroRNA-494 downregulates KIT and inhibits gastrointestinal stromal tumor cell proliferation. Clin Cancer Res 2011;17(24):7584–7594. doi:10.1158/1078-0432.CCR-11-0166 1078-0432.CCR-11-0166 [pii].

47. Akcakaya P, Caramuta S, Ahlen J, Ghaderi M, Berglund E, Ostman A et al. microRNA expression signatures of gastrointestinal stromal tumours: associations with imatinib resistance and patient outcome. Br J Cancer 2014;111(11):2091–2102. doi:10.1038/bjc.2014.548 bjc2014548 [pii].

48. Gits CM, van Kuijk PF, Jonkers MB, Boersma AW, van Ijcken WF, Wozniak A et al. MiR-17-92 and miR-221/222 cluster members target KIT and ETV1 in human gastrointestinal stromal tumours. Br J Cancer 2013;109(6):1625–1635. doi:10.1038/bjc.2013.483 bjc2013483 [pii].

49. Cheng G. Circulating miRNAs: roles in cancer diagnosis, prognosis and therapy. Adv Drug Deliv Rev 2015;81:75–93. doi:10.1016/j.addr.2014.09.001 S0169-409X(14)00199-9 [pii].

50. Ono S, Lam S, Nagahara M, Hoon DS. Circulating microRNA biomarkers as liquid biopsy for cancer patients: pros and cons of current assays. J Clin Med 2015;4(10):1890–1907. doi:10.3390/jcm4101890 jcm4101890 [pii].

51. Carninci P, Kasukawa T, Katayama S, Gough J, Frith MC, Maeda N et al. The transcriptional landscape of the mammalian genome. Science. 2005;309(5740):1559–1563. doi:10.1126/science.1112014 309/5740/1559 [pii].

52. Wang KC, Chang HY. Molecular mechanisms of long noncoding RNAs. Mol Cell 2011;43(6):904–914. doi:10.1016/j.molcel.2011.08.018 S1097-2765(11)00636-8 [pii].

53. Chen X, Yan CC, Zhang X, You ZH. Long non-coding RNAs and complex diseases: from experimental results to computational models. Brief Bioinform. 2016. doi:10.1093/bib/bbw060 bbw060 [pii].

54. Yu B, Shan G. Functions of long noncoding RNAs in the nucleus. Nucleus. 2016;7(2):155–66. doi:10.1080/19491034.2016.1179408.

55. Ponting CP, Oliver PL, Reik W. Evolution and functions of long noncoding RNAs. Cell 2009;136(4):629–641. doi:10.1016/j.cell.2009.02.006 S0092-8674(09)00142-1 [pii].

56. Lee NK, Lee JH, Kim WK, Yun S, Youn YH, Park CH et al. Promoter methylation of PCDH10 by HOTAIR regulates the progression of gastrointestinal stromal tumors. Oncotarget 2016;7(46):75307–75318. doi:10.18632/oncotarget.12171 12171 [pii].

Liquid Biopsies in Malignant Melanoma: From Bench to Bedside

17

Estíbaliz Alegre, Leyre Zubiri, Juan Pablo Fusco,
Natalia Ramírez, Álvaro González,
and Ignacio Gil-Bazo

Abbreviations

APP	Amyloid-beta precursor protein
BEAMing	Beads, emulsions, amplification and magnetics
Bp	Base pairs
BRAF	B-Raf proto-oncogene, serine/threonine kinase
CD 125	Cluster differentiation 125
CDKN2a	Cyclin-dependent kinase inhibitor 2A
CDK4	Cyclin-dependent kinase 4
ctDNA	Cell-free circulating tumour DNA
CTCs	Circulating tumour cells
CTLA-4	Cytotoxic T lymphocyte-associated antigen 4
DFS	Disease-free survival
FDA	Food and drug administration
HGF	Hepatocyte growth factor
HGFR/MET	Hepatocyte growth factor receptor
HR	Hazard ratio
IFN-α	Interferon alpha
IGF-1R	Insulin-like growth factor 1 receptor
LDH	Lactate dehydrogenase
MAPK	Mitogen-activated protein kinase
MEK	MAP kinase-ERK kinase
MGMT	O6-Methylguanine-DNA methyltransferase
MITF	Microphthalmia transcription factor
NK	Natural killer
NRAS	Neuroblastoma RAS viral (v-ras) oncogene homolog
OS	Overall survival
PCR	Polymerase chain reaction
PD1	Programmed cell death protein 1
PDGFR-β	Beta-type platelet-derived growth factor receptor
PDL-1	Programmed death-ligand 1
PFS	Progression-free survival
PI3K	Phosphatidylinositol 3-kinase
PIP2	Phosphatidylinositol 4,5-biphosphate
PIP3	Phosphatidylinositol 3,4,5-triphosphate
PTEN	Phosphatase and tensin homolog
qPCR	Quantitative polymerase chain reaction

E. Alegre • A. González
Department of Biochemistry, Clínica Universidad de Navarra, IDISNA, Pamplona, Spain

L. Zubiri • J.P. Fusco
Department of Oncology, Clínica Universidad de Navarra, IDISNA, Pamplona, Spain

N. Ramírez
Oncohematology Research Group, Navarrabiomed, Miguel Servet Foundation, IDISNA (Navarra's Health Research Institute), Pamplona, Spain

I. Gil-Bazo (✉)
Department of Oncology, Clínica Universidad de Navarra, IDISNA, Pamplona, Spain

Program of Solid Tumors and Biomarkers, Center for Applied Medical Research, IDISNA, Pamplona, Spain
e-mail: igbazo@unav.es

© Springer International Publishing AG 2017
A. Giordano et al. (eds.), *Liquid Biopsy in Cancer Patients*, Current Clinical Pathology,
DOI 10.1007/978-3-319-55661-1_17

RAR-β   Retinoic acid receptor beta
RASSF1   Ras association (RalGDS/AF-6)
             domain family member 1
RECIST   Response evaluation criteria in solid
             tumours
RTK   Receptor tyrosine kinases
SCF   Stem cell factor
SOCS1   Suppressor of cytokine signalling 1
SOCS2   Suppressor of cytokine signalling 2
TILs   Tumour-infiltrating lymphocytes

Epidemiology and Molecular Biology of Malignant Melanoma

Epidemiology and Molecular Biology of Malignant Melanoma

Melanoma is a neoplastic disorder that is originated from a malignant transformation of melanocytes, the pigment-producing cells of the body. Almost half of melanomas are diagnosed before the sixth decade of life [1], so understanding the underlying biology of melanoma is a fundamental element to predict its clinical course and develop new therapies to improve survival. In this section, we will concentrate on cutaneous melanoma.

An increasing incidence of cutaneous melanoma in white population has been observed during the last few decades, whereas its incidence remains low in populations of African or Asian origin with darker pigmentation. In Europe, the incidence is 10–15 new cases per 100,000 inhabitants/year and in the USA reaches 18 new annual cases per 100,000 inhabitants. However, the highest incidence has been reported in Australian and New Zealand population ranging from 40 to 60 annual new cases per 100,000 inhabitants [2, 3].

Around 82–85% of patients with melanoma are diagnosed with a localized stage, and treatment consists of surgery alone. If there is lymph node involvement, treatment options also include the administration of high doses of interferon alpha (IFN-α) and radiotherapy. Finally, in a context of metastatic melanoma, traditional approach consisted of chemotherapy with dacarbazine, an agent that induces the methylation of the N7 position of guanine on DNA and cross-links DNA strands, so that inhibition of DNA, RNA and protein synthesis is produced. Historically, this treatment has resulted in a very limited efficacy with an 8% objective response rate and without a demonstrated improvement in overall survival in metastatic melanoma [4]. The advanced discoveries in cell signalling in the last years have provided a better understanding of the molecular mechanisms underlying metastatic melanoma [5] and have led to the discovery of new therapies with the consequent improvement in the prognosis of this disease. These therapies include specific agents for the recently discovered molecular targets (anti-BRAF therapies) and immune-mediated treatments, derived from the research in this field, too.

The traditional classification of different types of melanoma distinguishes four histogenetic groups (superficial spreading, lentigo maligna, nodular and acral lentiginous melanoma). However, it has also been stated that there are different pathways that predominate in the distinct subtypes of melanoma, founding the notion that the different phenotypes of melanoma are supported by different genetic mechanisms [6]. The fundamental pathways related to melanoma tumorigenesis are discussed below.

Molecular Biology

MAPK Pathway

Mitogen-activated protein kinases (MAPK) are serine-threonine kinases that mediate intracellular signalling (Fig. 17.1) leading to a variety of cellular activities including cell proliferation, differentiation, survival, death and transformation [7]. MAPK signalling cascade has been implicated in the pathogenesis of a variety of human disorders including cancer. This oncogenic pathway is essential for the pathogenesis of cutaneous melanoma [8] and is composed by different proteins: RAS, RAF, MEK and ERK, all of which transfer signals from the cell surface to the nucleus, through protein phosphorylation, and activate the genes that induce cell proliferation and apoptosis (Myc, cyclin D1, p21, NF-κB).

One of the possible ways of initiating the signalling cascade is through the association between growth factor receptor tyrosine kinases

Fig. 17.1 MAPK pathway

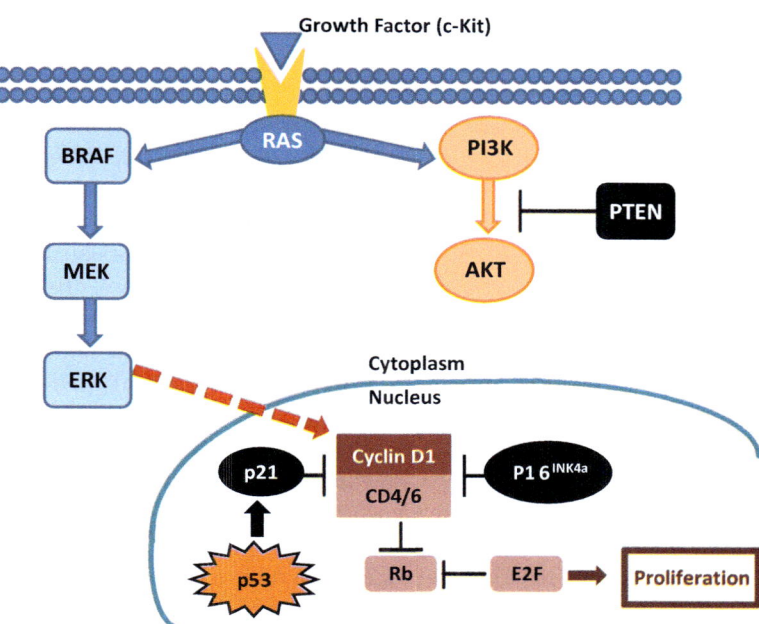

(RTK) and RAS. The complex RTK-RAS induces the activation of BRAF, MEK and ERK in the cytoplasm. Finally, ERK is phosphorylated and translocates to the nucleus to induce cell differentiation. In melanoma, MAPK pathway can be activated by oncogenic mutations, such as *N-RAS* and *BRAF*, and by mutations in membrane receptors, such as KIT (Fig. 17.1).

N-RAS is mutated in 25–35% of melanomas, and the most common mutation is a glutamine (Q) to arginine (R) substitution at position 61 (Q61R) [9]. The other two members of the *RAS* proto-oncogene family include HRAS and KRAS, all with GTPase activity. These mutations induce the constitutive activation of RAF proteins enhancing its signalling through the MAPK pathway and leading to proliferation, survival, invasion and angiogenesis in melanoma. The phosphatidylinositol 3-kinase (PI3K) cascade can also be activated by the MAPK pathway, but this phenomenon is much less common, being mutations in RAF the most common genetic alterations and main drivers in MAPK activation [8].

There are three different RAF isoforms in humans, ARAF, BRAF and CRAF, with different genetic events and activation mechanisms. BRAF shows constitutive phosphorylation of the N-terminus, as opposed to ARAF or CRAF, which can be one of the causes why BRAF is mutated in a higher proportion of patients, as it can be directly activated by RAS [10].

The most frequently mutated element of MAPK pathway is *BRAF*, which has been reported to be mutated in as many as 66% of cutaneous melanomas [11]. Ninety percent of these mutations consist of a substitution of a glutamic acid (E) for valine (V) (BRAF V600E) at the codon 600 (GTG to GAG) in exon 15 [11]. However, there are other less common activating mutations that are known and clinically relevant too, such as *BRAF* V600 K, the second most common *BRAF* mutation (present in 16% of all melanomas), and, thirdly, *BRAF* V600R, which is present in 3% of the patients [12]. *BRAF* V600E mutation constitutively activates the MEK and ERK cascade, independent of upstream RAS activation (Fig. 17.1).

After the discovery of the role of aberrant activation of the RAS/RAF/MEK/ERK pathway in tumorigenesis, great efforts have been made to look for drugs that selectively target this pathway. The development of targeted therapies represents the main achievement in systemic therapy for metastatic melanoma in the last decade. In this context, PLX4720 (vemurafenib), a selective BRAF inhibitor [13], demonstrated significant activity in metastatic melanoma patients, with an

84% overall survival rate after 6 months, a progression-free survival of 5.3 months and a 48% objective response rate, compared to the poor 8% response rate of dacarbazine. After the confirmation of its activity in other randomized studies, it was approved (together with other later similar drugs) for its use in the treatment of metastatic melanoma.

PI3K/AKT Pathway

The PI3K/AKT pathway can be activated due to growth factor receptors, so that the phosphoinositide-3-OH kinase (PI3K) phosphorylates phosphatidylinositol 4,5-biphosphate (PIP2) to phosphatidylinositol 3,4,5-triphosphate (PIP3), provoking its downstream activation and consequently promoting cell proliferation and survival. In a great proportion of melanomas, this signalling pathway is hyperactivated, sometimes due to *PI3K* mutations, but most times in response to loss of PTEN function.

PTEN causes dephosphorylation of PIP3, and, as a result, it negatively regulates the pathway [14]. PTEN is deleted in approximately 45% of melanomas, and the inhibition of PTEN function causes *Akt* gene amplification [15]. Both, deregulation of the PI3K signalling and loss of PTEN function, lead to an increase in the expression of Akt3, which at the same time is associated with a shorter survival [16]. As aforementioned, RAS can simultaneously activate PI3K and MAPK pathways, so the two signalling cascades can be co-activated in many melanomas [17]. Therefore, therapies with BRAF inhibitors can result ineffective, due to the escape mechanism of PI3K/AKT pathway activation. The understanding of these molecular concepts has settled the fundaments for the combined therapy with inhibition in the MAPK pathway and the PI3K/AKT cascade.

Furthermore, PI3K/AKT can be activated through RAS independent signalling, a statement that is confirmed with the fact that PTEN somatic mutations are seen in melanomas with mutations in *BRAF* but not *NRAS* [18]. Herein, when oncogenic NRAS is present, additional mutations in *BRAF* and *PTEN* are not necessary [19], as NRAS can activate both MAPK and PI3K/AKT pathways.

p16(INK4a)-Rb Pathway

The p16(INK4a)-Rb pathway acts through the p53 pathway to provoke cycle arrest or apoptosis [20]. When Cdk4/6 is hypophosphorylated, Rb binds the E2F transcription factor provoking its repression and, so, avoiding the progression through the S phase [21]. On the contrary, in the phosphorylated state, cells progress through G1 to S phase, driven by Rb. The tumour suppressor p16(INK4a) binds to the cyclin-D-Cdk4/6 complex and inhibits it, stopping cell cycle [20]. When p16(INK4a) is inactivated, cell proliferation is stimulated, inducing tumour progression. Germ line mutations in p16(INK4a) are associated with familial melanoma, and, in fact, these mutations have been found in approximately 20–40% of melanoma-prone families worldwide [22]. Similarly, somatic mutations in *p16(INK4a)* are also found in sporadic melanomas [23].

It is known that, after a limited number of divisions, normal somatic cells enter a state called senescence. This state also takes place in response to oncogenic stress, acting as a protector factor against cancer [24]. Thus, independent activation of proliferative pathways in melanoma can promote senescence, inhibiting cellular growth [25]. In fact, BRAF V600E has been found to induce p16(INK4a) expression and senescence [26].

Activating mutations in cyclin-dependent kinase 4 (*CDK4*) can disrupt p16(INK4a) binding [27] and, thus, be related to the development of resistance to BRAF-targeted therapy.

Microphthalmia transcription factor (MITF) is a component which is also related to melanoma pathogeny, as its transcription leads to pigment production. Activation of pERK, due to mutated *BRAF*, provokes a decrease in levels of MITF and induces melanoma cell proliferation, through interaction with CDKN2a and BCL-2 [28], among other mechanisms. Nevertheless, further work is necessary to better characterize the role of this pathway in the development of BRAF-targeted therapy.

The Role of c-Kit

c-KIT mutations are rare in melanoma (10%) and are mainly associated with tumours located in mucosal and acral areas and genital regions or melanomas that have been originated in sun-damaged skin. MAPK pathway can be activated by the mutational activation of growth factor receptors such c-KIT. KIT is a transmembrane receptor with tyrosine kinase activity. When KIT binds to its ligand, stem cell factor (SCF), it induces dimerization and autophosphorylation of the receptor, resulting in the activation of pathways (MAPK and PI3K/AKT) that stimulate cell survival and proliferation (Fig. 17.1). c-Kit is also involved in the melanocyte pigmentary pathway through activation of MITF.

Imatinib mesylate is a tyrosine kinase inhibitor active against BCR-abl in chronic myelogenous leukaemia. It also blocks downstream c-KIT signalling in gastrointestinal stromal tumours. A phase II study [29] was conducted to analyse the effect of the therapy with imatinib in 43 patients diagnosed with KIT-mutant metastatic melanoma. An ORR of 23% was demonstrated with stable disease observed in 30.2% patients, and median PFS was 3.5 months. Additional analysis of the correlation of responses to *c-Kit* aberrations demonstrated that patients with mutations in exon 11 or exon 13 of *c-Kit* may be most sensitive to imatinib [29]. Thus, there is a rationale for using imatinib in the subset of patients whose melanoma overexpresses or carries mutations in c-Kit. It appears that *NRAS* mutations can be related to c-Kit-targeted therapy resistance [30].

Immunotherapy

The best treatment option for metastatic melanoma depends on several factors, including *BRAF* mutation status, the natural history of the disease and the presence of symptoms. Regulation and control of the immune system is another essential aspect in melanoma. Patients with low tumour burden and few symptoms are good candidates for immune therapy: ipilimumab or IL-2, as there is probably time for a lasting immune response. The only therapies which have shown clinical benefit in the adjuvant setting after surgery are IFN-α 2b and peg-IFN-α 2b, when given to patients with high risk of recurrence [31]. Ipilimumab, a monoclonal antibody directed to the receptor of the immune checkpoint termed "cytotoxic T lymphocyte-associated antigen 4 (CTLA-4)" was approved by the FDA for metastatic melanoma in March 2011 [32]. This drug stimulates T cells and is associated with secondary immune reactions (diarrhoea is the most common). T cells need two signals for activation: the one provided by the complex TCR-CD3 and another one derived from the binding CD28-B7 on antigen-presenting cells [33]. CTLA-4 can bind to B7 with a 50- to 100-fold higher avidity than CD28. Engagement of CTLA-4 provokes the termination of the T-cell response (Fig. 17.2).

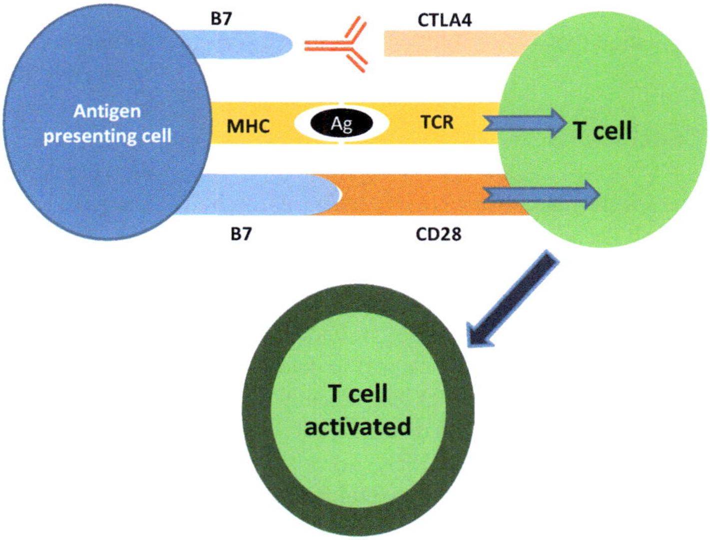

Fig. 17.2 Interaction between B7 and CTLA-4 in T-cell activation and the mechanism of action of ipilimumab

Generally, it has been stated that immune therapy has no efficacy for melanoma patients with brain metastasis. However, 7-month median OS was shown when ipilimumab was administered at 10 mg/kg every 3 weeks for 24 weeks to 72 patients with melanoma brain metastases in a phase II study [34]. That was the first evidence of immune therapy benefit for melanoma patients showing brain metastases.

On 4 September 2014, the FDA granted accelerated approval to pembrolizumab, a PD-1 checkpoint inhibitor, for patients with advanced or unresectable melanoma following treatment with ipilimumab. For melanoma harbouring BRAF V600 mutations, it is intended after treatment with ipilimumab and a BRAF inhibitor. Pembrolizumab is an antibody that specifically blocks PD-1, thereby overcoming immune resistance (since tumour cells express PD-L1, an immunosuppressive PD-1 ligand, inhibition of the interaction between PD-1 and PD-L1 can enhance T-cell responses and mediate antitumour activity).

As it has been shown, a combination of multiple therapies, including surgery, radiation, chemotherapy and target and immune therapies, is plausible in the context of melanoma. Recent studies support the possibility to combine immune and targeted treatments in patients with metastatic melanoma. Again, the understanding of molecular biology and immune pathways in cancer is essential to achieve the best approach directed to induce immune activation and stop regulation [35].

Conclusions

The spectacular advance in molecular research of the last decade has provided a new scenario with a wide spectrum of different strategies of treatment in patients diagnosed with metastatic melanoma. The understanding of underlying biologic pathogenesis and the specific details of the distinct signalling cascades has radically changed the natural history of this disease.

The RAS/RAF/MEK/ERK signalling pathway has shown to be fundamental for melanoma growth and proliferation, and the possibility of targeting the elements of this cascade with inhibitors has supposed a clear clinical benefit for patients with metastatic melanoma. However, despite the excellent responses, 50% of metastatic BRAF-mutated melanoma patients develop resistance to BRAF inhibitors after months on therapy, making further approaches necessary to improve the perspectives of the illness and the clinical outcomes.

Clinical Management of Advanced Malignant Melanoma

Introduction

In the last 5 years, the better understanding of the molecular aberrations and the immunogenicity of melanoma has allowed to improve our ability to develop rational and effective new treatments with the subsequent improvement in the expected overall survival and quality of life for patients with advanced disease. The new agents recently approved for the treatment of advanced melanoma are represented in Fig. 17.3.

Clinical Management

Chemotherapy

Different chemotherapy agents have been classically used alone or in combination with limited antitumour activity and unclear benefit over best supportive care. Although no randomized controlled clinical trials have shown improvement in overall survival, dacarbazine has been considered the standard therapy for advanced disease [36]. Dacarbazine treatment renders a 7–12% response rate and median overall survival of 6–7 months [4, 37]. In a clinical trial, temozolomide was compared with dacarbazine. Temozolomide arm was associated with a non-significant improvement in overall survival [38]. Biochemotherapy combining cisplatin, vinblastine and dacarbazine plus interleukin-2 and interferon α 2b has been evaluated as well, showing no evidence of superiority over single-agent dacarbazine or temozolomide [39].

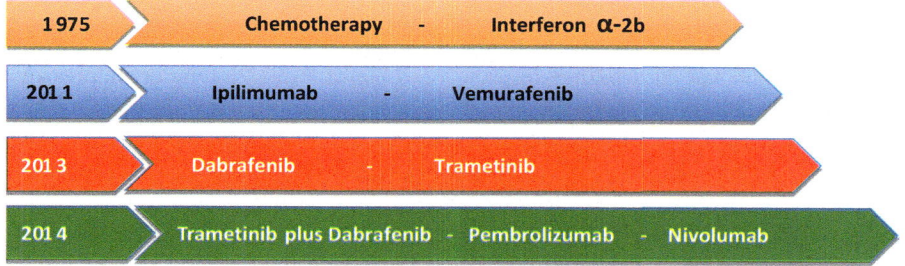

Fig. 17.3 FDA (US Food and Drug Administration) approval of novel agents for advanced melanoma treatment

Target Therapy

One of the most relevant signalling pathways in tumour cells is the mitogen-activated protein kinase (MAPK) pathway or RAS/RAF/MEK/ERK pathway, which regulates cell growth, proliferation and differentiation. *BRAF* mutations constitutively activate BRAF and the downstream signal transduction in the MAPK pathway. When this protein was targeted in BRAF-mutant melanoma cell lines with specific BRAF inhibitors, the cell growth and proliferation were significantly inhibited [40]. The frequency of *BRAF* mutations in metastatic cutaneous melanoma ranges from 42% to 55% [41, 42]. The 80–90% of BRAF-mutant melanomas show that V^{600E} mutation (glutamic acid is substituted by valine), V^{600K} mutation and other *BRAF* mutations (V^{600D}, V^{600R}) are less frequent [43, 44].

BRAF Inhibitors

Vemurafenib

Vemurafenib is a highly specific inhibitor of the tyrosine kinase domain in mutant *BRAF*. This drug has notable antitumour effects against *BRAF*-mutant melanoma cell lines but not against *BRAF* wild-type cell lines [45, 46].

The maximum tolerated dose of vemurafenib established in the phase I clinical trial was 960 mg twice daily. This trial showed a spectacular clinical activity associated with vemurafenib, showing an unprecedented response rate (complete plus partial tumour responses) of 81% in the extension cohort [47].

In the phase II trial with the same drug, 132 BRAF V600-mutant metastatic melanoma patients were treated with vemurafenib 960 mg twice daily. The confirmed overall response rate was 53% (complete responses in 6% and partial responses in 47% of the patients). In most patients, the time to response was 6 weeks. The median progression-free survival was 6.8 months, and the overall survival reached 15.9 months [48].

The phase III randomized clinical trial compared vemurafenib (960 mg twice daily) with dacarbazine (1000 mg/m^2) in 675 untreated patients with diagnosis of metastatic melanoma harbouring *BRAF* V600E mutation. The primary endpoints of the study included overall survival (OS) and progression-free survival (PFS). Treatment with vemurafenib showed a relative reduction of 63% in the risk of death and 74% in the risk of tumour progression compared to the control arm ($p < 0.01$ for both comparisons). After a follow-up of 12.5 months, vemurafenib was associated with improved efficacy compared with dacarbazine showing a response rate of 57% and a median time to response of 1.45 months. Overall survival was significantly superior in the vemurafenib arm compared to dacarbazine (13.6 vs. 9.7 months; HR 0.70; $p < 0.001$). Progression-free survival was 6.9 months vs. 1.6 months for vemurafenib and dacarbazine arms, respectively (HR 0.36, $p < 0.001$) [49, 50]. Vemurafenib demonstrated to be active in patients carrying either BRAF V600E or BRAF V600 K mutations [51].

The most frequent adverse events in relation with vemurafenib were arthralgia, rash, fatigue and photosensitivity. It is important to notice that skin toxicity represented by keratoacanthoma and the development of squamous cell carcinoma were reported in 18% of the patients; these lesions were resolved with surgery. Discontinuations due to adverse events were observed in 7% and 2% of the patients on vemurafenib and dacarbazine, respectively. A potential mechanism of the induction of cutaneous tumours seems to be the paradoxical activation of the MAPK pathway in wild-type *BRAF* skin cells [52, 53].

Dabrafenib

Dabrafenib is a highly active inhibitor of V600-mutant *BRAF* that showed similar efficacy to vemurafenib [54]. The dabrafenib dose of 150 mg orally twice daily was demonstrated to be safe [55].

In a phase II clinical trial, 92 patients with advanced melanoma were enrolled. All of them harboured BRAF V600 mutations, 83% V600E and 17% V600 K. Median PFS for BRAF V600E and BRAF V600 K groups was 6.3 months and 4.5 months, and median OS was 13.1 months and 12.9 months, respectively [56].

A phase III clinical trial enrolled 250 metastatic melanoma patients with demonstrated BRAF V600E mutations. Patients were randomized to receive dabrafenib 150 mg twice daily or i.v. dacarbazine 1000 mg/m^2 every 3 weeks. Dabrafenib significantly improved median PFS compared to dacarbazine [5.1 months for dabrafenib and 2.7 months for dacarbazine, with a hazard ratio of 0.30 (95% CI 0·18–0·51; $p < 0.0001$)]. The more common adverse events associated with dabrafenib were erythrodysesthesia, pyrexia and fatigue [54]. The efficacy of dabrafenib was observed independently of the *BRAF* mutation subtype presented [57].

Resistance to BRAF Inhibitors

BRAF inhibitors have shown, as aforementioned, improvement in terms of response rate, progression-free survival and overall survival, compared to standard chemotherapy in patients with *BRAF*-mutant metastatic melanoma. However, despite of its remarkable efficacy, almost all patients receiving BRAF inhibitors experience progression after weeks to months of therapy due to acquired resistance (secondary resistance) in which tumour progression is preceded by an initial response. There are also some *BRAF*-mutant melanoma patients never responding to BRAF inhibitors by initial refractoriness (primary resistance).

Loss of PTEN, a tumour suppressor gene that normally inhibits Akt signalling pathway, was found in tumour samples of a cohort of patients with *BRAF*-mutant melanoma, resulting in Akt activation. In melanoma patients, loss of PTEN function is observed in 10–27% of the cases and may play a role in intrinsic BRAF inhibitor resistance [58].

Cyclin D1, a protein required for progression through the G1 phase of the cell cycle, may contribute to BRAF inhibitor resistance of melanoma cells. In some studies, melanoma cell lines showed increased cyclin D1 expression with subsequent intrinsic resistance to BRAF inhibitors [59].

The tumour microenvironment may also play a role in innate tumour resistance to therapy. Stromal cells produce hepatocyte growth factor (HGF), which activates MAPK and PI3K/Akt signalling pathways through its receptor (HGFR or MET) in *BRAF*-mutant melanoma cells [60, 61].

Similarly, multiple mechanisms are associated with acquired resistance to BRAF inhibitors such as the activation of different signalling pathways through several receptors such as insulin-like growth factor 1 receptor (IGF-1R) and beta-type platelet-derived growth factor receptor (PDGFR-β) [62, 63]. The overexpression of MAP3K8 (COT) and the presence of activating KRAS (Q61K) and *MEK* mutations may also produce reactivation of the mitogen-activated protein kinase (MAPK), conferring secondary resistance to BRAF inhibitors [64–66].

Finally, BRAF amplification and BRAF alternative splicing generating truncated BRAF isoforms that permit its dimerization in the presence of BRAF inhibitors are other mechanisms responsible for activating the MAPK pathway [67, 65].

MEK Inhibitors

MEK protein (MEK1 and MEK2) is a protein downstream BRAF in the MAPK pathway that is constitutively active in patients with *BRAF* mutations. Thus, MEK inhibition is an attractive mechanism for blocking reactivation of the MAPK pathway.

Trametinib

Trametinib is an oral selective allosteric inhibitor of MEK1 and MEK2. In vitro trametinib shows cell proliferation decrease and apoptosis induction [68]. The recommended dose based on safety and pharmacokinetic and pharmacodynamic data was 2 mg once daily [55]. In the phase I and II clinical trials, trametinib showed clinical activity in BRAF-inhibitor-naïve patients and minimal clinical activity in patients previously treated with BRAF inhibitors suggesting that BRAF and MEK inhibitors share the same resistance mechanisms.

In the phase III open-label trial, trametinib was evaluated in 322 patients diagnosed with metastatic melanoma harbouring a V600E or V600 K BRAF mutation, not previously treated with BRAF inhibitors, MEK inhibitors or ipilimumab. Patients received either trametinib 2 mg once daily or chemotherapy (dacarbazine or paclitaxel). Overall response rate including partial or complete responses was 22% and 8% ($p = 0.01$) in the trametinib arm compared to the chemotherapy group, respectively. Median PFS was 4.8 months in the trametinib arm and 1.5 months in the chemotherapy group (HR for disease progression or death in the trametinib group was 0.45; $p < 0.001$). At 6 months, median OS was 81% in the trametinib group and 67% in the chemotherapy arm [69].

Combined BRAF and MEK Inhibitors

Considering that MEK is an important escape route allowing treatment resistance, it is rational to think that combination therapy delays the appearance of resistance to BRAF inhibitors.

The combination treatment with dabrafenib 150 mg twice daily and trametinib 2 mg once daily was safe and showed antitumour activity [69]. Combination therapy was compared to vemurafenib monotherapy in a phase III clinical trial, showing a significantly improved OS in untreated metastatic melanoma patients carrying *BRAF* V600E or V600 K mutations, with an acceptable toxicity profile [70].

Immunotherapy

Immunotherapy has changed the natural history of advanced melanoma. At the end of the nineteenth century, Coley observed a spontaneous tumour regression due to postsurgical fever, relating the observed tumour response with the immune system activation [71]. Dynamic interactions exist between the host and the tumour, and the ability of the tumour to evade the recognition of the immune system and determine the clinical course of the disease has been proven. Therefore, in the last several years, immunomodulation has become one of the main characters in the treatment of advanced melanoma.

Anti-CTLA-4 Agents

Cytotoxic T lymphocyte-associated antigen 4 (CTLA-4, also known as CD125) is expressed on the surface of T cells. Its activation induces an inhibition of T-cell activity [72].

Ipilimumab is a fully human (immunoglobulin G1) antagonist antibody recognizing human CTLA-4 [73]. After the observation of an improved OS in two clinical trials testing this drug, the FDA approved ipilimumab 3 mg/kg for the treatment of patients with untreatable or metastatic melanoma.

A randomized, double-blind phase III clinical trial evaluated 676 patients with advanced melanoma. This study compared three different treatment arms: ipilimumab at a dose of 3 mg/kg every 3 weeks for four doses, gp 100 peptide vaccine alone and gp 100 peptide vaccine plus ipilimumab. Ipilimumab arm conferred an improved median OS (10.1 vs. 6.4 months, $p = 0.003$) [32].

A second randomized phase III clinical trial comparing dacarbazine plus ipilimumab against dacarbazine plus placebo was conducted in 502 patients with metastatic melanoma. Patients received ipilimumab at a dose of 10 mg/kg every 3 weeks for four doses, followed by maintenance treatment of ipilimumab every 3 months. In the ipilimumab arm, a clear benefit in median OS was observed (11.2 vs. 9.1 months, $p = <0.001$) [74].

Anti-PD-1 Agents

The PD-1 (programmed cell death protein 1) receptor is a transmembrane glycoprotein expressed in activated T cells, activated B cells, activated NK cells, TILs (tumour-infiltrating lymphocytes) and different tumour types, where it exerts its immune system inhibitory function over its receptor [75]. In normal conditions, this receptor is important for maintaining self-tolerance and avoiding tissue injury due to the immune response to pathogenic infection. However, in patients with cancer, the activation of the PD-1 in the tumour microenvironment produces a tumour resistance to the inhibition of the cytotoxic tumour-specific T cells [76].

Pembrolizumab

Pembrolizumab was the first PD-1 inhibitor to be approved at a dose of 2 mg/kg every 3 weeks. It is a humanized monoclonal IgG4 antibody against PD-1. Pembrolizumab showed antitumour activity in patients with advanced melanoma who progressed to ipilimumab. The treatment was well tolerated, with a similar safety profile for both administrations [77].

Pembrolizumab showed better results compared with ipilimumab in terms of objective rate response, PFS and OS [78].

Nivolumab

Nivolumab is a fully human IgG4 PD-1 immune checkpoint inhibitor antibody. In the phase I clinical trial, an objective response rate was observed at a dose of 3.0 mg/kg in 41% of the patients (7/17 patients) [79].

Based on those data, the efficacy and safety of nivolumab were assessed in a randomized, controlled, open-label, phase III clinical trial with 405 patients with advanced melanoma who progressed after anti-CTLA-4 treatment. Nivolumab (3 mg/kg) was compared to chemotherapy (dacarbazine or paclitaxel 175 mg/m² combined with carboplatin), showing a higher rate response (31.7 vs. 10.6%) [80].

In a different phase III clinical trial, nivolumab was compared to dacarbazine 1000 mg in previously untreated melanoma patients without *BRAF* mutations. Nivolumab showed a significant improvement in OS and PFS, when compared to dacarbazine [70]. Nivolumab shows similar clinical activity regardless of patient's *BRAF* mutation status [81].

On the basis of these reports, pembrolizumab and nivolumab received accelerated approval for the treatment of patients with advanced melanoma

and disease progression after ipilimumab and a BRAF inhibitor in case of the presence of a BRAF V600 mutation, in September 2014 and December 2014, respectively.

Predictive Biomarkers of Response to Immunotherapy

Currently, there is not a predictive biomarker for anti-PD-1 therapy in metastatic melanoma. PD-L (ligand)-1 expression by immunohistochemical analysis in tumour tissue has been intensively studied in clinical trials as a potential biomarker. Patients, who show tumour PDL-1 overexpression, tend to have better responses than negative PDL-1 individuals. However, some responses have been shown despite low levels of PDL-1 expression that make the interpretation of this biomarker difficult [82].

Combined Immunotherapy

The development of therapies to enhance tumour immunity is a rational treatment strategy. Preclinical studies in mouse models have shown that CTLA-4 and PD-1 combination blockade has a synergistic antitumour activity [83, 84].

Ipilimumab Plus Nivolumab

The combined therapy with nivolumab and ipilimumab has been shown to be safe and active against advanced melanoma [85, 86].

In a phase II clinical trial, combined therapy was evaluated using ipilimumab 3 mg/kg and nivolumab 1 mg/kg or placebo every 3 weeks for four doses, followed for nivolumab 3 mg/kg or placebo. The confirmed objective response rate was 61% for the combination arm and 11% for the ipilimumab monotherapy group. The combined therapy showed an acceptable safety profile. The response observed was independent of baseline PDL-1 expression and *BRAF* status.

Currently, we are witnessing an enormous advance in the therapeutic options against metastatic melanoma. On the one hand, it seems evident that the combination is better than monotherapy. On the other hand, it is unclear the best sequence of treatment in some patients, in which there are several treatment options. One important point will be to find immuno-biomarkers to help selecting the proper drug or combination of drugs in the more adequate patient as well as the appropriate sequence of different treatment options.

Clinical Need of Liquid Biopsies in Malignant Melanoma

The better knowledge of tumour biology and the signalling pathways involved in cancer progression and metastasis, along with the emergence of new targeted therapies against certain tumour types, has motivated the intense investigation of tumour markers in cancer [87].

Malignant melanoma is one of the solid tumours in which this aspect is being intensively investigated to provide better tools for less invasive disease management [88]. Historically, the lack of effective therapies against advanced melanoma has limited the utility of these markers. However, encouraging results obtained with new therapeutic strategies, such as BRAF inhibitors or different immune checkpoint inhibitors, have stimulated a renewed interest in this field [89].

Melanoma cells are able to release a number of substances into circulation either by active secretion or as result of cell death. Other compounds are endogenously produced in response to the disease process [88].

Logically, the concentration of those substances, as biomarkers, is a dynamic variable and can vary and be modified during the disease course as a result of tumour response and tumour progression or due to a certain therapeutic intervention. These soluble markers include nucleic acids, proteins, metabolites and microvesicles [90]. Moreover, during disease progression, some cells can detach from the primary tumour, enter the circulatory compartment and, therefore, serve as true biomarkers [91].

As ideal tumour markers, their general properties should include the following characteristics [92]:

1. Their specific production by premalignant or malignant tissue early in the progression of disease

2. To be produced at detectable levels in all patients with a specific malignancy, expression in an organ site-specific manner, evidence of presence in bodily fluids obtained noninvasively, levels related quantitatively to tumour volume, biological behaviour or disease progression

3. Their relatively short half-life, reflecting temporal changes in tumour burden and response to therapy

4. The existence of a standardized, reproducible and validated objective and quantitative assay

In addition, these soluble biomarkers should show high sensitivity and specificity. Blood is a very accessible specimen that can be obtained repeatedly providing a more dynamic picture of the disease process vs. a tissue biopsy that implies a single point in time.

Potentially, circulating biomarkers in melanoma patients may offer a complete information related to not only the diagnosis, staging and prognosis but also to monitoring the disease process during periods on and off treatment.

Exosomes and miRNAs

Exosomes

Exosomes Biogenesis and Characteristics

Several types of vesicles can be found in the extracellular space: apoptotic bodies, microvesicles, exosomes, etc. Although exosomes were first defined as vesicles of around 40–100 nm, this definition originated a misunderstanding because different types of vesicles share that range of size. For that reason, it was stablished that exosomes correspond to vesicles of that size, exclusively originated from endosomal membrane. This specific origin differentiates them from microvesicles that are originated by budding from the plasma membrane [93].

During their biogenesis, exosomes are first intraluminal vesicles (ILV) originated inside multivesicular bodies (MVBs). Subsequent fusion of MVBs with the plasma membrane releases those intraluminal vesicles to the extracellular space as exosomes. During ILV biogenesis from the MVB membrane, there is an accumulation of cholesterol; sphingomyelin; ceramide; lysobisphosphatidic acid, which is a phospholipid specific of this membrane; and ubiquitinated proteins incorporated by the endosomal sorting complex required for transport (ESCRT). There are also other mechanisms involved in ILV biogenesis independent of ESCRT, such as oligomerization of tetraspanin complexes or ceramide, whose structure favours membrane invaginations. Regarding exosome release, as in other vesicle trafficking, proteins of Rab family seem to play a role in its regulation. Similarly, p53 protein seems also to be involved in exosome release [94], and its dysregulation in cancer might translate into a higher release of exosomes in cancer. Interestingly enough, there is a feedback regulatory mechanism where exosomes present in the cellular microenvironment of the source cells inhibit the release of new exosomes [95].

Multiple cellular types are able to release exosomes. First observations of exosomes were accomplished during reticulocyte differentiation, in lymphocytes and dendritic cells [96]. Later, these observations extended to several cellular types including neurons and epithelial cells [97] and also multiple types of cancer such as melanoma [50], prostatic [98], breast [99], ovarian [100], lung [101] or pancreatic [102]. In fact, higher levels of exosomes have been detected in cancer patients than in healthy controls, associated with tumour staging [103] and with a shorter survival [104]. As a consequence of their secretion from such a wide range of cellular types, exosomes have been detected in several body fluids including blood, urine, semen, breast milk, bile and organic fluids such as amniotic fluid or cerebrospinal fluid [96]. Once in the extracellular compartment, exosomes can either be incorporated by cells of vicinity by endocytosis [105] or enter into systemic circulation that allows exosomes to reach distant cells. Even more, they can participate in tropism mechanism responsible of the preference of tumours to metastasize certain specific organs [106].

Exosomes, independent of the cell they originate from, contain proteins related to their biogenesis such as Alix and Rab proteins and tetraspanin such as CD9, CD81 and CD63 [97]. Along these proteins, exosomes also contain proteins specific of the cell they are derived from such as MHC-II in exosomes derived from antigen-presenting cells [107] or CD86 in those derived from dendritic cells [108]. In case of cancer, traditionally used markers have been also detected in exosomes. For example, carcinoembryonic antigen (CEA) has been detected in colon carcinoma-derived exosomes isolated in ascites [109] or CA125 [100] and other proteins in exosomes from ovarian carcinoma. Even more, the detection of these proteins allows us to identify exosomes derived specifically from the tumour and not from other sources. Given the diversity of proteins identified in exosomes, a useful tool in exosome research has been developed recently, Exocarta (www.exocarta.org), which is a growing database containing data about exosome characterization in humans and other species [110].

Exosomes Isolation

Multiple techniques have been used to isolate exosomes [111]. Ultracentrifugation is one of the preferentially employed methods especially for the isolation of exosomes derived from cell culture supernatants. Ultracentrifugation requires previous steps of centrifugation and filtration to remove cellular debris and other types of extracellular vesicles. This methodology presents some reproducibility issues as exosome recovery is affected by rotor type, angle of centrifugation and viscosity of the solution among other factors. A strategy to achieve a stricter isolation is to perform the ultracentrifugation within a sucrose gradient, as exosome density is fixed in the range of 1.1–1.19 g/mL. Although the ultracentrifugation usually lasts around 16 h, some studies reflect that this time should be prolonged to 60–90 h to avoid the contamination of exosome fraction. In any case, ultracentrifugation is clearly time-consuming and requires quite large sample sizes, which are usually reduced in the case of clinical samples. Both reasons limit ultracentrifugation application to clinical routine, and alternative methods have been developed. One of them is exosome precipitation with solutions containing polymers such as polyethylene glycol. One of the most used is ExoQuick™ solution, which allows exosome isolation in a much shorter time, easily and without requirements of special instrumentation. However, these polymers do not remove lipoproteins, and when using them, we should consider their potential interference in the subsequent analysis to be performed in those isolated exosomes. Another recent approach is exosome capture based on immunoaffinity, using antibodies immobilized in beads or plates that target common exosome antigens, mainly tetraspanin such as CD63. This procedure seems to achieve a higher level of exosome than ultracentrifugation with or without sucrose gradient [112].

Exosomes in Cancer

As aforementioned, some proteins traditionally used as biomarkers in cancer have been detected in exosomes. For that reason, exosomes and their content have been proposed as potential markers, and, in some cancer, their utility has been already proved. For example, prostate-specific antigen in urinary exosomes reflects responses to treatment in prostate cancer patients [113], or glypycan-1 in serum exosomes is useful for early pancreatic cancer detection and as prognostic factor [114].

Exosomes constitute an important mechanism of communication between cells and can be a vehicle to transfer tumour characteristics from cancer cells to non-cancer cells [115]. Thus, in cancer, exosome importance is not limited to their role as disease markers, but also as a collaborating part involving in cancer pathogenesis itself, being involved in tumour progression and spreading through different mechanisms that include favouring angiogenesis, tumour growth, invasiveness and niche adequation [93, 116].

Furthermore, exosomes can regulate immune response and, as a consequence, play a role in tumour immune escape: exosomes have been proven responsible for the expansion of regula-

tory T cells [117], the apoptosis of T cells through the Fas/FasL system [118, 119] and the reduction of NK cell cytotoxicity by different mechanisms including downregulation of NKG2D in cell surface [120]. On the other hand, exosomes containing MHC molecules can present antigens to T cells and initiate an immune response. Exosomes are also involved in immunotherapy resistance. B-cell lymphoma cell-derived exosomes contain CD20, which bind therapeutic anti-CD20 antibodies, resulting in complement consumption and target cell escape from antibody attack [121]. For that reason, it is crucial to keep on with exosome investigation on this field.

Exosomes in Melanoma

Exosomes have been also detected in melanoma. In fact, Logozzi et al. described an increase in exosomes expressing CD63 and caveolin-1 in plasma from melanoma patients when compared with healthy controls [122]. Later, another comprehensive study of Peinado et al. reported no differences in exosome number or size, but a higher exosomal protein content in melanoma stage IV patients associated with a shorter survival [50]. The same study described a specific exosomal signature in stage IV melanoma patients including very late antigen 4, heat shock protein 70, an HSP90 isoform, MET oncoprotein and tyrosinase-related protein-2 (TYRP2). Even more, exosomal TYRP2 levels predicted disease progression in patients with stage III melanoma. Regarding metastasis detection, increase in MDA-9 and GRP78 proteins in exosomes identifies melanoma patients with lymph node metastasis [123], and in the case of uveal melanoma, an increase in exosome total protein levels has been described in metastatic patients [124]. Melanoma cells also release exosomes containing HLA-G, an immunosuppressive molecule [125] that in exosomes can be detected and ubiquitinated [126]. Recently, S100B and MIA melanoma markers have been also detected in exosomes from melanoma patients, with better diagnostic efficiency than their measurements in serum and with prognostic value [88].

miRNAs

miRNA Biogenesis and Incorporation into Exosomes

Besides proteins, exosomes also carry different types of nucleic acids: functional mRNAs that result in the detection of proteins previously not detected in the acceptor cells [127], double-stranded DNA presenting same mutations than source cell [128] and microRNAs (miRNAs) which are small noncoding RNA transcripts of 20–24 nucleotides. These miRNAs regulate certain gene expressions post-transcriptionally by inducing mRNA degradation or inhibiting its translation. In fact, although miRNAS can be transported by HDL lipoproteins [129], the main proportion of circulating miRNAs are contained inside exosomes [130] where they are protected from degradation by RNAses [131]. This protection contributes to miRNAs high stability when maintained at room temperature or even when subjected to multiple freeze-thawing cycles [132].

miRNA biogenesis is a complex and regulated process review by Ha et al. [133]. miRNAs are first transcribed by RNA polymerase II as long primary transcripts (pri-miRNAs), which undergo subsequent maturation processes within the nucleus. First of all, RNase III Drosha and its cofactor DGCR8 form a complex called microprocessor that cleaves pri-miRNA, to render a fragment with a hairpin structure of about 70 nucleotides that constitutes pre-miRNA. Then, pre-miRNAs form a complex with exportin-5/Ran-GTP that is translocated to the cytoplasm. Once there, GTP is hydrolysed, and pre-miRNA is released from the complex. In the cytoplasm, Dicer hydrolyses pre-miRNA loop rendering a double-stranded RNA that is loaded in AGO protein to form the complex called RNA-induced silencing complex (RISC), where one of the strands stands (guide), whereas the other one (passenger) is degraded. This mature miRNA is already able to control gene expression by affecting mRNA translation and degradation.

Currently, there are four proposed mechanisms for miRNA loading into exosomes: neutral sphingomyelinase 2 [134], sumoylated heteroge-neous nuclear ribonucleoproteins (hnRNPs) that recognize the 3′ miRNA sequences [135], the uridylated 3′ end of miRNA itself [136] and the AGO2 protein included in RISC complex [137]. miRNAs are not randomly incorporated in exosomes. On the contrary, there are some miRNAs that preferentially enter exosomes in different cellular types, including miRNA-150, miRNA-142-3p and miRNA-451 [137]. Nevertheless, pathological processes affecting the source cell such as cancer affect miRNAs profile in exosomes [138].

miRNA Quantification

As mentioned before, miRNAs present high stability making them candidates for cancer marker research. Nevertheless, pre-analytical and analytical considerations should be taken into account when quantifying miRNAs. For example, heparin plasma is not a suitable sample for miRNA quantification by qRT-PCR [139], and although serum and plasma miRNA levels correlate, mixing specimen types is not recommended [139], because levels can be different [140]. Special caution should be taken with haemolysed samples. Haemolysis affects miRNAs levels, since some miRNAs such as miR-16 or miR-15b are also present inside erythrocytes. Most of imprecision observed in miRNA quantification is due to miRNA isolation process itself [140]. For that reason, it is essential to introduce internal standards consisting in spiked *C. elegans* miRNAs such as cel-miR-39 or cel-miR-54 [139]. Some authors even recommend to use an endogenous normalizer such as miR-16 in the case of melanoma, once haemolysis has been ruled out [141]. These endogenous normalizers allow us to avoid variability due to different rates of exosome release, which in fact has been proven to be elevated in melanoma. Obviously, miRNA candidates for endogenous normalizer must be ubiquitously expressed and with stable levels as miR-16 in the case of melanoma [141].

miRNAs in Cancer

miRNAs are involved in several malignancies at different levels [142]. For example, in non-small cell lung cancer, exosomes deliver miRNA-21 and miRNA-29a to tumour-associated macrophages provoking an activation of NF-κB that traduces in an IL-6 and TNF-α pro-inflammatory cytokines, which in turn favours tumour growth and metastasis [143]. In gastric cancer, miR-25 promotes progression by directly downregulating TOB1 expression [144], whereas miR-129 presents anti-proliferative properties, by downregulating Cdk6 [145]. On the contrary, let-7 is a tumour suppressor miRNA that reduces proliferation and metastasis capability [142], and miR-27b inhibits colorectal cancer progression and angiogenesis [146]. Concerning chemoresistance, in breast cancer, exosome-contained miRNAs can transfer chemoresistance to Adriamycin [53] and docetaxel to acceptor cells, with miR-100, miR-222, miR-30a and miR-17 being probably involved [54]. Neuroblastoma exosomes also transfer miRNA-21 to monocytes. In this case, NF-κB activation provokes miRNA-155 transcription which is then shuttled back to neuroblastoma cells resulting in an alteration in telomerase activity and resistance to cisplatin [147]. Contrary to that, miRNA-134 transference by exosomes in breast cancer provokes an increased sensitivity to anti-Hsp90 drugs [55].

miRNAs in Melanoma

miRNAs are also involved in melanoma development and metastasis [148]. For that reason, several studies have compared miRNA profile between melanoma cell lines and normal melanocyte cell lines [149]. When comparing melanoma and normal melanocyte biopsies, a cluster of 14 miRNAs (miR-506-514 cluster) is overexpressed in melanoma tissue independently of N-RAS or B-RAF mutational status [150]. On the contrary, 57 miRNAs have been detected downregulated, many of them included in a large miRNA cluster on human chromosome 14q32 [151]. miRNA profile has been also probed to differentiate melanoma subtypes [152]. However, although differences in miRNA profile are frequently detected in multiple studies, there are few miRNAs consistently upregulated or downregulated across the different studies [149].

An enrichment of certain miRNAs and downregulation of others were observed in exosomes when comparing their miRNA profile with the profile of cells they are derived from, both melanocytes and melanoma cells. Similarly comparison between melanoma-derived and melanocyte-derived exosomes rendered differences in miRNA profile [153]. Many of these miRNAs differentially expressed are associated with cancer, cell cycle, cellular growth and proliferation. These miRNAs include let-7c, miR-138, miR-125b, miR-130a, miR-34a, miR-613, miR-205 and miR-149 [153]. Even more, treatment of melanocyte cells with melanoma-derived exosomes results in a higher invasiveness capability which suggests functional mRNA and miRNA transfer via exosomes.

In the case of circulating miRNAs, Kanemaru et al. demonstrated higher serum levels of miRNA-221 in melanoma patients when compared to healthy controls [154], whereas Friedman et al. proposed a risk model based on five circulating miRNA levels (miR-150, miR-15b, miR-199a-5p, miR-33a, miR-424) to identify patients with a higher recurrence risk [155]. In a more recent study, miR-150 and miR-15b were also able to predict recurrence along with two other miRNAs: miR-425 and miR-30d [156], the latter of them associated with melanoma invasion and metastasis [157]. Regarding miR-15b, its presence in melanoma tissues has been associated with poorer recurrence-free and overall survival [158]. Some of these miRNAs have also been described in other malignancies. For example, miR-150 reduces migration and invasion in pancreatic cancer [159], miR-15b reduced expression is associated with chemotherapy resistance and poor prognosis in tongue squamous cell carcinoma [160], and miR-424 expression in endothelial cells promotes angiogenesis [161]. Related to metastasis detection, miRNAs have also probed their usefulness in melanoma. miR-9, miR-145, miR-150, miR-155 and miR-205 levels distinguish patients with metastasis from those without it, being the combination of the five even more sensitive than any of the individual measurements [162].

It has been reported that miR-125 is downregulated in melanoma biopsies [153] and its circulating levels have been probed of interest in other cancers. Alegre et al. compared both in serum and serum-derived exosomes, miR-125 levels from healthy controls and melanoma patients [141], which has been observed down-regulated in melanoma biopsies [153] and whose circulating levels have been probed of interest in other cancers. As in melanoma tissue, miR-125 levels were lower in exosomes but not in serum from melanoma patients, suggesting exosomes as a more accurate material for measuring miRNA levels. In the case of uveal melanoma, miR-146a levels were increased in both serum and serum exosomes [163].

Circulating DNA

Circulating Nucleic Acids as Biomarkers

The Nature of Cell-Free Circulating DNA

The presence of cell-free DNA in plasma was unveiled long time ago, in 1948, by Mandel and Metais [164], but it was not until much later, in 1973, that Koffler et al. [165] showed that patients with cancer, especially those suffering metastasis, had increased levels of cell-free DNA. Later, in 1989, Stroun et al. reported the presence of neoplastic characteristics in this cell-free DNA, demonstrating that part of this DNA comes from cancer cells [166]. Since then, many studies showed in cell-free DNA similar alterations

reported for tumour DNA, such as mutations, microsatellite variances or changes in DNA methylation.

The release of DNA from cells into circulation can be passive from apoptotic and necrotic cells [167], as illustrated in Fig. 17.4. Apoptosis would produce fragments with sizes multiples of 180 pb, corresponding to the size of the DNA wrapped around the nucleosome. Necrosis would result in more irregular and larger-sized cell-free DNA. Alternatively, large fragments higher than 10kB of DNA can be actively secreted included into exosomes [168]. Different analyses of the size of cell-free DNA suggest that most of it is released mainly from apoptotic cells, but is subsequently fragmented by the action of nucleases, mononucleosome breakdown, or by phagocytosis resulting in predominant circulating fragments of about 60 pb [169, 170]. The size of the fragments of cell-free DNA can be different between healthy subjects and cancer patients. Pinzani et al. analysed by PCR four amplicons of 67, 180, 306 and 476 bp of the *APP* gene in cutaneous melanoma. They showed that the most abundant fragments in plasma of melanoma patients were those comprised between 181 and 307 bp, while in healthy subjects, there was a prevalence of shorter fragments (Fig. 17.4) [171].

As mentioned before, alterations observed in primary tumours can be also observed in cell-free DNA, so the analysis of these molecular markers could be a very valuable information

Fig. 17.4 Circulating DNA graphic

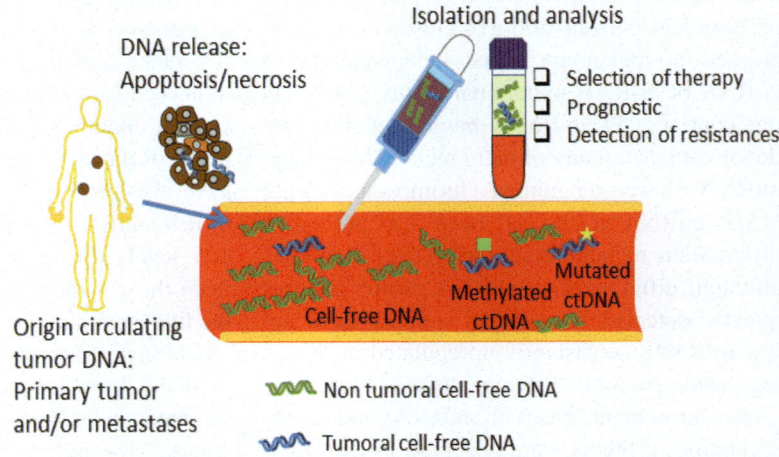

tool with respect to diagnosis, progression and selection of the therapy. Tumour-associated molecular alterations, such as microsatellite alterations, single-nucleotide mutations or epigenetic modifications, have been detected in cell-free DNA from melanoma patients, as we resume in this chapter. In addition, serial measurements in blood can be useful for monitoring tumour changes and resistance to therapy (Fig. 17.4) [172].

Cell-Free DNA Isolation and Analysis

Cell-free DNA levels in healthy individuals are in the order of few ng/mL, while in cancer patients range widely, with concentrations overlapping with healthy people or be as elevated as thousands of ng/mL [172, 173]. Also, cell-free DNA concentration varies even in healthy individuals during short period of times due to different situations, such as stress, disease or exercise [174]. The variability of cell-free DNA levels in cancer patients also depends on the kinetic of apparition and disappearance into the bloodstream. Some factors influence the cell-free DNA spilling into the bloodstream such as the location and irrigation of tumour, size and metastases, vascularity and state of the tumour. Others affect the capability for cell-free DNA clearance in some disease, such as liver or kidney diseases.

The conditions for sample processing and storage are very important to obtain reliable results [173], but there is no consensus with a high variability between laboratories. Cell-free DNA levels in plasma are lower and less variable than in serum because serum also contains genomic DNA released from leukocytes and haematopoietic cells during the clotting process. Additionally some particles that carry cell-free DNA, such as exosomes, can associate with fibrin resulting in the loss of some fractions. Consequently plasma is the type of specimen preferred, especially for mutation analysis, due to the lower level of background achieved.

Samples should be properly centrifuged to sediment all cells that could falsely increase cell-free DNA levels. Prolonged plasma storage leads to an annual DNA degradation rate of 30% [175]. In addition, repeated freeze-thaw cycles could

not result in the loss of cell-free DNA concentration, but result in increased fragmentation.

Due to the low concentration and the high degree of fragmentation of cell-free DNA, extraction methods strongly influence the DNA yield, and different procedures can produce differences in cell-free DNA quantity as high as 50%. Furthermore, the same extraction method can produce different results in different laboratories. There is no consensus in the best method, and most researches use commercial kits with very different results. Traditionally, cell-free DNA measurements have been performed using fluorescent probes or spectrophotometry, but housekeeping gene quantification through qPCR is increasingly used although it is more expensive and time-consuming.

The detection of cancer mutation in circulation is a very challenging issue, which can be compared to "finding a needle in a haystack". All nucleated cells have DNA, which can be released to circulation. Additionally, even tumour cells can release non-mutant DNA resulting in a great dilution of the mutant copies. Therefore, although DNA mutant copies can be proportionally abundant related to wild-type DNA, they normally constitute a very small fraction of the total circulating copies, usually less than 1–0.1% [176]. Most works performed before this decade suffer from the lack of enough analytical sensitivity to detect this low tumour cell-free DNA in the bloodstream. Methods used only a few years ago had a low sensitivity, such as COLD-PCR (sensitivity of 3.1%) [177], allele-specific TaqMan-based real-time PCR (sensitivity of 0.3%) [178] or amplification refractory mutation system (sensitivity of 0.1%) [179]. Nevertheless, new techniques have been developed to quantifying very small amounts of mutated DNA, such as BEAMing or digital PCR (sensitivity of 0.01%). Next-generation sequencing is technically challenging and not sensitive enough but probably in the future may allow detection of many tumourspecific mutations in the patient's blood. However, the analysis of single-nucleotide mutation (one or several in case of possible tumour heterogeneity) should be sufficient for tumour monitoring, either during treatment or as a control of recurrence after excision of the primary tumour [180]. In the last few years, some platforms have appeared providing automatization to the cell-free DNA analysis, focusing in hotspot mutations.

Quantitative cell-free DNA analysis using new PCR technologies is a very sensitive and specific biomarker in diagnosis and dynamic evaluation of tumours during treatment [181]. Cell-free DNA has a very rapid turnover, with a half-life of less than 30 min [182], being very appropriate for the monitoring of tumour response to therapy. Changes in cell-free DNA levels have shown to be very interesting biomarkers in patients with lung [183] and breast [184] cancers and also melanoma [180].

Clinical Utility of Cell-Free DNA in Melanoma

Detection of Cell-Free *BRAF* Mutation in the Blood

Almost all studies addressing single point mutation in melanoma have focused on *BRAF* V600E mutation as approximately half of melanoma tumours harbour *BRAF* mutations and the majority (80–90%) corresponds to *BRAF* V600E mutation. Therefore, the high frequency of hotspot mutations in *BRAF* makes ctDNA analysis by high sensitive techniques particularly attractive for the follow-up of patients with metastatic cutaneous melanoma.

While in some studies no *BRAF* V600E mutations were detected in healthy donors [183], in others, low numbers of copies were detected in some of them [180]. Moreover, benign lesions harbour *BRAF* V600E mutations, and so it can be found in benign nevus cells [185]. These data evidently affect the diagnostic specificity, and some caution should be applied when used as a screening test, although we do not know yet the clinical significance of the presence of this mutation in the blood from otherwise healthy people.

There is a high degree of agreement with the *BRAF* V600E mutation in tissue [180]. Considering patients in advanced stages and positive for *BRAF* mutations in tumour, *BRAF* mutations can be detected in cell-free DNA in more than 80% of blood samples using droplet digital PCR assays [180, 186]. Similar sensitivity in relation to positive tumour biopsy was obtained when V600 K was analysed [187]. Other earlier studies reported a sensitivity of 38–57%, probably due to the use of a less technically sensitive method [188–190]. However, when biopsy is easily available, cell-free DNA may not be appropriate as the unique sample for evaluating *BRAF* status as some patients with *BRAF* mutation-positive tumours are negative when analysed in plasma.

The concentration of mutant copies of *BRAF* V600E in blood has a high dynamic range and a high correlation with tumour burden [180]. Additionally, *BRAF V600E* correlated with the other serological circulating melanoma tumour markers MIA and S100B, in addition to LDH. This enzyme is the only approved biomarker in melanoma [191], but cell-free DNA is a better indicator of tumour burden than LDH [186] and also presents a higher sensitivity and specificity. Chang et al. showed that in patients with RECIST scores <5 cm prior to treatment initiation, cell-free DNA levels were elevated in 71% of the patients compared to LDH which was elevated in only 8% of them. In earlier stages, however, *BRAF* V600E cell-free DNA analysis seems to be less sensitive, but this topic should be revaluated using new more sensitive experimental techniques. Analysing 103 melanoma patients, Shinozaki et al. detected *BRAF V600E* in serum from 32% AJCC stage I/II patients [192].

Patient's selection for treatment with *BRAF/MEK* inhibitors is mainly based on the analysis of the *BRAF* V600 mutation in the tumour biopsy. However, *BRAF* discordant status between the distinct samples can be found in almost 14% significant proportion of melanoma patients [193]. This can be probably due to the existence of different subclones in the melanoma tumour causing heterogeneity on *BRAF* status. Also, *BRAF* mutation detection in biopsy can be missed in cases of samples with lower numbers of tumour cells or widespread necrosis. Consequently, *BRAF* wild type in one tumour biopsy sample may not be a definitive result, and therefore, it is important to retest in other tumour lesions and during the evolution of the disease. Therefore, the fact that cell-free DNA can reflect the *BRAF* status in any lesion of the body suggests that the analysis of cell-free *BRAF* V600E mutation in the blood could help to select melanoma patients for *BRAF* inhibitor therapy.

The presence of *BRAF* mutation in serum also has prognostic significance. Shinozaki et al. showed in a group of patients treated with chemotherapy plus IL2 and IFN-α 2b that patients with undetectable serum levels of *BRAF* mutation had a significant better overall survival compared with patients in which serum *BRAF* mutations were detected [192]. Furthermore, cell-free DNA *BRAF* V600E mutation levels in patients treated with *BRAF* inhibitors have predictive value. Sanmamed et al. showed that patients with less than 216 mutant copies/mL before treatment had significantly longer overall survival and progression-free survival than those patients with higher levels of mutation [180]. In a recent study including 836 *BRAF* V600E mutation-positive melanoma patients, those negative for *BRAF* mutations in cell-free DNA had longer progression-free survival and overall survival compared with patients with detectable cell-free DNA *BRAF* mutations [187].

While *BRAF* mutation analysis in biopsy would continue as a gold standard in the future for initial treatment selection, cell-free DNA *BRAF* V600E analysis probably will be essential in the patient's follow-up, especially for monitoring the response to the therapy providing dynamic information of the tumour response [180, 183]. It has been observed that the decrease in the number of detectable mutant copies is associated with a response, and in some cases, the mutation can become even undetectable in plasma. On the contrary, increased concentration of mutant copies observed during disease progression reflects treatment resistance. Importantly, it has been observed that the increase in cell-free *BRAF* V600E levels precedes the clinical progression as determined by RECIST, which could help in an early adoption of an alternative therapy [180, 194]. Tsao et al. described increasing ctDNA levels in one patient with enlarging brain metastases while LDH measurements failed to rise above

normal [194]. Similar data were reported by Chang et al. where these authors also observed that ctDNA is more sensitive than LDH to detect metastatic disease at low RECIST levels and at times of non-RECIST disease progression [186]. ctDNA outperforms LDH as a biomarker in cases of new or increasing brain metastases (83% vs. 50%, respectively).

Taking together all these data, we could conclude that cell-free *BRAF* determination in the blood of patients with advanced stage melanoma can offer clinically relevant information concerning tumour burden and prognosis. Furthermore, ctDNA could help in the clinical management of these patients during disease monitoring and in treatment decisions. Importantly, a rebound cell-free *BRAF* V600E level correlates with treatment resistance and can precede imaging detection of progressive disease.

Other Cell-Free DNA Tumour Analysis

NRAS mutations, primarily Q61R, Q61H and Q61K, occur in 15–20% of the melanoma patients and mutually exclusive with BRAF mutations. A few studies analysed cell-free NRASQ61K/R/L by droplet digital PCR, although the number of melanoma patients included was quite short. In patients harbouring this mutation in biopsy, one study detected cell-free *NRAS* mutations in seven out of nine patients [186], while another detected this mutation in all patients (n = 4) [195]. The analysis of *NRAS* mutations can be of utility in the monitoring of the immunotherapy response [194]. In addition, the emergence of *NRAS* mutations is one of the mechanisms of resistance to BRAF inhibitor therapy. Gray et al. found in three out of seven patients with BRAF mutation that during treatment with BRAF/MEK inhibitors, the amount of mutant cell-free *NRAS* increased (being negative at baseline) as the *BRAF*-mutant ctDNA rebounded during progressive disease [195].

Some epigenetic alterations such as genomic promoter region methylation of CpG islands or histone modification have been shown to be important in melanoma progression. These epigenetic changes observed in tumour tissues have also been detected in circulating cell-free DNA

[196]. Methylation status was analysed using methylation-specific polymerase chain reaction, and aberrant methylation of CpG promoter regions has been detected in plasma from melanoma patients. However, Hoon et al. showed that the concordance of plasma gene hypermethylation status to respective paired tumours is not very high: 33% for O6-methylguanine-DNA methyltransferase (MGMT), 24% for RASSF1A and 18% for RAR-β2. This difference could be due to degradation or limited technical sensitivity. Interestingly, in two patients, hypermethylation of RASSF1A was present in plasma but absent in tumours [197].

Marini et al. [198] in a group of 41 melanoma patients at different stages showed that most frequently methylated genes in the serum were SOCS1 (75%) and CDKN2a (75%), followed by RASSF1A (64%), MGMT (64%) and SOCS2 (43%). Also, 83% of these patients had one hypermethylated gene. The analysis of epigenomic alterations in cell-free DNA has reported to be of utility for melanoma as prognostic marker and to monitor the response to biochemotherapy for metastatic melanoma [199, 200]. Mori et al. showed that methylated *RASSF1A* was significantly less frequent in responders to biochemotherapy than in non-responders and that increased methylation correlated with a poorer overall survival and resistance to therapy.

Finally, other few authors studied in blood other DNA alterations, such as DNA integrity [171] and allelic instability [201]. One group demonstrated free circulating DNA microsatellites with loss of heterozygosity in the blood of melanoma patients. The loss of heterozygosity incidence and frequency correlated with advancing stage and has prognostic utility [201]. The presence of loss of heterozygosity was associated with disease progression in metastatic melanoma patients treated with biochemotherapy [202].

Circulating Tumour Cells

Circulating tumour cells (CTCs) are cancer cells that have detached from the primary or metastatic tumour, subsequently entering the bloodstream.

CTCs were first observed among patients with melanoma by molecular techniques [203]. CTCs have been investigated intensively in the last decade as potential biomarkers due to their potential usefulness when compared to tissue biopsy and are not only feasible for transcriptomic and genomic profiling as biomarkers, but they may also provide new insights into the metastatic mechanisms in melanoma while monitoring disease progression. These cells in transit can be obtained by simple venipuncture in contrast to invasive surgical resection or percutaneous tissue biopsy. In the case of melanoma with a high potential for systemic dissemination, the utility of CTC assessment in these patients is particularly beneficial. In fact, in the last several years, this aspect has been supported by different studies revealing the prognostic value of CTCs as true biomarkers in terms of disease-free survival (DFS) and OS [91, 204, 205]. Nonetheless, CTCs in melanoma patients are heterogeneous. Some of them show characteristics of tumour stem cells with a true metastatic capacity, while others survive and circulate with limited or no metastatic ability. The special subpopulation of malignant melanoma stem cells is characterized by their preferential ability to initiate and propagate tumour growth and their selective capacity for self-renewal and differentiation into less tumorigenic melanoma cells [206]. PCR has been the predominant method used for melanoma CTC analysis [207]. This fact differs from other epithelium-originated malignancies in which CTC assays are mainly based on immunocapture enrichment of CTC through the expression of several cell surface antigens. In melanoma cells, the pattern of antigenic expression results unique. Melanoma-associated antigens (MAAs), such as MART-1, MAGE-A3, PAX3 and ganglioside GM2/GD2 glycosyltransferase (GalNAc-T), are absent in normal peripheral blood leukocytes (PBL) [207, 208]. This condition favours the detection of melanoma CTCs by direct quantitative reverse transcription PCR (qRT-PCR) assays, and CTCs do not need to be isolated or enriched. However, melanoma is heterogeneous in terms of transcriptomic expression and genomic alterations, and therefore, it results critical to use to improve sensitivity in the assessment of CTCs [209, 210]. Direct qRT-PCR (non-capturing) for melanoma CTC assessment based on the expression of multiple MAAs is logistically consistent, and it shows high sensitivity. Studies on CTC MAA biomarkers using qRT-PCR have shown that the presence of CTC markers was correlated with advanced stages [205], as well as decreased DFS and OS [204, 205, 211]. On the other hand, melanoma has limited unique cell surface antigens for CTC isolation by an immunomagnetic bead capture method [208, 212]. Recently, a HMW-MAA-dependent CellSearch platform that uses CD146 (MelCAM) and HMM-MAA antibodies for melanoma CTC capture and detection, respectively, has shown that CTC detection may provide prognostic relevance in metastatic melanoma [213]. Due to their role in invasion and dissemination, CTCs represent an important analytical target for the early diagnosis and assessment of metastatic risk.

Methods for CTC Enrichment and Detection in Melanoma

Different methodologies have evolved in the last decades for enrichment and detection of melanoma CTCs. Methods for enrichment are mainly based on their physical properties or antigenic characteristics [214]. Although in most studies CTCs are obtained from 5 to 15 mL of peripheral blood [215], others have used larger sample volumes [216]. Following enrichment, CTCs may be characterized by immunologic or molecular techniques.

An easy and inexpensive method to extract melanoma CTCs is based on density-gradient centrifugation using commercial separation mediums, such as Ficoll-Paque™ or Lymphoprep™, by which CTCs are obtained from the mononuclear fraction [217]. Despite its advantages, this approach lacks specificity and possesses low sensitivity as some CTCs are lost during centrifugation. The OncoQuick™ device uses a specially developed separation medium for melanoma tumour cells and can enrich CTCs up to 400-fold [218]. Using this method, the authors [215] iden-

tified two subpopulations, one of which was consistent with leukocyte/macrophage-tumour hybrids. Interestingly enough, this cell type had only been previously detected in tissues. Melanoma CTCs have been also isolated by filtration using an ISET assay (isolation by size of epithelial tumour cells, ISET Block™, Rarecells Diagnostics) [219]. This method is based on the fact that lymphocytes are smaller than melanoma CTCs and can be readily filtered through a membrane with pores of 8 μm, while melanoma CTCs, having a cell size >16 μm, are retained without damaging their morphology.

In the last few years, other methods based on physical properties have been developed to isolate CTCs, but their usefulness has not been demonstrated with melanoma CTCs [220]. CTCs in melanoma patients are frequently isolated using antibody-coated immunomagnetic beads. Purification is positive if antibodies are directed against tumour antigens or negative if they bind leukocytes and/or endothelial cells [221].

Melanoma CTCs are heterogeneous regarding the expression of melanoma-associated antigens not only from patient to patient but also from one tumour lesion to another in the same patient. Thus, a better approach may be to use marker panels [221]. However, more recently, some studies found that a combination of two methods may produce better melanoma CTC enrichment. Keeping an absolute specificity, the highest sensitivities were achieved when Ficoll-Hypaque/red blood cell lysis was combined with immunomagnetic enrichment and subsequent multimarker detection.

However, the only FDA-approved method for CTC detection in clinical practice is the CellSearch™ system (Veridex, Raritan, NJ, USA) [222]. It is a semiautomated procedure for CTC extraction and identification. This approach combines immunomagnetic tumour cell purification via anti-MCAM and identification with anti-MCSP. The nucleus is stained with DAPI (40,6-diamino-2-phenylindole) and cells co-stained with CD34 and CD45 to distinguish melanoma CTCs from endothelial cells or leukocytes, respectively. Melanoma cells are then viewed and enumerated by automated digital fluorescent microscopy. However, tumour cells with low marker expression may be missed.

Unfortunately, this approach tends to be less efficient than the ISET isolation method combined with immunocytochemical analysis [221].

Target Genes in Melanoma CTC Detection

Melanoma CTC identification may be achieved via analysis of melanoma-associated transcripts using RT-PCR. These indirect methods, however, cannot quantify melanoma CTC or provide information regarding morphology or vitality. Tyrosinase transcript is the earliest [203] and widely used mRNA marker. This enzyme, responsible for the first two steps of melanin biosynthesis, is a very specific melanocytic marker, being only expressed in melanocytes, melanoma cells and Schwann cells [223].

In the last few years, large discrepancies have been described in the success rate of the tyrosinase reverse transcription polymerase chain reaction (RT-PCR) for detecting melanoma cells in the peripheral blood of melanoma patients. De Vries et al. reported a quality control study in which they analysed the reproducibility of detection of tyrosinase and MART-1 transcripts in 106 blood samples from 68 melanoma patients (stages III and IV) [224]. With this study, they aimed to improve insight in the reproducibility of a RT-PCR for the detection of minimal amounts of melanoma CTCs. In their study, the majority of blood samples was negative for tyrosinase (80%) or MART-1 (66%). Only four samples were positive in four different determinations for tyrosinase and seven for MART-1. Variable results (1–3 times positive results) were obtained for tyrosinase and MART-1 in 16% and 27%, respectively. MART-1 PCR showed a better performance than tyrosinase PCR. Sensitivity increased when both markers were used [224]. More interestingly, when applying real-time quantitative PCR for tyrosinase and MART-1, the authors found that a low amount of SK-MEL-28 cell equivalents was present in the blood of melanoma patients, with a higher number of equivalents in

the group with a consistently positive result. According to their results, it could be concluded that low reproducibility of a repeated assay for the detection of melanoma CTCs is not caused by differences in mRNA quality between the samples, but due to low numbers of amplifiable target mRNA molecules in the mRNA sample. Use of more than one marker and repetition of the assay might increase the probability of finding positive PCR results.

In fact, there is a wide methodological variation when melanoma-associated gene transcripts are analysed. For instance, when analysing tyrosinase by RT-PCR in uveal melanoma, the detection frequency of CMC varies from negative [225] to higher than 50% of patients [226]. In fact, among patients with hypomelanotic melanoma, tyrosinase expression can be negative [227]. To increase CMC detection rate, tyrosinase mRNA has been combined with other mRNA targets [228]. These include melanoma antigen recognized by T cells (Melan-A/MART-1) [229], microphthalmia-associated transcription factor (MITF) [230], gp100, MAGE-3 [231] and p97 (melanotransferrin).

Clinical Utility of CTC in Melanoma

Detection of melanoma CTCs in the peripheral blood can serve not only as a liquid biopsy approach but also as a source of valuable tumour markers [232]. CTCs are generally rare, and thus their detection, enumeration and molecular characterization is extremely challenging. CTCs have the unique characteristic of being noninvasively isolated from blood and can be used to monitor patients during targeted treatment and follow-up [233]. In fact, these cells may provide significant information to better understand tumour biology and tumour cell dissemination [234].

At the same time, a thorough molecular characterization of melanoma CTCs may offer the unique potential to better understand the biology of metastasis and how primary and acquired resistance occurs [235]. That decisive knowledge may aid to develop new therapies, and their analysis currently presents a promising field for both advanced- and early-stage patients.

However, melanoma CTCs are more frequently detected as disease progresses [236]. In fact, the detection rate in patients with localized disease is usually very low [88]. Positivity is more frequent in patients with more advanced disease, but even in metastatic melanoma CTCs, detection is often not very high [213]. In fact, a meta-analysis of 1799 patients in 23 studies based on tyrosinase mRNA detection by RT-PCR found an overall positivity of 18% in stage I, 28% in stage II, 19% in stage I/II localized, 30% in stage III and 45% in stage IV disease [237].

Interestingly enough, sequential sampling is able to improve CTC detection rate in melanoma patients. In a study analysing tyrosinase expression in stage III patients, the authors showed that rate of detection substantially increased from 11.8% in patients analysed at baseline to 49% when multiple sampling was performed [217].

However, CTC count is a dynamic variable, and the detection rate can significantly vary depending of the disease stage, response or progression to treatment and the treatments administered. Thus, positive patients can become negative and vice versa. Fusi et al. [238] have reported similar findings. In this study, positivity increased from 5.6% at baseline to 36.6% during the 60-month study.

Moreover, CTC detection has been proposed as a new prognostic parameter in malignant melanoma patients. According to this hypothesis, the presence of these cells in the peripheral blood may be associated with poorer prognosis (shorter DFS and/or OS) [239]. Hoon et al., for example [240], studied the recurrence of melanoma after radical surgery with no clinical evidence of residual disease at the time of blood collection. They employed a multimarker CTC detection approach using RT-PCR of tyrosinase, p97, MUC-18 and MAGE-3. The authors found that the probability of recurrent disease in a 60-month follow-up period increased from 25% in patients with 0–2 positive markers to 56% in patients with 3–4 positive markers [240].

In a different study by Klinac et al., CTCs were captured by targeting the melanoma-associated markers MCSP and MCAM as well as the melanoma stem cell markers ABCB5 and CD271 [235]. Melanoma CTCs were quantified in 27 metastatic melanoma patients treated with surgery or with vemurafenib, ipilimumab or dacarbazine. Patients were enrolled prospectively and CTC counts performed at baseline (prior to treatment), during and after treatment. In contrast with the previously mentioned report by Hoon et al., baseline CTC counts were not found to be prognostic of OS nor of PFS. However, interestingly enough, a low baseline CTC number was associated with a rapid response to vemurafenib therapy. Additionally, a decrease in CTCs after treatment initiation was associated with response to treatment and prolonged OS in vemurafenib-treated patients [235]. Another study examined melanoma stem cells after negative CTC enrichment from 32 metastatic melanoma patients [216]. Multiparameter cytometry was performed with CD133 and nestin. This study found that nestin expression was increased in stage IV patients vs. stages III–IV patients with no evidence of disease and correlated to tumour burden and number of metastatic sites. In addition, the authors found that melanoma CTCs expressed stem cell-associated markers NES and CD133, proposing a higher expression of NES on CMCs as a potential index of poor prognosis.

Challenges and Clinical Implementation

CTC analysis is a promising diagnostic and prognostic tool for melanoma patients. However, there are still many analytical and technical challenges that must be solved before a wide clinical implementation could be envisioned [215]. The underlying cause for explaining the inconsistency in previous reports is most likely due to variability of assay approaches [207, 214, 220], melanoma heterogeneity [209, 221, 241], patients' disease status [204, 238] and poor sensitivity and specificity of melanoma CTC detection system [223, 229, 237]. As aforementioned, the level of CTCs in early- and late-stage melanoma patients varies. Tumour burden is also a factor that is often ignored in assay assessment. In addition, it is important that assessment of CTC assay efficiency be performed by only using the disease-free and disease recurrence analysis of the same patient.

Nonetheless, melanoma CTC detection will likely improve due to the massive parallel sequencing-based newly developed approaches, along with establishment of more sensitive molecular assays [233]. The advantage of direct qRT-PCR CTC assay outweighs antibody (Ab) capture approaches as cell surface MAAs are limited and infrequent on all stages of melanoma [212]. This is an inherent problem for epithelial solid tumour analysis in Ab capture assay, since all tumour cell subsets are not detected. Recently, the use of a size or mass isolation platform followed by multimarker detection or molecular characterization has become a favourable method of isolation and detection of melanoma CTC, owing to its autonomy from surface antigen expression for CTC enrichment [221].

Past approaches using antibody-based capture are known for limited specificity and select tumour cell capture [212]. In the last few years, the FDA has approved a relevant number of new agents and combinations for treating stage III and IV melanoma patients, making the utility of melanoma CTC significantly more important in the near future [34, 51, 54, 70, 78, 80, 242].

Future Perspectives and Conclusions

Circulating tumour cells (CTCs), circulating tumour DNA (ctDNA) and messenger RNA (mRNA), collectively termed circulating tumour products (CTPs) or liquid biopsy, represent areas of immense interest from scientists' and clinicians' perspectives.

In melanoma, liquid biopsy analysis may have clinical utility in many areas, from screening and diagnosis to clinical decision-making aids, as surveillance biomarkers or sources of real-time genetic or molecular characterization. In addition, CTP analysis can be useful in the discovery of new biomarkers, patterns of treatment resistance and mechanisms of metastasis development.

Scientific advancement has enabled the rapid development of tools to analyse circulating tumour cells, tumour DNA and messenger RNA, collectively termed circulating tumour products (CTPs). A variety of techniques has emerged to detect and characterize melanoma CTPs; however, only a fraction has been applied to human subjects.

Melanoma is highly heterogeneous, and multiple markers have been shown to improve assay sensitivity, thus contributing to its clinical impact. Liquid biopsy assessment based on the combination of CTC, different forms of ctDNA and/or cmiRNA may have potential to improve the diagnostic and prognostic performance in melanoma patients, but this requires further investigation.

In fact, two relevant clinical unmet needs are to identify metastatic melanoma prior to exhibition of clinical evidence of relapse and monitor the progression of disease during treatment. It is evident that liquid biopsy utilizing CTC, ctDNA and cmiRNA holds prognostic and diagnostic potentials by dynamically monitoring biomarkers that can detect the tumour progression and genomic or epigenomic alterations. For early-stage melanoma patients, the liquid biopsy approach may identify patients at high risk of relapse and be useful in stratifying high-risk patients for adjuvant therapy or close monitoring of disease progression. For late-stage melanoma patients, the CTP approach may help to predict treatment response, stratify patients for adequate treatment or monitor the response during treatment for evolving tumour biology, particularly those pertinent to mechanisms of drug resistance or identification of new targets for treatment.

References

1. Merrill RM. Risk-adjusted melanoma skin cancer incidence rates in whites (United States). Melanoma Res. 2011;21(6):535–40.
2. Garbe C, Peris K, Hauschild A, Saiag P, Middleton M, Spatz A, et al. Diagnosis and treatment of melanoma: European consensus-based interdisciplinary guideline. Eur J Cancer. 2010;46(2):270–83.

3. Garbe C, Leiter U. Melanoma epidemiology and trends. Clin Dermatol. 2009;27(1):3–9.
4. Chapman PB, Einhorn LH, Meyers ML, Saxman S, Destro AN, Panageas KS, et al. Phase III multicenter randomized trial of the Dartmouth regimen versus dacarbazine in patients with metastatic melanoma. J Clin Oncol. 1999;17(9):2745–51.
5. Hill VK, Gartner JJ, Samuels Y, Goldstein AM. The genetics of melanoma: recent advances. Annu Rev Genomics Hum Genet. 2013;14:257–79.
6. Curtin JA, Fridlyand J, Kageshita T, Patel HN, Busam KJ, Kutzner H, et al. Distinct sets of genetic alterations in melanoma. N Engl J Med. 2005; 353(20):2135–47.
7. McCubrey JA, Lahair MM, Franklin RA. Reactive oxygen species-induced activation of the MAP kinase signaling pathways. Antioxid Redox Signal. 2006;8(9–10):1775–89.
8. McCubrey JA, Steelman LS, Chappell WH, Abrams SL, Wong EW, Chang F, et al. Roles of the Raf/MEK/ERK pathway in cell growth, malignant transformation and drug resistance. Biochim Biophys Acta. 2007;1773(8):1263–84.
9. Ellerhorst JA, Greene VR, Ekmekcioglu S, Warneke CL, Johnson MM, Cooke CP, et al. Clinical correlates of NRAS and BRAF mutations in primary human melanoma. Clin Cancer Res. 2011;17(2): 229–35.
10. Mason CS, Springer CJ, Cooper RG, Superti-Furga G, Marshall CJ, Marais R. Serine and tyrosine phosphorylations cooperate in Raf-1, but not B-Raf activation. EMBO J. 1999;18(8):2137–48.
11. Davies H, Bignell GR, Cox C, Stephens P, Edkins S, Clegg S, et al. Mutations of the BRAF gene in human cancer. Nature. 2002;417(6892):949–54.
12. Long GV, Menzies AM, Nagrial AM, Haydu LE, Hamilton AL, Mann GJ, et al. Prognostic and clinicopathologic associations of oncogenic BRAF in metastatic melanoma. J Clin Oncol. 2011;29(10): 1239–46.
13. Liu Y, Gray NS. Rational design of inhibitors that bind to inactive kinase conformations. Nat Chem Biol. 2006;2(7):358–64.
14. Hennessy BT, Smith DL, Ram PT, Lu Y, Mills GB. Exploiting the PI3K/AKT pathway for cancer drug discovery. Nat Rev Drug Discov. 2005;4(12): 988–1004.
15. Stahl JM, Sharma A, Cheung M, Zimmerman M, Cheng JQ, Bosenberg MW, et al. Deregulated Akt3 activity promotes development of malignant melanoma. Cancer Res. 2004;64(19):7002–10.
16. Fecher LA, Cummings SD, Keefe MJ, Alani RM. Toward a molecular classification of melanoma. J Clin Oncol. 2007;25(12):1606–20.
17. Russo AE, Torrisi E, Bevelacqua Y, Perrotta R, Libra M, McCubrey JA, et al. Melanoma: molecular pathogenesis and emerging target therapies (review). Int J Oncol. 2009;34(6):1481–9.
18. Tsao H, Goel V, Wu H, Yang G, Haluska FG. Genetic interaction between NRAS and BRAF mutations and PTEN/MMAC1 inactivation in melanoma. J Invest Dermatol. 2004;122(2):337–41.
19. Gray-Schopfer V, Wellbrock C, Marais R. Melanoma biology and new targeted therapy. Nature. 2007; 445(7130):851–7.
20. Serrano M, Gomez-Lahoz E, DePinho RA, Beach D, Bar-Sagi D. Inhibition of ras-induced proliferation and cellular transformation by p16INK4. Science. 1995;267(5195):249–52.
21. Harbour JW, Dean DC. The Rb/E2F pathway: expanding roles and emerging paradigms. Genes Dev. 2000;14(19):2393–409.
22. Goldstein AM, Chan M, Harland M, Gillanders EM, Hayward NK, Avril MF, et al. High-risk melanoma susceptibility genes and pancreatic cancer, neural system tumors, and uveal melanoma across GenoMEL. Cancer Res. 2006;66(20):9818–28.
23. Walker GJ, Flores JF, Glendening JM, Lin AH, Markl ID, Fountain JW. Virtually 100% of melanoma cell lines harbor alterations at the DNA level within CDKN2A, CDKN2B, or one of their downstream targets. Genes Chromosomes Cancer. 1998;22(2):157–63.
24. Bartkova J, Rezaei N, Liontos M, Karakaidos P, Kletsas D, Issaeva N, et al. Oncogene-induced senescence is part of the tumorigenesis barrier imposed by DNA damage checkpoints. Nature. 2006;444(7119):633–7.
25. Madhunapantula SV, Robertson GP. Is B-Raf a good therapeutic target for melanoma and other malignancies? Cancer Res. 2008;68(1):5–8.
26. Gray-Schopfer VC, Cheong SC, Chong H, Chow J, Moss T, Abdel-Malek ZA, et al. Cellular senescence in naevi and immortalisation in melanoma: a role for p16? Br J Cancer. 2006;95(4):496–505.
27. Hayward NK. Genetics of melanoma predisposition. Oncogene. 2003;22(20):3053–62.
28. Wellbrock C, Rana S, Paterson H, Pickersgill H, Brummelkamp T, Marais R. Oncogenic BRAF regulates melanoma proliferation through the lineage specific factor MITF. PLoS One. 2008;3(7):e2734.
29. Guo J, Si L, Kong Y, Flaherty KT, Xu X, Zhu Y, et al. Phase II, open-label, single-arm trial of imatinib mesylate in patients with metastatic melanoma harboring c-kit mutation or amplification. J Clin Oncol. 2011;29(21):2904–9.
30. Minor DR, Kashani-Sabet M, Garrido M, O'Day SJ, Hamid O, Bastian BC. Sunitinib therapy for melanoma patients with KIT mutations. Clin Cancer Res. 2012;18(5):1457–63.
31. Bottomley A, Coens C, Suciu S, Santinami M, Kruit W, Testori A, et al. Adjuvant therapy with pegylated interferon alfa-2b versus observation in resected stage III melanoma: a phase III randomized controlled trial of health-related quality of life and symptoms by the European Organisation for

Research and Treatment of Cancer melanoma group. J Clin Oncol. 2009;27(18):2916–23.

32. Hodi FS, O'Day SJ, McDermott DF, Weber RW, Sosman JA, Haanen JB, et al. Improved survival with ipilimumab in patients with metastatic melanoma. N Engl J Med. 2010;363(8):711–23.

33. Kalland ME, Oberprieler NG, Vang T, Tasken K, Torgersen KM. T cell-signaling network analysis reveals distinct differences between CD28 and CD2 costimulation responses in various subsets and in the MAPK pathway between resting and activated regulatory T cells. J Immunol. 2011;187(10):5233–45.

34. Margolin K, Ernstoff MS, Hamid O, Lawrence D, McDermott D, Puzanov I, et al. Ipilimumab in patients with melanoma and brain metastases: an open-label, phase 2 trial. Lancet Oncol. 2012;13(5): 459–65.

35. Schwarzer A, Wolf B, Fisher JL, Schwaab T, Olek S, Baron U, et al. Regulatory T-cells and associated pathways in metastatic renal cell carcinoma (mRCC) patients undergoing DC-vaccination and cytokine-therapy. PLoS One. 2012;7(10):e46600.

36. Crosby T, Fish R, Coles B, Mason MD. Systemic treatments for metastatic cutaneous melanoma. Cochrane Database Syst Rev. 2000;2:CD001215.

37. Avril MF, Aamdal S, Grob JJ, Hauschild A, Mohr P, Bonerandi JJ, et al. Fotemustine compared with dacarbazine in patients with disseminated malignant melanoma: a phase III study. J Clin Oncol. 2004; 22(6):1118–25.

38. Middleton MR, Grob JJ, Aaronson N, Fierlbeck G, Tilgen W, Seiter S, et al. Randomized phase III study of temozolomide versus dacarbazine in the treatment of patients with advanced metastatic malignant melanoma. J Clin Oncol. 2000;18(1):158–66.

39. Atkins MB. Cytokine-based therapy and biochemotherapy for advanced melanoma. Clin Cancer Res. 2006;12(7 Pt 2):2353s–8s.

40. Joseph EW, Pratilas CA, Poulikakos PI, Tadi M, Wang W, Taylor BS, et al. The RAF inhibitor PLX4032 inhibits ERK signaling and tumor cell proliferation in a V600E BRAF-selective manner. Proc Natl Acad Sci U S A. 2010;107(33):14903–8.

41. Houben R, Becker JC, Kappel A, Terheyden P, Brocker EB, Goetz R, et al. Constitutive activation of the ras-Raf signaling pathway in metastatic melanoma is associated with poor prognosis. J Carcinog. 2004;3(1):6.

42. Ugurel S, Thirumaran RK, Bloethner S, Gast A, Sucker A, Mueller-Berghaus J, et al. B-RAF and N-RAS mutations are preserved during short time in vitro propagation and differentially impact prognosis. PLoS One. 2007;2(2):e236.

43. Jakob JA, Bassett Jr RL, Ng CS, Curry JL, Joseph RW, Alvarado GC, et al. NRAS mutation status is an independent prognostic factor in metastatic melanoma. Cancer. 2012;118(16):4014–23.

44. Bucheit AD, Syklawer E, Jakob JA, Bassett Jr RL, Curry JL, Gershenwald JE, et al. Clinical characteristics and outcomes with specific BRAF and NRAS

mutations in patients with metastatic melanoma. Cancer. 2013;119(21):3821–9.

45. Bollag G, Hirth P, Tsai J, Zhang J, Ibrahim PN, Cho H, et al. Clinical efficacy of a RAF inhibitor needs broad target blockade in BRAF-mutant melanoma. Nature. 2010;467(7315):596–9.

46. Tsai J, Lee JT, Wang W, Zhang J, Cho H, Mamo S, et al. Discovery of a selective inhibitor of oncogenic B-Raf kinase with potent antimelanoma activity. Proc Natl Acad Sci U S A. 2008;105(8):3041–6.

47. Flaherty KT, Puzanov I, Kim KB, Ribas A, McArthur GA, Sosman JA, et al. Inhibition of mutated, activated BRAF in metastatic melanoma. N Engl J Med. 2010;363(9):809–19.

48. Sosman JA, Kim KB, Schuchter L, Gonzalez R, Pavlick AC, Weber JS, et al. Survival in BRAF V600-mutant advanced melanoma treated with vemurafenib. N Engl J Med. 2012;366(8):707–14.

49. Chapman PB, Hauschild A, Robert C, Haanen JB, Ascierto P, Larkin J, et al. Improved survival with vemurafenib in melanoma with BRAF V600E mutation. N Engl J Med. 2011;364(26):2507–16.

50. Peinado H, Aleckovic M, Lavotshkin S, Matei I, Costa-Silva B, Moreno-Bueno G, et al. Melanoma exosomes educate bone marrow progenitor cells toward a pro-metastatic phenotype through MET. Nat Med. 2012;18(6):883–91.

51. McArthur GA, Chapman PB, Robert C, Larkin J, Haanen JB, Dummer R, et al. Safety and efficacy of vemurafenib in BRAF(V600E) and BRAF(V600K) mutation-positive melanoma (BRIM-3): extended follow-up of a phase 3, randomised, open-label study. Lancet Oncol. 2014;15(3):323–32.

52. Heidorn SJ, Milagre C, Whittaker S, Nourry A, Niculescu-Duvas I, Dhomen N, et al. Kinase-dead BRAF and oncogenic RAS cooperate to drive tumor progression through CRAF. Cell. 2010;140(2): 209–21.

53. Su F, Viros A, Milagre C, Trunzer K, Bollag G, Spleiss O, et al. RAS mutations in cutaneous squamous-cell carcinomas in patients treated with BRAF inhibitors. N Engl J Med. 2012;366(3): 207–15.

54. Hauschild A, Grob JJ, Demidov LV, Jouary T, Gutzmer R, Millward M, et al. Dabrafenib in BRAF-mutated metastatic melanoma: a multicentre, open-label, phase 3 randomised controlled trial. Lancet. 2012;380(9839):358–65.

55. Falchook GS, Lewis KD, Infante JR, Gordon MS, Vogelzang NJ, DeMarini DJ, et al. Activity of the oral MEK inhibitor trametinib in patients with advanced melanoma: a phase 1 dose-escalation trial. Lancet Oncol. 2012;13(8):782–9.

56. Ascierto PA, Minor D, Ribas A, Lebbe C, O'Hagan A, Arya N, et al. Phase II trial (BREAK-2) of the BRAF inhibitor dabrafenib (GSK2118436) in patients with metastatic melanoma. J Clin Oncol. 2013;31(26):3205–11.

57. Long GV, Trefzer U, Davies MA, Kefford RF, Ascierto PA, Chapman PB, et al. Dabrafenib in

patients with Val600Glu or Val600Lys BRAF-mutant melanoma metastatic to the brain (BREAK-MB): a multicentre, open-label, phase 2 trial. Lancet Oncol. 2012;13(11):1087–95.

58. Paraiso KH, Xiang Y, Rebecca VW, Abel EV, Chen YA, Munko AC, et al. PTEN loss confers BRAF inhibitor resistance to melanoma cells through the suppression of BIM expression. Cancer Res. 2011;71(7):2750–60.

59. Smalley KS, Lioni M, Dalla Palma M, Xiao M, Desai B, Egyhazi S, et al. Increased cyclin D1 expression can mediate BRAF inhibitor resistance in BRAF V600E-mutated melanomas. Mol Cancer Ther. 2008;7(9):2876–83.

60. Straussman R, Morikawa T, Shee K, Barzily-Rokni M, Qian ZR, Du J, et al. Tumour micro-environment elicits innate resistance to RAF inhibitors through HGF secretion. Nature. 2012;487(7408):500–4.

61. Sullivan RJ, Flaherty KT. Resistance to BRAF-targeted therapy in melanoma. Eur J Cancer. 2013; 49(6):1297–304.

62. Villanueva J, Vultur A, Lee JT, Somasundaram R, Fukunaga-Kalabis M, Cipolla AK, et al. Acquired resistance to BRAF inhibitors mediated by a RAF kinase switch in melanoma can be overcome by cotargeting MEK and IGF-1R/PI3K. Cancer Cell. 2010;18(6):683–95.

63. Nazarian R, Shi H, Wang Q, Kong X, Koya RC, Lee H, et al. Melanomas acquire resistance to B-RAF(V600E) inhibition by RTK or N-RAS upregulation. Nature. 2010;468(7326):973–7.

64. Johannessen CM, Boehm JS, Kim SY, Thomas SR, Wardwell L, Johnson LA, et al. COT drives resistance to RAF inhibition through MAP kinase pathway reactivation. Nature. 2010;468(7326):968–72.

65. Fedorenko IV, Paraiso KH, Smalley KS. Acquired and intrinsic BRAF inhibitor resistance in BRAF V600E mutant melanoma. Biochem Pharmacol. 2011;82(3):201–9.

66. Wagle N, Emery C, Berger MF, Davis MJ, Sawyer A, Pochanard P, et al. Dissecting therapeutic resistance to RAF inhibition in melanoma by tumor genomic profiling. J Clin Oncol. 2011;29(22): 3085–96.

67. Poulikakos PI, Persaud Y, Janakiraman M, Kong X, Ng C, Moriceau G, et al. RAF inhibitor resistance is mediated by dimerization of aberrantly spliced BRAF(V600E). Nature. 2011;480(7377):387–90.

68. Gilmartin AG, Bleam MR, Groy A, Moss KG, Minthorn EA, Kulkarni SG, et al. GSK1120212 (JTP-74057) is an inhibitor of MEK activity and activation with favorable pharmacokinetic properties for sustained in vivo pathway inhibition. Clin Cancer Res. 2011;17(5):989–1000.

69. Flaherty KT, Robert C, Hersey P, Nathan P, Garbe C, Milhem M, et al. Improved survival with MEK inhibition in BRAF-mutated melanoma. N Engl J Med. 2012;367(2):107–14.

70. Robert C, Karaszewska B, Schachter J, Rutkowski P, Mackiewicz A, Stroiakovski D, et al. Improved overall survival in melanoma with combined dabrafenib and trametinib. N Engl J Med. 2015;372(1):30–9.

71. Coley WB. The treatment of malignant tumors by repeated inoculations of erysipelas. With a report of ten original cases. 1893. Clin Orthop Relat Res. 1991;(262):3–11.

72. Schwartz RH. Costimulation of T lymphocytes: the role of CD28, CTLA-4, and B7/BB1 in interleukin-2 production and immunotherapy. Cell. 1992;71(7): 1065–8.

73. Phan GQ, Yang JC, Sherry RM, Hwu P, Topalian SL, Schwartzentruber DJ, et al. Cancer regression and autoimmunity induced by cytotoxic T lymphocyte-associated antigen 4 blockade in patients with metastatic melanoma. Proc Natl Acad Sci U S A. 2003;100(14):8372–7.

74. Robert C, Thomas L, Bondarenko I, O'Day S, Weber J, Garbe C, et al. Ipilimumab plus dacarbazine for previously untreated metastatic melanoma. N Engl J Med. 2011;364(26):2517–26.

75. Merelli B, Massi D, Cattaneo L, Mandala M. Targeting the PD1/PD-L1 axis in melanoma: biological rationale, clinical challenges and opportunities. Crit Rev Oncol Hematol. 2014;89(1):140–65.

76. Pardoll DM. The blockade of immune checkpoints in cancer immunotherapy. Nat Rev Cancer. 2012; 12(4):252–64.

77. Robert C, Ribas A, Wolchok JD, Hodi FS, Hamid O, Kefford R, et al. Anti-programmed-death-receptor-1 treatment with pembrolizumab in ipilimumab-refractory advanced melanoma: a randomised dose-comparison cohort of a phase 1 trial. Lancet. 2014; 384(9948):1109–17.

78. Robert C, Long GV, Brady B, Dutriaux C, Maio M, Mortier L, et al. Nivolumab in previously untreated melanoma without BRAF mutation. N Engl J Med. 2015;372(4):320–30.

79. Topalian SL, Hodi FS, Brahmer JR, Gettinger SN, Smith DC, McDermott DF, et al. Safety, activity, and immune correlates of anti-PD-1 antibody in cancer. N Engl J Med. 2012;366(26):2443–54.

80. Weber JS, D'Angelo SP, Minor D, Hodi FS, Gutzmer R, Neyns B, et al. Nivolumab versus chemotherapy in patients with advanced melanoma who progressed after anti-CTLA-4 treatment (CheckMate 037): a randomised, controlled, open-label, phase 3 trial. Lancet Oncol. 2015;16(4):375–84.

81. Weber JS, Kudchadkar RR, Yu B, Gallenstein D, Horak CE, Inzunza HD, et al. Safety, efficacy, and biomarkers of nivolumab with vaccine in ipilimumab-refractory or -naive melanoma. J Clin Oncol. 2013;31(34):4311–8.

82. Patel SP, Kurzrock R. PD-L1 expression as a predictive biomarker in cancer immunotherapy. Mol Cancer Ther. 2015;14(4):847–56.

83. Korman A, Chen B, Wang C, Wu L, Cardarelli P and Selby M. Activity of anti-PD-1 in murine tumor models: role of "host" PD-L1 and synergistic effect of anti-PD-1 and anti-CTLA-4. J Immunol 2007;178(1 Supple):S82.

84. Curran MA, Montalvo W, Yagita H, Allison JP. PD-1 and CTLA-4 combination blockade expands infiltrating T cells and reduces regulatory T and myeloid cells within B16 melanoma tumors. Proc Natl Acad Sci U S A. 2010;107(9):4275–80.

85. Callahan MK, Postow MA, Wolchok JD. CTLA-4 and PD-1 pathway blockade: combinations in the clinic. Front Oncol. 2014;4:385.

86. Wolchok JD, Kluger H, Callahan MK, Postow MA, Rizvi NA, Lesokhin AM, et al. Nivolumab plus ipilimumab in advanced melanoma. N Engl J Med. 2013;369(2):122–33.

87. Gion M, Daidone MG. Circulating biomarkers from tumour bulk to tumour machinery: promises and pitfalls. Eur J Cancer. 2004;40(17):2613–22.

88. Alegre E, Sammamed M, Fernandez-Landazuri S, Zubiri L, Gonzalez A. Circulating biomarkers in malignant melanoma. Adv Clin Chem. 2015;69: 47–89.

89. Davey RJ, Westhuizen A, Bowden NA. Metastatic melanoma treatment: combining old and new therapies. Crit Rev Oncol Hematol. 2016;98:242–53.

90. Neagu M, Constantin C, Manda G, Margaritescu I. Biomarkers of metastatic melanoma. Biomark Med. 2009;3(1):71–89.

91. Khoja L, Lorigan P, Dive C, Keilholz U, Fusi A. Circulating tumour cells as tumour biomarkers in melanoma: detection methods and clinical relevance. Ann Oncol. 2015;26(1):33–9.

92. Jain KK. Cancer biomarkers: current issues and future directions. Curr Opin Mol Ther. 2007;9(6):563–71.

93. Brinton LT, Sloane HS, Kester M, Kelly KA. Formation and role of exosomes in cancer. Cell Mol Life Sci. 2015;72(4):659–71.

94. Yu X, Harris SL, Levine AJ. The regulation of exosome secretion: a novel function of the p53 protein. Cancer Res. 2006;66(9):4795–801.

95. Riches A, Campbell E, Borger E, Powis S. Regulation of exosome release from mammary epithelial and breast cancer cells – a new regulatory pathway. Eur J Cancer. 2014;50(5):1025–34.

96. Raposo G, Stoorvogel W. Extracellular vesicles: exosomes, microvesicles, and friends. J Cell Biol. 2013;200(4):373–83.

97. Simons M, Raposo G. Exosomes--vesicular carriers for intercellular communication. Curr Opin Cell Biol. 2009;21(4):575–81.

98. Duijvesz D, Luider T, Bangma CH, Jenster G. Exosomes as biomarker treasure chests for prostate cancer. Eur Urol. 2011;59(5):823–31.

99. Staubach S, Razawi H, Hanisch FG. Proteomics of MUC1-containing lipid rafts from plasma membranes and exosomes of human breast carcinoma cells MCF-7. Proteomics. 2009;9(10):2820–35.

100. Peng P, Yan Y, Keng S. Exosomes in the ascites of ovarian cancer patients: origin and effects on anti-tumor immunity. Oncol Rep. 2011;25(3):749–62.

101. Li Y, Zhang Y, Qiu F, Qiu Z. Proteomic identification of exosomal LRG1: a potential urinary bio-marker for detecting NSCLC. Electrophoresis. 2011;32(15):1976–83.

102. Adamczyk KA, Klein-Scory S, Tehrani MM, Warnken U, Schmiegel W, Schnolzer M, et al. Characterization of soluble and exosomal forms of the EGFR released from pancreatic cancer cells. Life Sci. 2011;89(9–10):304–12.

103. Szajnik M, Derbis M, Lach M, Patalas P, Michalak M, Drzewiecka H, et al. Exosomes in plasma of patients with ovarian carcinoma: potential biomarkers of tumor progression and response to therapy. Gynecol Obstet (Sunnyvale). 2013;Suppl 4:3.

104. Silva J, Garcia V, Rodriguez M, Compte M, Cisneros E, Veguillas P, et al. Analysis of exosome release and its prognostic value in human colorectal cancer. Genes Chromosomes Cancer. 2012;51(4):409–18.

105. Morelli AE, Larregina AT, Shufesky WJ, Sullivan ML, Stolz DB, Papworth GD, et al. Endocytosis, intracellular sorting, and processing of exosomes by dendritic cells. Blood. 2004;104(10):3257–66.

106. Hoshino A, Costa-Silva B, Shen TL, Rodrigues G, Hashimoto A, Tesic Mark M, et al. Tumour exosome integrins determine organotropic metastasis. Nature. 2015;527(7578):329–35.

107. Raposo G, Nijman HW, Stoorvogel W, Liejendekker R, Harding CV, Melief CJ, et al. B lymphocytes secrete antigen-presenting vesicles. J Exp Med. 1996;183(3):1161–72.

108. Delcayre A, Shu H, Le Pecq JB. Dendritic cell-derived exosomes in cancer immunotherapy: exploiting nature's antigen delivery pathway. Expert Rev Anticancer Ther. 2005;5(3):537–47.

109. Dai S, Wei D, Wu Z, Zhou X, Wei X, Huang H, et al. Phase I clinical trial of autologous ascites-derived exosomes combined with GM-CSF for colorectal cancer. Mol Ther. 2008;16(4):782–90.

110. Mathivanan S, Fahner CJ, Reid GE, Simpson RJ. ExoCarta 2012: database of exosomal proteins, RNA and lipids. Nucleic Acids Res. 2012;40(Database issue):D1241–4.

111. Taylor DD, Shah S. Methods of isolating extracellular vesicles impact down-stream analyses of their cargoes. Methods. 2015;87:3–10.

112. Tauro BJ, Greening DW, Mathias RA, Ji H, Mathivanan S, Scott AM, et al. Comparison of ultracentrifugation, density gradient separation, and immunoaffinity capture methods for isolating human colon cancer cell line LIM1863-derived exosomes. Methods. 2012;56(2):293–304.

113. Mitchell PJ, Welton J, Staffurth J, Court J, Mason MD, Tabi Z, et al. Can urinary exosomes act as treatment response markers in prostate cancer? J Transl Med. 2009;7:4.

114. Melo SA, Luecke LB, Kahlert C, Fernandez AF, Gammon ST, Kaye J, et al. Glypican-1 identifies cancer exosomes and detects early pancreatic cancer. Nature. 2015;523(7559):177–82.

115. O'Brien K, Rani S, Corcoran C, Wallace R, Hughes L, Friel AM, et al. Exosomes from triple-negative

breast cancer cells can transfer phenotypic traits representing their cells of origin to secondary cells. Eur J Cancer. 2013;49(8):1845–59.

116. Guo L, Guo N. Exosomes: potent regulators of tumor malignancy and potential bio-tools in clinical application. Crit Rev Oncol Hematol. 2015;95(3):346–58.

117. Wieckowski EU, Visus C, Szajnik M, Szczepanski MJ, Storkus WJ, Whiteside TL. Tumor-derived microvesicles promote regulatory T cell expansion and induce apoptosis in tumor-reactive activated CD8+ T lymphocytes. J Immunol. 2009;183(6):3720–30.

118. Taylor DD, Gercel-Taylor C, Lyons KS, Stanson J, Whiteside TL. T-cell apoptosis and suppression of T-cell receptor/CD3-zeta by Fas ligand-containing membrane vesicles shed from ovarian tumors. Clin Cancer Res. 2003;9(14):5113–9.

119. Andreola G, Rivoltini L, Castelli C, Huber V, Perego P, Deho P, et al. Induction of lymphocyte apoptosis by tumor cell secretion of FasL-bearing microvesicles. J Exp Med. 2002;195(10):1303–16.

120. Ashiru O, Boutet P, Fernandez-Messina L, Aguera-Gonzalez S, Skepper JN, Vales-Gomez M, et al. Natural killer cell cytotoxicity is suppressed by exposure to the human NKG2D ligand MICA*008 that is shed by tumor cells in exosomes. Cancer Res. 2010;70(2):481–9.

121. Aung T, Chapuy B, Vogel D, Wenzel D, Oppermann M, Lahmann M, et al. Exosomal evasion of humoral immunotherapy in aggressive B-cell lymphoma modulated by ATP-binding cassette transporter A3. Proc Natl Acad Sci U S A. 2011;108(37):15336–41.

122. Logozzi M, De Milito A, Lugini L, Borghi M, Calabro L, Spada M, et al. High levels of exosomes expressing CD63 and caveolin-1 in plasma of melanoma patients. PLoS One. 2009;4(4):e5219.

123. Guan M, Chen X, Ma Y, Tang L, Guan L, Ren X, et al. MDA-9 and GRP78 as potential diagnostic biomarkers for early detection of melanoma metastasis. Tumour Biol. 2015;36(4):2973–82.

124. Eldh M, Olofsson Bagge R, Lasser C, Svanvik J, Sjostrand M, Mattsson J, et al. MicroRNA in exosomes isolated directly from the liver circulation in patients with metastatic uveal melanoma. BMC Cancer. 2014;14:962.

125. Riteau B, Faure F, Menier C, Viel S, Carosella ED, Amigorena S, et al. Exosomes bearing HLA-G are released by melanoma cells. Hum Immunol. 2003;64(11):1064–72.

126. Alegre E, Rebmann V, Lemaoult J, Rodriguez C, Horn PA, Diaz-Lagares A, et al. In vivo identification of an HLA-G complex as ubiquitinated protein circulating in exosomes. Eur J Immunol. 2013;43(7):1933–9.

127. Deregibus MC, Cantaluppi V, Calogero R, Lo Iacono M, Tetta C, Biancone L, et al. Endothelial progenitor cell derived microvesicles activate an angiogenic program in endothelial cells by a horizontal transfer of mRNA. Blood. 2007;110(7):2440–8.

128. Thakur BK, Zhang H, Becker A, Matei I, Huang Y, Costa-Silva B, et al. Double-stranded DNA in exosomes: a novel biomarker in cancer detection. Cell Res. 2014;24(6):766–9.

129. Vickers KC, Palmisano BT, Shoucri BM, Shamburek RD, Remaley AT. MicroRNAs are transported in plasma and delivered to recipient cells by high-density lipoproteins. Nat Cell Biol. 2011;13(4):423–33.

130. Gallo A, Tandon M, Alevizos I, Illei GG. The majority of microRNAs detectable in serum and saliva is concentrated in exosomes. PLoS One. 2012;7(3):e30679.

131. Cheng L, Sharples RA, Scicluna BJ, Hill AF. Exosomes provide a protective and enriched source of miRNA for biomarker profiling compared to intracellular and cell-free blood. J Extracell Vesicles. 2014;3

132. Mitchell PS, Parkin RK, Kroh EM, Fritz BR, Wyman SK, Pogosova-Agadjanyan EL, et al. Circulating microRNAs as stable blood-based markers for cancer detection. Proc Natl Acad Sci U S A. 2008;105(30):10513–8.

133. Ha M, Kim VN. Regulation of microRNA biogenesis. Nat Rev Mol Cell Biol. 2014;15(8):509–24.

134. Kosaka N, Iguchi H, Hagiwara K, Yoshioka Y, Takeshita F, Ochiya T. Neutral sphingomyelinase 2 (nSMase2)-dependent exosomal transfer of angiogenic microRNAs regulate cancer cell metastasis. J Biol Chem. 2013;288(15):10849–59.

135. Villarroya-Beltri C, Gutierrez-Vazquez C, Sanchez-Cabo F, Perez-Hernandez D, Vazquez J, Martin-Cofreces N, et al. Sumoylated hnRNPA2B1 controls the sorting of miRNAs into exosomes through binding to specific motifs. Nat Commun. 2013;4:2980.

136. Koppers-Lalic D, Hackenberg M, Bijnsdorp IV, van Eijndhoven MA, Sadek P, Sie D, et al. Nontemplated nucleotide additions distinguish the small RNA composition in cells from exosomes. Cell Rep. 2014;8(6):1649–58.

137. Guduric-Fuchs J, O'Connor A, Camp B, O'Neill CL, Medina RJ, Simpson DA. Selective extracellular vesicle-mediated export of an overlapping set of microRNAs from multiple cell types. BMC Genomics. 2012;13:357.

138. Zhang J, Li S, Li L, Li M, Guo C, Yao J, et al. Exosome and exosomal microRNA: trafficking, sorting, and function. Genomics Proteomics Bioinformatics. 2015;13(1):17–24.

139. Kroh EM, Parkin RK, Mitchell PS, Tewari M. Analysis of circulating microRNA biomarkers in plasma and serum using quantitative reverse transcription-PCR (qRT-PCR). Methods. 2010;50(4):298–301.

140. McDonald JS, Milosevic D, Reddi HV, Grebe SK, Algeciras-Schimnich A. Analysis of circulating microRNA: preanalytical and analytical challenges. Clin Chem. 2011;57(6):833–40.

141. Alegre E, Sanmamed MF, Rodriguez C, Carranza O, Martin-Algarra S, Gonzalez A. Study of circulating microRNA-125b levels in serum exosomes in advanced melanoma. Arch Pathol Lab Med. 2014;138(6):828–32.

142. Mishra S, Yadav T, Rani V. Exploring miRNA based approaches in cancer diagnostics and therapeutics. Crit Rev Oncol Hematol. 2016;98:12–23.

143. Fabbri M, Paone A, Calore F, Galli R, Gaudio E, Santhanam R, et al. MicroRNAs bind to toll-like receptors to induce prometastatic inflammatory response. Proc Natl Acad Sci U S A. 2012;109(31):E2110–6.

144. Li BS, Zuo QF, Zhao YL, Xiao B, Zhuang Y, Mao XH, et al. MicroRNA-25 promotes gastric cancer migration, invasion and proliferation by directly targeting transducer of ERBB2, 1 and correlates with poor survival. Oncogene. 2015;34(20):2556–65.

145. Wu J, Qian J, Li C, Kwok L, Cheng F, Liu P, et al. miR-129 regulates cell proliferation by downregulating Cdk6 expression. Cell Cycle. 2010;9(9):1809–18.

146. Ye J, Wu X, Wu D, Wu P, Ni C, Zhang Z, et al. miRNA-27b targets vascular endothelial growth factor C to inhibit tumor progression and angiogenesis in colorectal cancer. PLoS One. 2013;8(4):e60687.

147. Challagundla KB, Wise PM, Neviani P, Chava H, Murtadha M, Xu T, et al. Exosome-mediated transfer of microRNAs within the tumor microenvironment and neuroblastoma resistance to chemotherapy. J Natl Cancer Inst. 2015;107(7)

148. Gajos-Michniewicz A, Duechler M, Czyz M. MiRNA in melanoma-derived exosomes. Cancer Lett. 2014;347(1):29–37.

149. Leibowitz-Amit R, Sidi Y, Avni D. Aberrations in the micro-RNA biogenesis machinery and the emerging roles of micro-RNAs in the pathogenesis of cutaneous malignant melanoma. Pigment Cell Melanoma Res. 2012;25(6):740–57.

150. Streicher KL, Zhu W, Lehmann KP, Georgantas RW, Morehouse CA, Brohawn P, et al. A novel oncogenic role for the miRNA-506-514 cluster in initiating melanocyte transformation and promoting melanoma growth. Oncogene. 2012;31(12):1558–70.

151. Zehavi L, Avraham R, Barzilai A, Bar-Ilan D, Navon R, Sidi Y, et al. Silencing of a large microRNA cluster on human chromosome 14q32 in melanoma: biological effects of mir-376a and mir-376c on insulin growth factor 1 receptor. Mol Cancer. 2012;11:44.

152. Chan E, Patel R, Nallur S, Ratner E, Bacchiocchi A, Hoyt K, et al. MicroRNA signatures differentiate melanoma subtypes. Cell Cycle. 2011;10(11):1845–52.

153. Xiao D, Ohlendorf J, Chen Y, Taylor DD, Rai SN, Waigel S, et al. Identifying mRNA, microRNA and protein profiles of melanoma exosomes. PLoS One. 2012;7(10):e46874.

154. Kanemaru H, Fukushima S, Yamashita J, Honda N, Oyama R, Kakimoto A, et al. The circulating microRNA-221 level in patients with malignant melanoma as a new tumor marker. J Dermatol Sci. 2011;61(3):187–93.

155. Friedman EB, Shang S, de Miera EV, Fog JU, Teilum MW, Ma MW, et al. Serum microRNAs as biomarkers for recurrence in melanoma. J Transl Med. 2012;10:155.

156. Fleming NH, Zhong J, da Silva IP, Vega-Saenz de Miera E, Brady B, Han SW, et al. Serum-based miRNAs in the prediction and detection of recurrence in melanoma patients. Cancer. 2015;121(1):51–9.

157. Gaziel-Sovran A, Segura MF, Di Micco R, Collins MK, Hanniford D, Vega-Saenz de Miera E, et al. miR-30b/30d regulation of GalNAc transferases enhances invasion and immunosuppression during metastasis. Cancer Cell. 2011;20(1):104–18.

158. Satzger I, Mattern A, Kuettler U, Weinspach D, Voelker B, Kapp A, et al. MicroRNA-15b represents an independent prognostic parameter and is correlated with tumor cell proliferation and apoptosis in malignant melanoma. Int J Cancer. 2010;126(11):2553–62.

159. Srivastava SK, Bhardwaj A, Singh S, Arora S, Wang B, Grizzle WE, et al. MicroRNA-150 directly targets MUC4 and suppresses growth and malignant behavior of pancreatic cancer cells. Carcinogenesis. 2011;32(12):1832–9.

160. Sun L, Yao Y, Liu B, Lin Z, Lin L, Yang M, et al. MiR-200b and miR-15b regulate chemotherapy-induced epithelial-mesenchymal transition in human tongue cancer cells by targeting BMI1. Oncogene. 2012;31(4):432–45.

161. Ghosh G, Subramanian IV, Adhikari N, Zhang X, Joshi HP, Basi D, et al. Hypoxia-induced microRNA-424 expression in human endothelial cells regulates HIF-alpha isoforms and promotes angiogenesis. J Clin Invest. 2010;120(11):4141–54.

162. Shiiyama R, Fukushima S, Jinnin M, Yamashita J, Miyashita A, Nakahara S, et al. Sensitive detection of melanoma metastasis using circulating microRNA expression profiles. Melanoma Res. 2013;23(5):366–72.

163. Ragusa M, Barbagallo C, Statello L, Caltabiano R, Russo A, Puzzo L, et al. miRNA profiling in vitreous humor, vitreal exosomes and serum from uveal melanoma patients: pathological and diagnostic implications. Cancer Biol Ther. 2015;16(9):1387–96.

164. Mandel P, Metais P. Les acides nucléiques du plasma sanguin chez l'homme. C R Seances Soc Biol Fil. 1948;142(3–4):241–3.

165. Koffler D, Agnello V, Winchester R, Kunkel HG. The occurrence of single-stranded DNA in the serum of patients with systemic lupus erythematosus and other diseases. J Clin Invest. 1973;52(1):198–204.

166. Stroun M, Anker P, Maurice P, Lyautey J, Lederrey C, Beljanski M. Neoplastic characteristics of the DNA found in the plasma of cancer patients. Oncology. 1989;46(5):318–22.

167. Jahr S, Hentze H, Englisch S, Hardt D, Fackelmayer FO, Hesch RD, et al. DNA fragments in the blood plasma of cancer patients: quantitations and evidence for their origin from apoptotic and necrotic cells. Cancer Res. 2001;61(4):1659–65.

168. Kahlert C, Melo SA, Protopopov A, Tang J, Seth S, Koch M, et al. Identification of double-stranded genomic DNA spanning all chromosomes with mutated KRAS and p53 DNA in the serum exosomes of patients with pancreatic cancer. J Biol Chem. 2014;289(7):3869–75.

169. Mouliere F, El Messaoudi S, Pang D, Dritschilo A, Thierry AR. Multi-marker analysis of circulating cell-free DNA toward personalized medicine for colorectal cancer. Mol Oncol. 2014;8(5):927–41.

170. Suzuki N, Kamataki A, Yamaki J, Homma Y. Characterization of circulating DNA in healthy human plasma. Clin Chim Acta. 2008;387(1–2):55–8.

171. Pinzani P, Salvianti F, Zaccara S, Massi D, De Giorgi V, Pazzagli M, et al. Circulating cell-free DNA in plasma of melanoma patients: qualitative and quantitative considerations. Clin Chim Acta. 2011;412(23–24):2141–5.

172. Schwarzenbach H, Hoon DS, Pantel K. Cell-free nucleic acids as biomarkers in cancer patients. Nat Rev Cancer. 2011;11(6):426–37.

173. El Messaoudi S, Rolet F, Mouliere F, Thierry AR. Circulating cell free DNA: preanalytical considerations. Clin Chim Acta. 2013;424:222–30.

174. Breitbach S, Tug S, Simon P. Circulating cell-free DNA: an up-coming molecular marker in exercise physiology. Sports Med (Auckland, NZ). 2012;42(7):565–86.

175. Sozzi G, Roz L, Conte D, Mariani L, Andriani F, Verderio P, et al. Effects of prolonged storage of whole plasma or isolated plasma DNA on the results of circulating DNA quantification assays. J Natl Cancer Inst. 2005;97(24):1848–50.

176. Diehl F, Schmidt K, Choti MA, Romans K, Goodman S, Li M, et al. Circulating mutant DNA to assess tumor dynamics. Nat Med. 2008;14(9):985–90.

177. Pinzani P, Santucci C, Mancini I, Simi L, Salvianti F, Pratesi N, et al. BRAFV600E detection in melanoma is highly improved by COLD-PCR. Clin Chim Acta. 2011;412(11–12):901–5.

178. Pinzani P, Salvianti F, Cascella R, Massi D, De Giorgi V, Pazzagli M, et al. Allele specific Taqman-based real-time PCR assay to quantify circulating BRAFV600E mutated DNA in plasma of melanoma patients. Clin Chim Acta. 2010;411(17–18):1319–24.

179. Board RE, Ellison G, Orr MC, Kemsley KR, McWalter G, Blockley LY, et al. Detection of BRAF mutations in the tumour and serum of patients enrolled in the AZD6244 (ARRY-142886) advanced melanoma phase II study. Br J Cancer. 2009;101(10):1724–30.

180. Sanmamed MF, Fernandez-Landazuri S, Rodriguez C, Zarate R, Lozano MD, Zubiri L, et al. Quantitative cell-free circulating BRAFV600E mutation analysis by use of droplet digital PCR in the follow-up of patients with melanoma being treated with BRAF inhibitors. Clin Chem. 2015;61(1):297–304.

181. Bettegowda C, Sausen M, Leary RJ, Kinde I, Wang Y, Agrawal N, et al. Detection of circulating tumor DNA in early- and late-stage human malignancies. Sci Transl Med. 2014;6(224):224ra24.

182. Lo YM, Zhang J, Leung TN, Lau TK, Chang AM, Hjelm NM. Rapid clearance of fetal DNA from maternal plasma. Am J Hum Genet. 1999;64(1):218–24.

183. Oxnard GR, Paweletz CP, Kuang Y, Mach SL, O'Connell A, Messineo MM, et al. Noninvasive detection of response and resistance in EGFR-mutant lung cancer using quantitative next-generation genotyping of cell-free plasma DNA. Clin Cancer Res. 2014;20(6):1698–705.

184. Wang P, Bahreini A, Gyanchandani R, Lucas PC, Hartmaier RJ, Watters RJ, et al. Sensitive detection of mono- and polyclonal ESR1 mutations in primary tumors, metastatic lesions and cell free DNA of breast cancer patients. Clin Cancer Res. 2016;22(5):1130–137.

185. De Giorgi V, Pinzani P, Salvianti F, Grazzini M, Orlando C, Lotti T, et al. Circulating benign nevus cells detected by ISET technique: warning for melanoma molecular diagnosis. Arch Dermatol. 2010;146(10):1120–4.

186. Chang GA, Tadepalli JS, Shao Y, Zhang Y, Weiss S, Robinson E, et al. Sensitivity of plasma BRAF and NRAS cell-free DNA assays to detect metastatic melanoma in patients with low RECIST scores and non-RECIST disease progression. Mol Oncol. 2016;10(1):157–65.

187. Santiago-Walker A, Gagnon R, Mazumdar J, Casey M, Long GV, Schadendorf D, et al. Correlation of BRAF mutation status in circulating-free DNA and tumor and association with clinical outcome across four BRAFi and MEKi clinical trials. Clin Cancer Res. 2016;22(3):567–74.

188. Yancovitz M, Yoon J, Mikhail M, Gai W, Shapiro RL, Berman RS, et al. Detection of mutant BRAF alleles in the plasma of patients with metastatic melanoma. J Mol Diagn: JMD. 2007;9(2):178–83.

189. Daniotti M, Vallacchi V, Rivoltini L, Patuzzo R, Santinami M, Arienti F, et al. Detection of mutated BRAFV600E variant in circulating DNA of stage III-IV melanoma patients. Int J Cancer. 2007;120(11):2439–44.

190. Gonzalez-Cao M, Mayo-de-Las-Casas C, Molina-Vila MA, De Mattos-Arruda L, Munoz-Couselo E, Manzano JL, et al. BRAF mutation analysis in circulating free tumor DNA of melanoma patients treated with BRAF inhibitors. Melanoma Res. 2015;25(6):486–95.

191. Diaz-Lagares A, Alegre E, Arroyo A, Gonzalez-Cao M, Zudaire ME, Viteri S, et al. Evaluation of multiple serum markers in advanced melanoma. Tumour Biol. 2011;32(6):1155–61.

192. Shinozaki M, O'Day SJ, Kitago M, Amersi F, Kuo C, Kim J, et al. Utility of circulating B-RAF DNA mutation in serum for monitoring melanoma patients receiving biochemotherapy. Clin Cancer Res. 2007; 13(7):2068–74.

193. Saint-Jean M, Quereux G, Nguyen JM, Peuvrel L, Brocard A, Vallee A, et al. Is a single BRAF wild-type test sufficient to exclude melanoma patients from vemurafenib therapy? J Invest Dermatol. 2014;134(5):1468–70.

194. Tsao SC, Weiss J, Hudson C, Christophi C, Cebon J, Behren A, et al. Monitoring response to therapy in melanoma by quantifying circulating tumour DNA with droplet digital PCR for BRAF and NRAS mutations. Sci Rep. 2015;5:11198.

195. Gray ES, Rizos H, Reid AL, Boyd SC, Pereira MR, Lo J, et al. Circulating tumor DNA to monitor treatment response and detect acquired resistance in patients with metastatic melanoma. Oncotarget. 2015;6(39):42008–18.

196. Greenberg ES, Chong KK, Huynh KT, Tanaka R, Hoon DS. Epigenetic biomarkers in skin cancer. Cancer Lett. 2014;342(2):170–7.

197. Hoon DS, Spugnardi M, Kuo C, Huang SK, Morton DL, Taback B. Profiling epigenetic inactivation of tumor suppressor genes in tumors and plasma from cutaneous melanoma patients. Oncogene. 2004; 23(22):4014–22.

198. Marini A, Mirmohammadsadegh A, Nambiar S, Gustrau A, Ruzicka T, Hengge UR. Epigenetic inactivation of tumor suppressor genes in serum of patients with cutaneous melanoma. J Invest Dermatol. 2006;126(2):422–31.

199. Mori T, O'Day SJ, Umetani N, Martinez SR, Kitago M, Koyanagi K, et al. Predictive utility of circulating methylated DNA in serum of melanoma patients receiving biochemotherapy. J Clin Oncol. 2005; 23(36):9351–8.

200. Mori T, Martinez SR, O'Day SJ, Morton DL, Umetani N, Kitago M, et al. Estrogen receptor-alpha methylation predicts melanoma progression. Cancer Res. 2006;66(13):6692–8.

201. Taback B, Fujiwara Y, Wang HJ, Foshag LJ, Morton DL, Hoon DS. Prognostic significance of circulating microsatellite markers in the plasma of melanoma patients. Cancer Res. 2001;61(15):5723–6.

202. Taback B, O'Day SJ, Boasberg PD, Shu S, Fournier P, Elashoff R, et al. Circulating DNA microsatellites: molecular determinants of response to biochemotherapy in patients with metastatic melanoma. J Natl Cancer Inst. 2004;96(2):152–6.

203. Smith B, Selby P, Southgate J, Pittman K, Bradley C, Blair GE. Detection of melanoma cells in peripheral blood by means of reverse transcriptase and polymerase chain reaction. Lancet. 1991;338(8777): 1227–9.

204. Hoshimoto S, Shingai T, Morton DL, Kuo C, Faries MB, Chong K, et al. Association between circulating tumor cells and prognosis in patients with stage III melanoma with sentinel lymph node metastasis in a

205. Koyanagi K, O'Day SJ, Gonzalez R, Lewis K, Robinson WA, Amatruda TT, et al. Serial monitoring of circulating melanoma cells during neoadjuvant biochemotherapy for stage III melanoma: outcome prediction in a multicenter trial. J Clin Oncol. 2005;23(31):8057–64.

206. Zimmerer RM, Matthiesen P, Kreher F, Kampmann A, Spalthoff S, Jehn P, et al. Putative CD133+ melanoma cancer stem cells induce initial angiogenesis in vivo. Microvasc Res. 2016;104:46–54.

207. Koyanagi K, Kuo C, Nakagawa T, Mori T, Ueno H, Lorico Jr AR, et al. Multimarker quantitative real-time PCR detection of circulating melanoma cells in peripheral blood: relation to disease stage in melanoma patients. Clin Chem. 2005;51(6):981–8.

208. Goto Y, Arigami T, Murali R, Scolyer RA, Tanemura A, Takata M, et al. High molecular weight-melanoma-associated antigen as a biomarker of desmoplastic melanoma. Pigment Cell Melanoma Res. 2010;23(1):137–40.

209. Gray ES, Reid AL, Bowyer S, Calapre L, Siew K, Pearce R, et al. Circulating melanoma cell subpopulations: their heterogeneity and differential responses to treatment. J Invest Dermatol. 2015;135(8): 2040–8.

210. Miyashiro I, Kuo C, Huynh K, Iida A, Morton D, Bilchik A, et al. Molecular strategy for detecting metastatic cancers with use of multiple tumor-specific MAGE-A genes. Clin Chem. 2001;47(3): 505–12.

211. Koyanagi K, Mori T, O'Day SJ, Martinez SR, Wang HJ, Hoon DS. Association of circulating tumor cells with serum tumor-related methylated DNA in peripheral blood of melanoma patients. Cancer Res. 2006;66(12):6111–7.

212. Kitago M, Koyanagi K, Nakamura T, Goto Y, Faries M, O'Day SJ, et al. mRNA expression and BRAF mutation in circulating melanoma cells isolated from peripheral blood with high molecular weight melanoma-associated antigen-specific monoclonal antibody beads. Clin Chem. 2009;55(4):757–64.

213. Khoja L, Lorigan P, Zhou C, Lancashire M, Booth J, Cummings J, et al. Biomarker utility of circulating tumor cells in metastatic cutaneous melanoma. J Invest Dermatol. 2013;133(6):1582–90.

214. Rodic S, Mihalcioiu C, Saleh RR. Detection methods of circulating tumor cells in cutaneous melanoma: a systematic review. Crit Rev Oncol Hematol. 2014;91(1):74–92.

215. Clawson GA, Kimchi E, Patrick SD, Xin P, Harouaka R, Zheng S, et al. Circulating tumor cells in melanoma patients. PLoS One. 2012;7(7):e41052.

216. Fusi A, Reichelt U, Busse A, Ochsenreither S, Rietz A, Maisel M, et al. Expression of the stem cell markers nestin and CD133 on circulating melanoma cells. J Invest Dermatol. 2011;131(2):487–94.

217. Osella-Abate S, Savoia P, Quaglino P, Fierro MT, Leporati C, Ortoncelli M, et al. Tyrosinase expression

in the peripheral blood of stage III melanoma patients is associated with a poor prognosis: a clinical follow-up study of 110 patients. Br J Cancer. 2003;89(8):1457–62.

218. Clawson GA. Cancer. Fusion for moving. Science. 2013;342(6159):699–700.

219. Vona G, Sabile A, Louha M, Sitruk V, Romana S, Schutze K, et al. Isolation by size of epithelial tumor cells: a new method for the immunomorphological and molecular characterization of circulating tumor cells. Am J Pathol. 2000;156(1):57–63.

220. Hou HW, Warkiani ME, Khoo BL, Li ZR, Soo RA, Tan DS, et al. Isolation and retrieval of circulating tumor cells using centrifugal forces. Sci Rep. 2013;3:1259.

221. Khoja L, Shenjere P, Hodgson C, Hodgetts J, Clack G, Hughes A, et al. Prevalence and heterogeneity of circulating tumour cells in metastatic cutaneous melanoma. Melanoma Res. 2014;24(1):40–6.

222. Onstenk W, Gratama JW, Foekens JA, Sleijfer S. Towards a personalized breast cancer treatment approach guided by circulating tumor cell (CTC) characteristics. Cancer Treat Rev. 2013;39(7): 691–700.

223. Max N, Wolf K, Thiel E, Keilholz U. Quantitative nested real-time RT-PCR specific for tyrosinase transcripts to quantitate minimal residual disease. Clin Chim Acta. 2002;317(1–2):39–46.

224. de Vries TJ, Fourkour A, Punt CJ, van de Locht LT, Wobbes T, van den Bosch S, et al. Reproducibility of detection of tyrosinase and MART-1 transcripts in the peripheral blood of melanoma patients: a quality control study using real-time quantitative RT-PCR. Br J Cancer. 1999;80(5–6):883–91.

225. Foss AJ, Guille MJ, Occleston NL, Hykin PG, Hungerford JL, Lightman S. The detection of melanoma cells in peripheral blood by reverse transcription-polymerase chain reaction. Br J Cancer. 1995;72(1):155–9.

226. Schuster R, Bechrakis NE, Stroux A, Busse A, Schmittel A, Thiel E, et al. Prognostic relevance of circulating tumor cells in metastatic uveal melanoma. Oncology. 2011;80(1–2):57–62.

227. Sarantou T, Chi DD, Garrison DA, Conrad AJ, Schmid P, Morton DL, et al. Melanoma-associated antigens as messenger RNA detection markers for melanoma. Cancer Res. 1997;57(7):1371–6.

228. Keilholz U, Willhauck M, Rimoldi D, Brasseur F, Dummer W, Rass K, et al. Reliability of reverse transcription-polymerase chain reaction (RT-PCR)-based assays for the detection of circulating tumour cells: a quality-assurance initiative of the EORTC melanoma cooperative group. Eur J Cancer. 1998; 34(5):750–3.

229. Xi L, Nicastri DG, El-Hefnawy T, Hughes SJ, Luketich JD, Godfrey TE. Optimal markers for real-time quantitative reverse transcription PCR detection of circulating tumor cells from melanoma, breast, colon, esophageal, head and neck, and lung cancers. Clin Chem. 2007;53(7):1206–15.

230. Samija I, Lukac J, Maric-Brozic J, Buljan M, Alajbeg I, Kovacevic D, et al. Prognostic value of microphthalmia-associated transcription factor and tyrosinase as markers for circulating tumor cells detection in patients with melanoma. Melanoma Res. 2010;20(4):293–302.

231. Reynolds SR, Albrecht J, Shapiro RL, Roses DF, Harris MN, Conrad A, et al. Changes in the presence of multiple markers of circulating melanoma cells correlate with clinical outcome in patients with melanoma. Clin Cancer Res. 2003;9(4):1497–502.

232. Hofman V, Ilie M, Long-Mira E, Giacchero D, Butori C, Dadone B, et al. Usefulness of immunocytochemistry for the detection of the BRAF(V600E) mutation in circulating tumor cells from metastatic melanoma patients. J Invest Dermatol. 2013;133(5): 1378–81.

233. Huang SK, Hoon DS. Liquid biopsy utility for the surveillance of cutaneous malignant melanoma patients. Oncotarget. 2015;6(39):42008–18.

234. Ma J, Frank MH. Isolation of circulating melanoma cells. Methods Mol Biol. 2015.

235. Klinac D, Gray ES, Freeman JB, Reid A, Bowyer S, Millward M, et al. Monitoring changes in circulating tumour cells as a prognostic indicator of overall survival and treatment response in patients with metastatic melanoma. BMC Cancer. 2014;14:423.

236. Voit C, Kron M, Rademaker J, Schwurzer-Voit M, Sterry W, Weber L, et al. Molecular staging in stage II and III melanoma patients and its effect on long-term survival. J Clin Oncol. 2005;23(6):1218–27.

237. Tsao H, Nadiminti U, Sober AJ, Bigby M. A meta-analysis of reverse transcriptase-polymerase chain reaction for tyrosinase mRNA as a marker for circulating tumor cells in cutaneous melanoma. Arch Dermatol. 2001;137(3):325–30.

238. Fusi A, Collette S, Busse A, Suciu S, Rietz A, Santinami M, et al. Circulating melanoma cells and distant metastasis-free survival in stage III melanoma patients with or without adjuvant interferon treatment (EORTC 18991 side study). Eur J Cancer. 2009;45(18):3189–97.

239. Xu MJ, Dorsey JF, Amaravadi R, Karakousis G, Simone 2nd CB, Xu X, et al. Circulating tumor cells, DNA, and mRNA: potential for clinical utility in patients with melanoma. Oncologist. 2016;21(1): 84–94.

240. Hoon DS, Bostick P, Kuo C, Okamoto T, Wang HJ, Elashoff R, et al. Molecular markers in blood as surrogate prognostic indicators of melanoma recurrence. Cancer Res. 2000;60(8):2253–7.

241. Ruiz C, Li J, Luttgen MS, Kolatkar A, Kendall JT, Flores E, et al. Limited genomic heterogeneity of circulating melanoma cells in advanced stage patients. Phys Biol. 2015;12(1):016008.

242. Robert C, Schachter J, Long GV, Arance A, Grob JJ, Mortier L, et al. Pembrolizumab versus ipilimumab in advanced melanoma. N Engl J Med. 2015; 372(26):2521–32.

Liquid Biopsies in Head and Neck Cancer Patients

Anthony H. Kong

Background

Head and neck cancers account for around 5% of all cancers and are the sixth most common malignancy worldwide [1, 2]. They comprise of cancers from several sites including paranasal sinuses, nasal cavity, oral cavity, larynx and pharynx. The majority of these tumours are squamous cell carcinoma (SCC), but other histologies include adenocarcinoma, adenoid cystic carcinoma, sarcoma, melanoma and lymphoma [1, 2]. The most important risk factors for head and neck squamous cell carcinoma (HNSCC) are tobacco and alcohol use although there has been an increasing incidence of oropharyngeal carcinoma due to human papillomavirus (HPV) infection, accounting for about 25% of all HNSCC cases [3, 4]. HPV has different subtypes and a few of which are considered to be high risk in inducing carcinogenesis including HPV-16, HPV-18 and HPV-31 which are implicated in cervical and anal cancers [4]. HPV-16 is the most important subtype for HNSCC and induces carcinogenesis through the viral oncoproteins E6 and E7 which bind to p53 and pRb, respectively, lead-

A.H. Kong (✉)
Institute of Head and Neck Studies (InHANSE),
Institute of Cancer and Genomic Sciences, University
of Birmingham, Robert Aitken Building, 2nd Floor,
Birmingham B15 2TT, UK
e-mail: a.h.kong@bham.ac.uk

ing to their inactivation and uncontrolled cellular growth [5].

At present, most of HNSCC patients are treated with either surgery, radiotherapy, chemotherapy and/or their combination [1]. Despite these intensive treatments, 5-year survival rate remains poor, at around 50% or less for high-risk patients who are HPV negative and heavy smokers [1]. In patients with metastatic cancers, the prognosis is less than 1 year [6]. Cetuximab, a monoclonal antibody to EGFR, is licensed in combination with platinum-based chemotherapy in recurrent or metastatic HNSCC, but the addition of cetuximab to chemotherapy only increased the median progression-free survival time from 3.3 to 5.6 months and the overall survival from 7.4 months to 10.1 months in these patients compared to platinum-based chemotherapy alone [6]. The EGFR expression does not predict response to cetuximab in HNSCC, and there is no known predictive factor that is used clinically [7].

There have been a few recent reports on the mutational landscape of HNSCC, and the most significantly mutated genes include TP53 (62%), CDKN2A (12%), NOTCH1 (14%), PTEN (7%) and PIK3CA (8%) [8–11]. There are clear differences between HPV-positive and HPV-negative tumours since HPV-positive tumours have a lower frequency of gene mutations and the majority of the mutations are in PI3K pathways [10, 12, 13]. Although HPV-positive status confers a favourable prognosis, patients with a >10 pack-year history have a poor prognosis and have a higher mutational burden including KRAS mutations. The HPV-negative HNSCCs have a similar mutation spectrum to lung and oesophageal SCC [11, 13]. These reports on the genetic analysis on HNSCC have revealed a high degree of intertumour heterogeneity and novel significantly mutated genes, confirming the complexity of head and neck biology. However, they also revealed targetable genetic aberrations in both HPV-positive and HPV-negative tumours, including FGFR and PI3K aberrations as potential therapeutic targets. Thus, it may be useful to use genetic molecular profile to guide treatment for individual patients. In addition, it may be useful to repeat biopsies following treatment to assess the genetic aberrations induced by the treatment causing drug resistance. However, repeated tumour biopsies to monitor treatment response and/or disease progression will be impractical and challenging in patients undergoing treatments. Repeated biopsies are inconvenient and invasive as well as can be painful and is associated with certain risks including haemorrhage and infection. Liquid biopsies may serve as useful alternatives to tissue biopsy, which include circulating tumour cells (CTCs), circulating tumour DNA (ctDNA) and circulating exosomes and microvesicles.

Circulating Tumour Cells (CTCs) and Circulating Tumour DNA (ctDNA)

Circulating tumour cells are intact tumour cells that have been shed into the bloodstream from a primary cancer, and it is thought to play a role in inducing metastasis in distant organs. They are rarely found in health individuals or patients with non-malignant diseases [14]. They can be detected in various advanced or metastatic cancers although the frequency is low, around 1–10 CTCc per ml of whole blood. CTCs are cells that are stained positive for epithelial cell markers, i.e. cytokeratin and epithelial cell adhesion molecule (EpCAM), but are negative for leucocyte

marker, CD45 [14]. To isolate CTC, most platforms require whole blood to be processed soon after the collection, and the CellSearch CTC test (FDA approved) requires the samples to be processed within 96 h of collection [14]. The definition of 'positive' test is defined differently for different cancers in the number of CTCs per 7.5 ml of blood, for example, ≥ 5 CTCs for metastatic breast and prostate cancers and ≥ 3 CTCs for metastatic colorectal cancer since these cutoff points are associated with decreased survivals in these patients [15–17].

The ctDNA is thought to be due to apoptosis or necrosis of the cells resulting in the small fragments of nuclei acid being released into the bloodstream [18, 19]. The fragments are around 150–180 bp in length but shorter in tumour-associated mutations (<150 bp). Due to background levels of wild-type DNA, the current available platforms cannot analyse the tumour RNA transcriptome or proteome but can detect the genetic or epigenetic changes in the tumour DNA such as mutations, amplifications, indels, translocations and methylation [18, 19].

CTC and ctDNA are two main sources of tumour DNA that can be assessed in bloods via non-invasive methods [18]. Many studies have shown that both CTCs and ctDNA can be present in advanced cancers although the mechanisms of how they are released into the circulation are still unclear. It is also unsure whether ctDNA definitely comes from the primary cancers or whether they are related to the CTCs. There have been a few studies that compared the frequency of the detection of ctDNA and CTC in the same patients of different cancer types and the conclusions have been mixed [16–23]. Part of the differences was thought to be due to the methods used to detect them [18].

Bettegowda et al. (2014) reported a study using digital polymerase chain reaction (PCR)-based technologies to detect circulating tumour DNA (ctDNA) in 640 patients with different tumour types [18]. The PCR-based assays were used to detect tumour-specific arrangements but not tumour-specific point mutations since the background level of the point mutations in these assays is too high. There were clear differences between the detection of ctDNA in those with metastatic disease compared to those with localized disease. The ctDNA was detected in >75% of patients with advanced disease (including head and neck cancers) but only 55% in patients with localized disease across all tumour types. It also varied with tumour types since ctDNA was detected in less than 50% in those with advanced renal, prostate, thyroid cancers and primary brain tumours. The study also compared the levels between ctDNA and CTCs, and it was found that the levels of ctDNA were always higher than that of CTCs [18]. Since ctDNA could be present in patients without detectable CTCs, it was suggested that these two biomarkers are distinct entities. In this study, it was shown that the detection of the clinically relevant KRAS gene mutations in the ctDNA had a sensitivity of 87.2% and a specificity of 99.2% in 206 patients with metastatic colorectal cancers. In addition, mutations in the genes involved in the mitogen-activated protein kinase pathway were found in 96% of the 24 patients who previously responded to EGFR therapy but subsequently relapsed [18]. Therefore, it was suggested that ctDNA may be used to monitor resistance to therapy.

CTCs and ctDNA in HNSCC

In a HNSCC study, CTCs were detected in 43% patients of around 1.7 CTCs per 3.75 ml blood, the frequency of which was higher in patients with a nodal stage of N2b or higher [24]. Interestingly, concurrent chemoradiation reduced the frequency of CTCs apart from 20% of cases [24]. In another prospective clinical follow-up study, 48 HNSCC patients were followed up for a mean of 19.0 months [25]. It was found that patients with no detectable CTCs per ml blood had a significantly higher probability of disease-free survival although there was no correlation between the presence of CTCs with any of the covariates including age, sex, tumour site, stage or nodal involvement [25].

In a study by Wang et al. (2014), DNA from saliva or plasma of 93 HNSCC patients was examined for tumour DNA consisting of somatic mutations or human papillomavirus genes [26]. The tumour DNA was detected in 96% of 47 patients when both plasma and saliva were used although there were differences according to the stage of disease and the tumour sites. The tumour DNA was detected in 100% in the early-stage disease and 95% in the late-stage disease [26]. The sensitivity for detection of tumour-derived DNA in the saliva was site dependent with the tumour DNA preferentially enriched in the saliva from the oral cavity because of the proximity. In a few patients, the tumour DNA in saliva was found postsurgically well in advance before clinical diagnosis of recurrence. There was an increased sensitivity (96%) when both saliva and plasma were available for the analysis, which is higher than those obtained with either saliva or plasma alone [26]. Thus, it seems that the tumour DNA in the saliva and plasma could potentially be valuable biomarker for detection and monitoring of treatment response in HNSCC.

Exosomes, Microvesicles and miRNAs

In addition to CTC and ctDNA, it has been shown that the exosomes isolated from patient blood samples could also serve as a non-invasive liquid biopsy that regularly updates and monitors relevant biomarkers or targets in cancers [27]. The exosomes are actively released vesicles ranging in size of 30–200 nm in diameter and can be isolated from all biofluids including serum, plasma, saliva, urine and cerebrospinal fluid [28]. The exosomes and other extracellular vesicles are stable carriers of proteins and genetic materials including DNAs and RNAs (including miRNAs) from the cells or origin [28]. The tumours can release exosomes to stimulate cell growth and induce angiogenesis and metastasis.

The miRNAs are short single-stranded non-coding RNA containing 18–22 nucleotides, which are known to have important roles at post-transcriptional and translational levels [29]. Most of the circulating miRNAs are included in lipid or lipoprotein complexes including exosomes or microvesicles to avoid degradation by RNAses [30]. The miRNAs are involved in the regulation and differentiation of normal cells as well as influencing the cancer cell progression and metastasis [31]. These miRNAs can regulate different gene functions and thus have different effects on the tumours. They can be broadly classified into either oncomiRs (oncogene) such as miR-21 or tsmiRs (tumour suppressors) such as let-7 [32]. One miRNA can regulate the transcription of multiple genes, and multiple miRNAs can target the mRNA of one gene [33].

Exosomal miRNAs in HNSCC

In a comprehensive mRNA profiling study of HNSCC, it was found that miR-21, miR-155, let-7i, miR-142-3p, miR-423, miR-106b, miR-20a and miR-16 were upregulated compared to normal tissues but there was downregulation of miR-125b, miR-375 and miR-10a [34]. In another study conducted by the same research team focusing on HPV-associated oropharyngeal carcinoma, it was found that miR-20b, miR-9 and miR-9* were significantly associated with HPV/p16 status [35]. In addition, miR-107, miR-151 and miR-492 were significantly associated with overall survival; miR-20b, miR-107, miR-151, miR-182 and miR-361 with disease-free survival; and miR-151, miR-152, miR-324-5p, miR-361 and miR492 with distant metastasis [35].

In another independent study, plasma miRNA expression was assessed in HNSCC, and it was found that miR-21 was significantly upregulated in plasma samples from HNSCC patients compared to healthy subjects [36]. In addition, the levels of miR-21 and miR-26b were reduced after the operation for HNSCC patients who survived for more than 1 year but not in those who died within 1 year. Therefore, these miRNAs could potentially be used as biomarkers for treatment response although the number of patients in this study was small [36]. Despite these aforementioned studies, no definite conclusion can be made on the role of these miRNAs in HNSCC. Further larger prospective studies are required to validate some of these miRNAs as prognostic and predictive biomarkers in HNSCC.

Conclusions

In the field of head and neck oncology, we are far from using patients' tumour genetic profile or liquid biopsies to guide clinical decision-making and patient management. This will require a complete paradigm shift from the current ways of the management of head and neck cancers, and it may take a long while before we ever implement liquid biopsies in the routine clinical practice. However, recent studies have established the proof of principle for using saliva and plasma as liquid biopsies to detect the presence of HNSCCs and other cancers with high sensitivity and specificity. Therefore, these tests using the biological fluids of patients could potentially be incorporated into routine investigations in the future to complement the current diagnostic methods in informing clinical decision-making in head and neck cancers.

References

1. Haddad RI, Shin DM. Recent advances in head and neck cancer. N Engl J Med. 2008;359(11):1143–54. PubMed PMID: 18784104.
2. Jemal A, Siegel R, Ward E, Hao Y, Xu J, Thun MJ. Cancer statistics, 2009. CA Cancer J Clin. 2009;59(4):225–49. PubMed PMID: 19474385.
3. Leemans CR, Braakhuis BJ, Brakenhoff RH. The molecular biology of head and neck cancer. Nat Rev Cancer. 2011;11(1):9–22. PubMed PMID: 21160525.
4. Zur Hausen H. Papillomaviruses and cancer: from basic studies to clinical application. Nat Rev Cancer. 2002;2(5):342–50. PubMed PMID: 12044010.
5. Braakhuis BJ, Snijders PJ, Keune WJ, Meijer CJ, Ruijter-Schippers HJ, Leemans CR, et al. Genetic patterns in head and neck cancers that contain or lack transcriptionally active human papillomavirus. J Natl Cancer Inst. 2004;96(13):998–1006. PubMed PMID: 15240783.
6. Vermorken JB, Mesia R, Rivera F, Remenar E, Kawecki A, Rottey S, et al. Platinum-based chemotherapy plus cetuximab in head and neck cancer. N

Engl J Med. 2008;359(11):1116–27. PubMed PMID: 18784101.

7. Arteaga CL. Epidermal growth factor receptor dependence in human tumors: more than just expression? Oncologist. 2002;7(Suppl 4):31–9. PubMed PMID: 12202786.

8. Stransky N, Egloff AM, Tward AD, Kostic AD, Cibulskis K, Sivachenko A, et al. The mutational landscape of head and neck squamous cell carcinoma. Science. 2011;333(6046):1157–60. PubMed PMID: 21798893. Pubmed Central PMCID: 3415217.

9. Agrawal N, Frederick MJ, Pickering CR, Bettegowda C, Chang K, Li RJ, et al. Exome sequencing of head and neck squamous cell carcinoma reveals inactivating mutations in NOTCH1. Science. 2011;333(6046):1154–7. PubMed PMID: 21798897. Pubmed Central PMCID: 3162986.

10. Cancer Genome Atlas N. Comprehensive genomic characterization of head and neck squamous cell carcinomas. Nature. 2015;517(7536):576–82. PubMed PMID: 25631445. Pubmed Central PMCID: 4311405.

11. Chung CH, Guthrie VB, Masica DL, Tokheim C, Kang H, Richmon J, et al. Genomic alterations in head and neck squamous cell carcinoma determined by cancer gene-targeted sequencing. Ann Oncol Off J Eur Soc Med Oncol/ESMO. 2015;26(6):1216–23. PubMed PMID: 25712460. Pubmed Central PMCID: 4516044.

12. Mountzios G, Rampias T, Psyrri A. The mutational spectrum of squamous-cell carcinoma of the head and neck: targetable genetic events and clinical impact. Ann Oncol Off J Eur Soc Med Oncol/ESMO. 2014;25(10):1889–900. PubMed PMID: 24718888.

13. Seiwert TY, Zuo Z, Keck MK, Khattri A, Pedamallu CS, Stricker T, et al. Integrative and comparative genomic analysis of HPV-positive and HPV-negative head and neck squamous cell carcinomas. Clin Cancer Res Off J Am Assoc Cancer Res. 2015;21(3):632–41. PubMed PMID: 25056374. Pubmed Central PMCID: 4305034.

14. Millner LM, Linder MW, Valdes Jr R. Circulating tumor cells: a review of present methods and the need to identify heterogeneous phenotypes. Ann Clin Lab Sci. 2013;43(3):295–304. PubMed PMID: 23884225.

15. Cristofanilli M, Budd GT, Ellis MJ, Stopeck A, Matera J, Miller MC, et al. Circulating tumor cells, disease progression, and survival in metastatic breast cancer. N Engl J Med. 2004;351(8):781–91. PubMed PMID: 15317891.

16. Danila DC, Heller G, Gignac GA, Gonzalez-Espinoza R, Anand A, Tanaka E, et al. Circulating tumor cell number and prognosis in progressive castration-resistant prostate cancer. Clin Cancer Res Off J Am Assoc Cancer Res. 2007;13(23):7053–8. PubMed PMID: 18056182.

17. Aggarwal C, Meropol NJ, Punt CJ, Iannotti N, Saidman BH, Sabbath KD, et al. Relationship among circulating tumor cells, CEA and overall survival in patients with metastatic colorectal cancer. Ann Oncol

Off J Eur Soc Med Oncol/ESMO. 2013;24(2):420–8. PubMed PMID: 23028040.

18. Bettegowda C, Sausen M, Leary RJ, Kinde I, Wang Y, Agrawal N, et al. Detection of circulating tumor DNA in early- and late-stage human malignancies. Sci Transl Med. 2014;6(224):224ra24. PubMed PMID: 24553385. Pubmed Central PMCID: 4017867.

19. Schwarzenbach H, Hoon DS, Pantel K. Cell-free nucleic acids as biomarkers in cancer patients. Nat Rev Cancer. 2011;11(6):426–37. PubMed PMID: 21562580.

20. Dawson SJ, Tsui DW, Murtaza M, Biggs H, Rueda OM, Chin SF, et al. Analysis of circulating tumor DNA to monitor metastatic breast cancer. N Engl J Med. 2013;368(13):1199–209. PubMed PMID: 23484797.

21. Maheswaran S, Sequist LV, Nagrath S, Ulkus L, Brannigan B, Collura CV, et al. Detection of mutations in EGFR in circulating lung-cancer cells. N Engl J Med. 2008;359(4):366–77. PubMed PMID: 18596266. Pubmed Central PMCID: 3551471.

22. Punnoose EA, Atwal S, Liu W, Raja R, Fine BM, Hughes BG, et al. Evaluation of circulating tumor cells and circulating tumor DNA in non-small cell lung cancer: association with clinical endpoints in a phase II clinical trial of pertuzumab and erlotinib. Clin Cancer Res Off J Am Assoc Cancer Res. 2012;18(8):2391–401. PubMed PMID: 22492982.

23. Sausen M, Leary RJ, Jones S, Wu J, Reynolds CP, Liu X, et al. Integrated genomic analyses identify ARID1A and ARID1B alterations in the childhood cancer neuroblastoma. Nat Genet. 2013;45(1):12–7. PubMed PMID: 23202128. Pubmed Central PMCID: 3557959.

24. Hristozova T, Konschak R, Stromberger C, Fusi A, Liu Z, Weichert W, et al. The presence of circulating tumor cells (CTCs) correlates with lymph node metastasis in nonresectable squamous cell carcinoma of the head and neck region (SCCHN). Ann Oncol Off J Eur Soc Med Oncol/ESMO. 2011;22(8):1878–85. PubMed PMID: 21525401.

25. Jatana KR, Balasubramanian P, Lang JC, Yang L, Jatana CA, White E, et al. Significance of circulating tumor cells in patients with squamous cell carcinoma of the head and neck: initial results. Arch Otolaryngol Head Neck surg. 2010;136(12):1274–9. PubMed PMID: 21173379. Pubmed Central PMCID: 3740520.

26. Wang Y, Springer S, Mulvey CL, Silliman N, Schaefer J, Sausen M, et al. Detection of somatic mutations and HPV in the saliva and plasma of patients with head and neck squamous cell carcinomas. Sci Transl Med. 2015;7(293):293ra104. PubMed PMID: 26109104. Pubmed Central PMCID: 4587492.

27. Martins VR, Dias MS, Hainaut P. Tumor-cell-derived microvesicles as carriers of molecular information in cancer. Curr Opin Oncol. 2013;25(1):66–75. PubMed PMID: 23165142.

28. Thery C, Zitvogel L, Amigorena S. Exosomes: composition, biogenesis and function. Nat Rev Immunol. 2002;2(8):569–79. PubMed PMID: 12154376.

29. Ono S, Lam S, Nagahara M, Hoon DS. Circulating microRNA biomarkers as liquid biopsy for cancer patients: pros and cons of current assays. J Clin Med. 2015;4(10):1890–907. PubMed Pubmed Central PMCID: 4626661.

30. Nagadia R, Pandit P, Coman WB, Cooper-White J, Punyadeera C. miRNAs in head and neck cancer revisited. Cell Oncol. 2013;36(1):1–7. PubMed PMID: 23338821.

31. Li M, Marin-Muller C, Bharadwaj U, Chow KH, Yao Q, Chen C. MicroRNAs: control and loss of control in human physiology and disease. World J Surg. 2009;33(4):667–84. PubMed PMID: 19030926. Pubmed Central PMCID: 2933043.

32. Garajova I, Le Large TY, Frampton AE, Rolfo C, Voortman J, Giovannetti E. Molecular mechanisms underlying the role of microRNAs in the chemoresistance of pancreatic cancer. Biomed Res Int. 2014;2014:678401. PubMed PMID: 25250326. Pubmed Central PMCID: 4163377.

33. John K, Wu J, Lee BW, Farah CS. MicroRNAs in head and neck cancer. Int J Dentistry. 2013;2013:650218. PubMed PMID: 24260035. Pubmed Central PMCID: 3821954.

34. Hui AB, Lenarduzzi M, Krushel T, Waldron L, Pintilie M, Shi W, et al. Comprehensive MicroRNA profiling for head and neck squamous cell carcinomas. Clin Cancer Res Off J Am Assoc Cancer Res. 2010;16(4):1129–39. PubMed PMID: 20145181.

35. Hui AB, Lin A, Xu W, Waldron L, Perez-Ordonez B, Weinreb I, et al. Potentially prognostic miRNAs in HPV-associated oropharyngeal carcinoma. Clin Cancer Res Off J Am Assoc Cancer Res. 2013; 19(8):2154–62. PubMed PMID: 23459718.

36. Hsu CM, Lin PM, Wang YM, Chen ZJ, Lin SF, Yang MY. Circulating miRNA is a novel marker for head and neck squamous cell carcinoma. Tumour Biol J Int Soc Oncodevelopmental Biol Med. 2012;33(6):1933–42. PubMed PMID: 22811001.

Clinical Practice Implications: Monitoring Drug Response and Resistance

Pasquale Pisapia, Umberto Malapelle, and Giancarlo Troncone

To date, for biomarker evaluation in predictive molecular pathology, tissue represents the gold standard. However, with the advent of the new therapeutic options, the number of actionable targets is steadily increasing, and tumor tissue sampled prior to treatment is not always sufficient for molecular testing [1]. In addition, under treatment pressure, clonal tumor dynamic evolution may modify the mutational status in relation to a treatment baseline assessment suggesting the need of monitoring the tumor genetic profile by serial samplings; as a matter of the fact, re-biopsy, after initial treatment, is not always feasible in patients with associated comorbidity. In these settings, liquid biopsy can represent a valid option [2].The term "liquid biopsy" is still debated by many pathologists that consider it as incorrect because it is not performed by a surgeon or a pneumologist and do not involve solid tissues but the extraction of blood or other body fluids [3]. Liquid biopsy cannot completely replace the tissue biopsies, but it may offer a valid alternative for patients with advanced disease who have no tissue availability or to refine the oncological decision-making process [1–3].

From a technical point of view, liquid biopsy represents a noninvasive and repeatable procedure that offers the possibility to detect in plasma and/or serum samples circulating tumor cells (CTCs) and/or circulating tumor DNA (ctDNA) (Fig. 19.1) [1–3]. In addition, exosomes and circulating tumor RNA (ctRNA) can also be analyzed. In particular, ctDNA and ctRNA are released from tumor cells, and their concentration raises in the advanced disease stage; CTCs are derived from the primary tumor mass and are crucial for the migration of tumor cells to secondary sites via the lymphatic and blood system. Exosomes are small membrane-derived vesicles that are released, from normal, diseased, and neoplastic cells, extracellularly following the fusion of multivesicular bodies or mature endosomes with the cellular membrane. They are characterized by a variety of molecules such as signal proteins and/or peptides, microRNAs, mRNAs, and lipids [2].

However, the implementation of liquid biopsy in clinical practice to monitor drug response and resistance is challenging, being CTCs, ctDNA, and ctRNA are present at a very low concentrations, thus requiring highly sensitive techniques, which in turn need a careful validation and integration in a complex algorithm, harmonizing with tissue-based molecular assessments [1]. In this landscape, targeted methods, such as real-time PCR (RT-PCR) or digital droplet PCR (ddPCR) adopted in many clinical trials, could not identify the whole spectrum of clinically relevant mutations [4, 5]. This limit can be

P. Pisapia • U. Malapelle • G. Troncone (✉)
Department of Public Health, University of Naples Federico II, Naples, Italy
e-mail: giancarlo.troncone@unina.it

© Springer International Publishing AG 2017
A. Giordano et al. (eds.), *Liquid Biopsy in Cancer Patients*, Current Clinical Pathology,
DOI 10.1007/978-3-319-55661-1_19

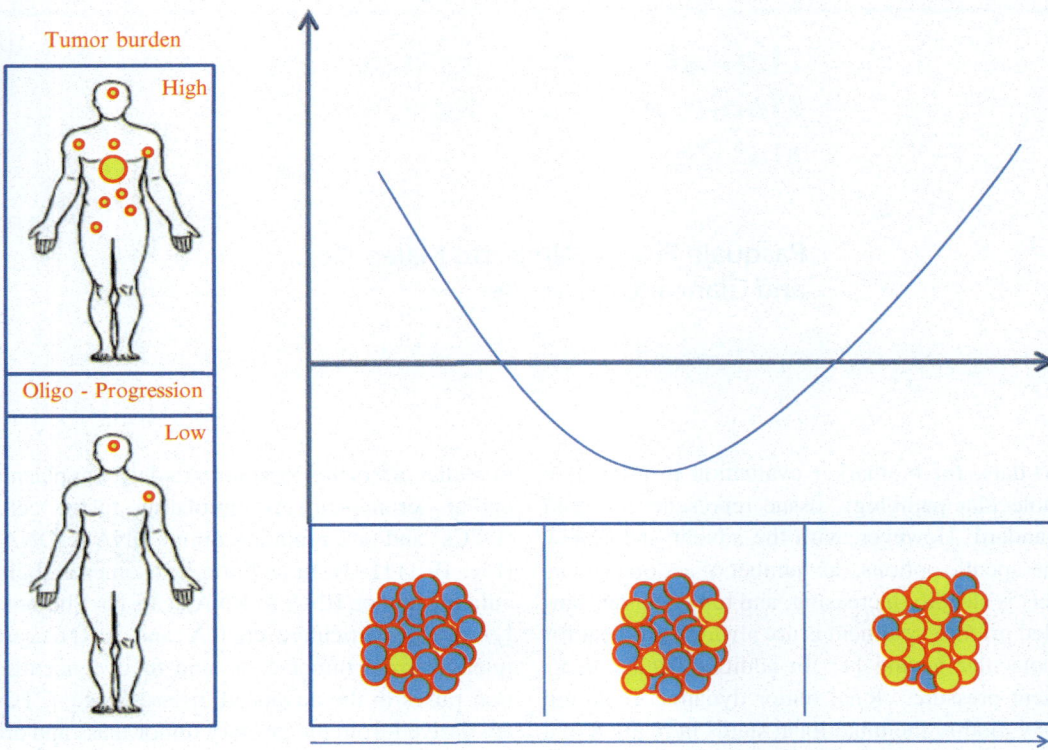

Fig. 19.1 Detection of genetic alteration in blood. Correlation between tumor burden (*y*-axis) and dynamic clonal evolution of the tumor in relation to the time and disease progression (*x*-axis). On the *left* is graphically represented the tumor burden and below (from *left* to *right*) the modification of genetic alteration quantity within the tumor

overcome by next-generation technologies, such as next-generation sequencing (NGS) or multiplex digital color-coded bar code hybridization technology (NanoString) which gives the possibility to simultaneously analyze the entire spectrum of clinically relevant alterations [1]. In the near future, these cultural and technological progresses may really change the clinical practice in monitoring drug response and resistance in cancer patients.

References

1. Malapelle U, Pisapia P, Rocco D, Smeraglio R, di Spirito M, Bellevicine C, Troncone G. Next generation sequencing techniques in liquid biopsy: focus on non-small cell lung cancer patients. Transl Lung Cancer Res. 2016;5:505–10.
2. Remon J, Caramella C, Jovelet C, Lacroix L, Lawson A, Smalley S, Howarth K, Gale D, Green E, Plagnol V, Rosenfeld N, Planchard D, Bluthgen MV, Gazzah A, Pannet C, Nicotra C, Auclin E, Soria JC, Besse B. Osimertinib benefit in EGFR-mutant NSCLC patients with T790M-mutation detected by circulating tumour DNA. Ann Oncol. 2017 Jan 18. pii: mdx017. doi: 10.1093/annonc/mdx017. [Epub ahead of print]
3. Molina-Vila MA, Mayo-de-Las-Casas C, Giménez-Capitán A, Jordana-Ariza N, Garzón M, Balada A, Villatoro S, Teixidó C, García-Peláez B, Aguado C, Catalán MJ, Campos R, Pérez-Rosado A, Bertran-Alamillo J, Martínez-Bueno A, Gil MD, González-Cao M, González X, Morales-Espinosa D, Viteri S, Karachaliou N, Rosell R. Liquid biopsy in non-small cell lung cancer. Front Med (Lausanne). 2016;3:69.
4. Wu YL, Sequist LV, Hu CP, Feng J, Lu S, Huang Y, Li W, Hou M, Schuler M, Mok T, Yamamoto N, O'Byrne K, Hirsh V, Gibson N, Massey D, Kim M, Yang JC. EGFR mutation detection in circulating cell-free DNA of lung adenocarcinoma patients: analysis of LUX-lung 3 and 6. Br J Cancer. 2017;116:175–85.
5. Valentino A, Reclusa P, Sirera R, Giallombardo M, Camps C, Pauwels P, Crispi S, Rolfo C. Exosomal microRNAs in liquid biopsies: future biomarkers for prostate cancer. Clin Transl Oncol. 2017 Jan 4. doi: 10.1007/s12094-016-1599-5. [Epub ahead of print] Review.

Erratum to: Liquid Biopsy in Cancer Patients: The Hand Lens for Tumor Evolution

Antonio Russo, Antonio Giordano, and Christian Rolfo

Erratum to:
A. Russo et al. (eds.), *Liquid Biopsy in Cancer Patients*, Current Clinical Pathology, DOI 10.1007/978-3-319-55661-1

The order of the volume editors in the published book was incorrect in the frontmatter and cover. The order has been revised to reflect the wishes of the editors.

The updated online version of this book can be found at.
http://dx.doi.org/10.1007/978-3-319-55661-1

Index

© Springer International Publishing AG 2017
A. Giordano et al. (eds.), *Liquid Biopsy in Cancer Patients*, Current Clinical Pathology,
DOI 10.1007/978-3-319-55661-1

The manufacturer's authorised representative in the EU is Springer
Nature Customer Service Centre GmbH, Europaplatz 3, 69115 Heidelberg,
Germany. If you have any concerns regarding our products, please
contact ProductSafety@springernature.com

Printed and bound by CPI Group (UK) Ltd, Croydon, CR0 4YY

23/04/2026

02095602-0008